Roderick McConchie
Discovery in Haste

LEXICOGRAPHICA

Series Maior

—

Supplementary Volumes to the International Annual
for Lexicography
Suppléments à la Revue Internationale
de Lexicographie
Supplementbände zum Internationalen Jahrbuch
für Lexikographie

Edited by
Rufus Hjalmar Gouws, Ulrich Heid, Thomas Herbst,
Anja Lobenstein-Reichmann, Oskar Reichmann,
Stefan J. Schierholz and Wolfgang Schweickard

Volume 156

Roderick McConchie

Discovery in Haste

English Medical Dictionaries and Lexicographers
1547 to 1796

DE GRUYTER

ISBN 978-3-11-063578-2
e-ISBN (PDF) 978-3-11-063918-6
e-ISBN (EPUB) 978-3-11-063602-4
ISSN 0175-9264

Library of Congress Control Number: 2019939538

Bibliographic information published by the Deutsche Nationalbibliothek
The Deutsche Nationalbibliothek lists this publication in the Deutsche Nationalbibliografie;
detailed bibliographic data are available on the Internet at http://dnb.dnb.de.

© 2019 Walter de Gruyter GmbH, Berlin/Boston
Printing and binding: CPI books GmbH, Leck

www.degruyter.com

Acknowledgments

I wish to thank Clare Hall, Cambridge, for the Visiting Fellowship in 2013–14 which provided a welcoming and encouraging atmosphere and without which this book would never have been written. I am also greatly indebted to Peter Jones, Librarian of Kings College, Cambridge, for his kindness, encouragement, and generosity. I also wish to record my heartfelt thanks to Professor John Considine of the University of Alberta, who has encouraged and assisted me in several projects and for many years in so many ways and helped with Latin in this book, and to Professor Ian Lancashire of the University of Toronto. Likewise for support from scholarships at the Cordell Dictionary Collection at ISU in Terre Haute, IND, and its former Director, David Vancil, for his unfailing expertise, generosity and friendship, as well as commenting on the Quincy chapter; Dr Jukka Tyrkkö for his continuing support and readiness to share ideas and information; the staff of the Munby Rare Book room at the Cambridge University Library, the Department of the History and Philosophy of Science at Cambridge University; Mr Phil Jenkins, who was kind enough to read my chapter on Robert James and whose help was invaluable; Dr Robert Adamson of Clare Hall, Cambridge; Dr Erik Nye and Mrs Andrea Cimoli for their generous help with genealogy;[1] Mrs Janet Payne, volunteer archivist at the Society of Apothecaries, who provided invaluable help with John Quincy; Dr Alexander Wright for his expertise on Robert James and for many discussions and his generosity; Susan Snell, Archivist and Records Manager of The Library and Museum of Freemasonry; as well as many friends and colleagues including Elizabeth Knowles, Professor Gabriele Stein, Peter Gilliver, Professor Lynda Mugglestone, Dr Frederic Dolezal, Professor Olga Timofeeva and Dr Debby Banham for their help with Latin, Seija Tiisala, Dr Mira Podhajecka, Dr Mark Kaunisto, Dr Trudy Tate, Dr Hannah Newton and many others whose encouragement and support has been indispensable sometimes simply because they were willing to listen, comment, and share ideas, a generosity which can hardly be overestimated. I must also thank the Varieng Centre of Excellence of the University of Helsinki for their financial support and providing a place to work while preparing some of the early material on George Motherby. Especial thanks are due to my wife, Aili Kämäräinen, who has supported me throughout and patiently listened to it all.

Finding funding for this book always been a problem; indeed, no research grant was ever obtained for it. This has meant that some of the archival resources which clamoured for my attention have been done only sporadically or not at all. Surely much remains therefore to be learnt from these resources. Whatever mistakes and omissions remain are my own responsibility.

---

1 It is my sad duty to record that Mrs Cimoli's untimely death occurred as this book was in its final stages of preparation.

https://doi.org/10.1515/9783110639186-202

Contents

1 Introduction

1.1 Lexicographical background

Lexicography as a means of compiling, organising, and disseminating information has been somewhat under-researched, especially the lexicography of the early modern period, during which knowledge expanded beyond the control of the individual and even the learned group. Medical terminology has been an area of dissent and dispute for centuries as competing languages, theories, and practices came and went, and the medical lexicon continued to expand. It is difficult to comprehend why so little attention has been paid to medical lexicography. Assembling, ordering, systematizing, and disseminating medical information has taken other and more obviously esteemed forms, however, whether these be introductions to the various medical and associated disciplines, popular handbooks, enchiridions and compendiums, recipe-books and, into the eighteenth century, taxonomies of various kinds, as well as nosologies. The problem of managing the dispersal of increasing quantities of information has been succinctly put by Malachy Postlethwayt in explaining the purpose of another specialist lexicographical work, his dictionary of trade and commerce:

> knowledge ... being scattered in an infinity of volumes, it is no easy matter to have immediate recourse to what may be occasionally requisite ... A subject of this extensive nature therefore being reduced to the form of a Dictionary, for alphabetical reference, seems the most naturally adapted to answer these desirable purposes (Postlethwayt 1749: 2; see Tarp 2013: 399)

The desired immediacy and access can be provided by a dictionary. Medical terminology has also formed significant components of encyclopaedias, dictionaries of arts and crafts, and herbals, not to mention the various lexical dictionaries of English which often claim to cover medicine specifically. To put lexicography into a more realistic perspective:

> lexicography is part–and an important part–of that interplay of technology and taxonomy which has helped our species to find means of storing information beyond the brain, our first and for an enormous length of time our only container of knowledge. The invention of writing, systems and adequate writing surfaces, the development of storage and presentational systems, the growth of techniques for classification (etc.) have all combined to provide us with a wide range of options in the kind of product or artefact we create, the kinds of layout that will animate them, the kinds of formats available for use, and the kinds of information poured into those formats. (McArthur 1998: 150)

Denis Diderot saw the advantages of an encyclopaedia clearly as inviting the expedited reconnaissance of an area of knowledge. "An encyclopedia" he argues, "is a rapid and disinterested exposition of the discoveries of men in all places, all kinds, and all centuries". (Diderot s.a.: s.v. *encylopedia*).

https://doi.org/10.1515/9783110639186-001

There had been a general historical change with the advent of printing from the fear of loss of knowledge in the era of scribal transmission to the problem of how to deal with the exponential growth of knowledge, and how to distinguish the good and useful from the worthless and spurious. What is regarded as spurious and what is not varies from one dictionary to another. The marked difference in defining scrofula between Robert James, who discusses it at length, and John Quincy, who dismisses it out of hand as not a genuine illness, has already been noted (French 1992: 98–99).

A complicating factor is the inherent tension between the compilers and the publishers of dictionaries, a tension which only increased as the period covered by this book proceeds. There is a large conceptual gulf between the dictionary compiled for personal use and then offered for publication, that which is assembled for the use of students, and the dictionary which is projected by a publisher or conger who then employs a hack to produce it for entirely commercial reasons. The hack may also employ a range of amanuenses. The end product of these various processes, however, may not seem to differ much on the page. It would be unwise to discount the influence of the publisher on the book itself and its contents; publishers had a very shrewd notion of what would sell: "Three-quarters of the vernacular medical books published between 1641 and 1740 appeared in multiple editions, underlining how accurately publishers knew what would sell" (Fissell 2007: 111). In such circumstances, one must also assume that publishers knew very well how to massage a text to ensure this outcome and were more than willing to do so.

> Over the longer early modern period, I suggest, print became a significant component of the medical marketplace in large cities such as London ... [where it] assumed an almost catalytic function in the later seventeenth century, permitting a range of practitioners to advertise and practice much more intensively than they had done a century before (Fissell 2007: 109–110)

Fissell has also produced figures for the publication of medical texts in the seventeenth century which suggest a large rise about the middle of the century and a lesser decline into the late century and the early eighteenth (Fissell 2007: 112–114).

Discovery in my title should not be taken in its contemporary sense of the act of revealing something previously entirely unknown but in the more mundane eighteenth-century sense of bringing something to light, whether previously known or not; restoring something overlooked or forgotten to notice (cf. OED sense 2b), a sense which then co-existed with the modern one. This sense is much closer to 'reveal', 'find', 'lay bare', as in someone who refuses to 'discover' what he or she knows. This kind of discovery may a repeatable event. The surgeon Daniel Turner, for example, writes of the hymen that "Columbus takes Notice that he never could discover it more than thrice in his numerous Dissections" (1714: 237). Motherby's dictionary under *castratio* that the surgeon Mr Gooch 'first slits the sheath of the cord ... then opens it further ... by which method the vessel is fairly discovered'; also the translation of Buffon's *Natural history*, on the subject of cats: "As the male has an inclination to devour the young, the female carefully conceals them; and, when apprehensive of a discovery, she takes them up, one by one, in her mouth, and hides them in holes, and in places which are inaccessible" (pt. 4: 51), or "There is no greater Mark nor Discovery of a Man, than to judge him by the Company he keeps" (Bulstrode 1715: 71). The idea is to show what was already known or to bring information to hand for immediate use when it becomes relevant.

Since almost nothing is known about the medical dictionaries, it stands to reason that as little is known about how they might fit into and reflect the larger scientific and cultural milieu of the period.[1] The still-stimulating volume published some decades ago by Rousseau and Porter (1980) offers so much which has not been taken up in the history of lexicography as yet. To take just one example, as the concept of the living world became temporalized in the course of the eighteenth century, moving away from the assumption that the creation had been once for all and was immutable (Roger 1980: 278–280), how was that reflected in dictionaries and glossaries? Was this a mediate reason for James Keir's failure to complete his chemical dictionary? Fixity meant fixed language, as in the attempt by Bishop John Wilkins and others to create a "universal character" in the seventeenth century (Wilkins 1668), but this increasingly flew in the face of the linguistic reality. Might the medical dictionary have simply have been understood as a practical ready reference in an emergency, as George Motherby suggested, to be used for the immediate purpose and hastily re-shelved?

Literature on the subject of medical dictionaries is very scanty. There are some dilettante pieces, such as that by Hadju (2005), which is really a very brief—and inadequate—account of the early medical dictionaries, accompanied by a list of entries from Motherby's dictionary presented as curiosities.[2] The egregiously disdainful piece by Mark Twain on Robert James's *A medicinal dictionary* falls into the same category, although in this case the author dwells in grisly and patronising detail on the horrors of eighteenth century medicine, deliberately eschewing any attempt to understand it in its own terms. Another modern article offers a translation of some entries in Blancard, as well as some comment, but the temptation to include entries for merely quaint notions alongside those which are historically revealing and useful proved irresistible (Jarcho 1982: esp. 568). There is certainly published research on medical terminology and medical terms in dictionaries, and this is an expanding area, but medical dictionaries themselves and those who compiled them remain an obscure subject. One still opens volume after volume on the history of early modern and eighteenth-century medicine, however, without finding so much a hint of the existence let

---

1 For a recent historical review of English medical dictionaries, see Charpy, Jean-Pierre (2011; in French). The early nineteenth century was rather better served; see the review of some then recent medical dictionaries and encyclopaedias in *Anon.* 1837.
2 Motherby's is not, as Hadju thinks, the first illustrated medical dictionary. Robert James's *A medicinal dictionary* (1743) had many large illustrations, and even Quincy's (1719) had some very modest diagrams. Surgical instruments had already been illustrated in the seventeenth century.

alone the role of medical dictionaries. As Sydenham claimed in 1676, diseases could be classified just as plants have been (see Bynum 1980: 216),[3] but we have been far more interested in the classifications themselves than in the works which contain them and the means of creating these works.[4]

We should also pause to ask what actually constitutes a dictionary rather than some other kind of reference work. A split had emerged by the eighteenth century between dictionaries, which were increasingly concerned with the world of words as lexical items, and that of encyclopaedias, concerned with the world of those things designated by words. Even into the seventeenth century, dictionaries were primarily concerned with glosses and lexical equivalence. While there is general agreement that a particular kind of work, usually lexical in nature, concerned with defining words, alphabetically arranged, and often containing linguistic information, constitutes a dictionary, there is a muzzy borderland between this and encyclopaedias, as well as other kinds of reference works which might exhibit some but not all of the characteristics associated with a dictionary, not to mention those works of reference which are called dictionaries without exhibiting many of the obvious defining features of one. The medical area has a number of these, and such works can be found going back well into the seventeenth century. It was not unusual at all for the increasingly common ready-reference medical handbooks for general non-professional use, for instance, to be alphabetically arranged without exhibiting any further lexicographical characteristics.

Encyclopaedias, on the other hand, while they may incorporate some lexicographical features, are less likely to contain linguistic information, and have information, often a great deal of it, over and above what a definition would require. A genus-species definition may be minimal or lacking altogether. There is nevertheless a cline in such works, rather than a clear division into types. Further, the influence of any one of them may be felt on dictionaries proper. Entitling a work a dictionary is not an indispensable guide either, since works which we can agree are dictionaries

---

3 Primò, expedit ut morbi omnes ad definitas as certas *species* revocentur, eâdem prorsus diligentiâ αχριζεια quâ id factum videmus à *Botanicis* scriptoribus in suis *Phytologiis*. Quippe reperiuntur morbi qui sub eodem genere ac Nomenclaturâ redacti, ac quoad nonnulla symptomata sibi invicem consimiles, tamen & naturâ inter se discreti diversum etiam medicandi modum postulant (Præfatio a2[r]). "First, it is convenient to reduce all diseases to certain and particular kinds, just as we see the botanical writers do in their phytologies. Naturally, diseases are found under the same genus and same name, and with some of the same symptoms, which nevertheless are of a different nature and require a different treatment."

4 Gerhard Fichtner's massive *Wissenschaftshistorische Bibliographie* (2009) only throws up a singleton modern edition of Castelli (no. 3014) from the various early modern medical lexicographers who might have received some scholarly attention among its 20,839 entries.

may have other descriptors, such as lexicon, thesaurus, repository, or glossary, and works which are not clearly dictionaries may employ the title.

While other compilations, such works as antidotaries and pharmacopœias, may use an elementary and partial alphabetical order, they do not qualify as dictionaries either, since these and dispensatories are organised more like nomenclators. John Banester's *An antidotarie chyrurgicall* (1589) is an example. Other forms of medical classification must remain peripheral to our subject, despite having some lexicographical characteristics as well as being a potential source of data for dictionaries. Nosology, pushed to the forefront by the belief that diseases, like plants, could be classified, reached its highest point in eighteenth-century Britain with the work of William Cullen (1710–1790). Despite the continuing drag of Hippocratic and Galenic medicine, "nosology became an Enlightenment enterprise of no small moment", as Bynum puts it (1980: 216).

As Jacyna pointed out many years ago, the 'great man' view of the history of science has died hard, perhaps because it involves such a simple but effective iconography (Jacyna 1983: 87). But lexicographers are rarely, if ever, seen as heroes or bring about change in any obvious way, despite the way they may have viewed their own labours.[5] The obverse of the 'great man' view is that the rest resist change and maintain the status quo, but a moment's reflection will show that this is a very reductive view as well, and slights many who brought less radical but still significant change. Many are reviled for their conservatism when it was in fact guarded and qualified by more progressive insights. Lexicographers are not associated with turning-points; indeed, early modern ones have often been reviled as mere plagiarists (see McConchie 2013), but we will see in this book that they can be more discriminating than might be imagined, and exert a quiet but still significant influence. As Jacyna also shows, professional, social and cultural context as well as achievement must be considered, especially as the one may to some extent determine the other.

Yeo deals with two of the radical shifts in the role of encyclopaedias and their compilers (2001: 84–85). The first is the shift towards loss of knowledge as the scientific world inspired by the Greeks passed into that of the later Roman era. In this process "each succeeding compiler quarried his immediate precursor, never returning to earlier sources, in spite of citing them as if he had" (2001: 84). The inevitable result was loss and degradation, but this process is not unique to this period, and instances can be found in almost any age. This is akin to the conventional image of the early modern lexicographer, uncritically appropriating the work of those who went before. The second stage which Yeo discusses is that brought about by the advent of printing, which meant the general transmission and dissemination of reliably reproduced

---

5 See, however, the introduction to Considine 2008 for a view of the lexicographer as hero, as well as the allusions to Cicero in Samuel Johnson's preface to his dictionary of 1755 pointed out by Nokes (2009: 150).

information for the first time. This was characterised by a shift from the "the need to gather the most essential knowledge in one place … to the need to select and distil" that knowledge to facilitate its availability. Even so, the impetus to preserve knowledge remained a powerful narrative throughout the early modern era (Yeo 2001: 84). This view derived its enduring force not only from the efforts of humanists to restore ancient texts, but also from the still-prevalent belief that the history of human culture was the history of decline from a golden age into the age of iron, and the assumption that the classical world offered the epitome of wisdom and knowledge to which all must inspire. The decline of these assumptions was very gradual, proceeded at a rate which varied from one discipline to another and from one author to another, and was almost as likely to revert as not, at least temporarily.

The flood of books coming from the presses of early-modern Europe eventually simply demanded that reference works like encyclopaedias and dictionaries be abridgements, which should be orderly and systematic (see Yeo 2001: 94). Copying was insufficient and inadequate to the task. Attention needed to be given to the quality of the information thus epitomised; indiscriminate plagiarism would miss the point entirely. The extent to which the various medical lexicographers acknowledged this point and dealt with it will occupy some of this book. At the same time, medical dictionaries needed to be so in an increasingly lexical sense (see Lancashire 2002); insofar as they were genuinely dictionaries, they needed to adjust to the changes taking place in early modern lexicography. This requirement was made considerably more urgent by the need to be bilingual dictionaries in a world which was seeing the decline of Latin as a language of science in general and Greek as contributing part of the core of medical terminology. Arabic had already largely been abandoned, although its vestiges remained in the medical lexicon. A significant development in language terms in the eighteenth century was the series issuing from the Medical Society of Edinburgh, *Medical essays and observations*, which was published in English, not Latin (Clark 1966 II: 554), the first appearing in 1733 (Craig 1976: 165). While slow, the trend to the use of English was of long standing, however, the *Philosophical transactions of the Royal Society*, a vehicle for much medical publication, having long been in the vernacular. The benefaction of Sir Thomas Gresham (1519–1579) at the end of the sixteenth century stipulated that lectures at Gresham College, including the medical ones, were to be given both in Latin and in English (see Clark I: 170–171).

A further sea-change taking place is evidenced by the sub-title of Robert Morris and James Kendrick's *The Edinburgh medical and physical dictionary* (1807), which is accompanied by "a Copious Glossary of Obsolete Terms Calculated to Assist Those who Have Occasion to Refer to the Writings of the Ancients", suggesting that the use of the ancients has by this time become a rather marginal activity. The bland assumption that "any dictionary reveals the state of knowledge extant in its time is likely to meet little objection" (Jarcho 1982: 568) precludes a more nuanced examination of what medical dictionaries have done in this regard, subject as they are to the vagaries of personal bias, inadequate information, the lumber of medical history, and the need to sell books. I hope that taking multiple, detailed approaches to these dictionaries will serve to call that assumption into question. The time for indulging in conspiratorial merriment with the readers against the early lexicographer is past.

The dictionaries discussed in this book will fit into this background in various ways. They are not all simply examples of the same artefact, but exhibit a broad variety of characteristics and approaches to the management of medical knowledge. They must also be seen against the background of the history of lexicography in England and on the continent, as well as being located as an integral part of medical thought and practice. Not only were practitioners availing themselves of such resources, patients were also becoming increasingly medically literate, especially since a good deal of the great wave of medical publishing which began in the later seventeenth century was directed at this market. Better informed patients were more able to negotiate the complexities of the "medical market" than ever before.[6]

Looking briefly at the various dictionaries which are the subject of this study might suggest that they all share the common and obvious intention of disseminating medical knowledge and informing a perceived market. The prefaces tend to invoke similar generalities about their aims, and are not always as revealing as they could be. We will see, however, that their often unstated agendas, which emerge from a study of what is on the page, are markedly individual and disparate. Blancard's was to provide a compendious alternative to the Latin-Greek dictionaries printed on the continent, James's was to be inclusive, a three-volume medical omnibus; Quincy's was to validate and advance the use of English in medicine in a compendious work and to advance Newtonian medicine, Barrow's was to introduce and to reinstate terminology from the three major sources of the medical lexicon and to foreground many of the new terms accruing from early modern exploration, while Motherby's was modestly proclaimed as a short-cut to both ancient wisdom and modern improvements, a means to "discover in haste" under the pressure of the immediate medical need (1775 Preface: vi). All shared a concern for what has been recently called "curation" to some degree; in this case "the work of composing texts that comprise collected, filtered, ordered information that must be rendered into a narrative, navigable form" (Kennedy 2016: 6), processes which stretched across and between editions of dictionaries and were always and necessarily incomplete. This has meant that my approach has not been uniform or predetermined; it has rather been a response to what seemed of primary interest to a particular lexicographer and dictionary.

The lives of those who compiled the various medical dictionaries are quite obscure, almost without exception. What Roy Porter wrote about the lives of quacks in early modern England might equally well be applied to medical lexicographers: "piecing together the jigsaw of their career structures, business ventures, the swings

---

6 See Jenner and Wallis, 2007 ch 1, for a discussion of research into the "medical market", as well as Mortimer 2007.

of their finances, fame and fortunes will require the assembling and assimilating of vast numbers of fragments of information from widely dispersed sources" (1987: 56). I can only sigh my agreement. In the present case, this has involved almost anything which might shed a little light on these people, including the forematter of various works, dedications, letters, archives, prints, wills, legal documents, contemporaneous comment, records of book sales, subscription lists, newspaper notices, advertisements, and so on. The exigencies of the *Lexicographica series maior* remit have necessarily meant that much of this biographical detail will remain in the background for now, but it has inevitably shaped my view of medical lexicography and of the particular dictionaries discussed here.

1.2 Ephraim Chambers on dictionaries

What then is a dictionary? We could do worse than ask Ephraim Chambers, who was acutely aware of his role as a lexicographer, not just as an encyclopaedist: "Were we … to give an absolute and consistent Definition of a Dictionary; we should say, 'It is a Collection of Definitions of the Words of a Language' " (1728: xxi). Since we are to consider definitions rather than the words as the sine qua non, dictionaries will vary greatly in nature. He also points out that the lexicographer

> was an Analyst; that his View was not to improve or advance Knowledge, but to teach, or convey it; and that he was hence led to unty the Complexions or Bundles of Ideas his Predecessors had made, and reduce 'em to their natural parity: which is all that is essential to a Dictionarist (1728 Preface: xxi).[7]

Chambers saw clearly that his job was not merely to record, but to analyse, interpret, and disseminate. Modern lexicographers are fond of stressing the task of description, but their work also involves a great deal of analysis as well. The hope is that the final analysis does not distort the perceived lexical reality. As Chambers shrewdly claims, although we perhaps cannot know the dictionary by the "condition" of the author, we can know something of the "condition" of the author by the dictionary (1728 Preface: xxi).

> Dictionarists are far from considering their Subject so closely, or confining themselves to so narrow, tho direct, a Channel: They must have more room; and think themselves privileg'd by the general Quality of Lexicographers, to use all kinds of Definitions promiscuously. 'Tis no wonder they should not keep to Views which they had not, and which could only arise from Researches they never made. While the Notions of Term and Art, remain'd yet in the Rubbish they were left

---

7 In the 1738 edition, there are two significant changes in this passage: "parity" has become "simplicity", suggesting a change in categorization, and "Dictionarist" now reads "lexicographer", a term which seems to have gained in frequency at the expense of *dictionarist* in this period.

by the Schoolmen; those of Definition and Dictionary must needs be vague and arbitrary enough; and the Dictionarists and Expositors, profited by an Embarrass it was their Business to have re-mov'd. (xxi)

The problem for Chambers then was compounded by the persistence of the dross of the schoolmen; a parallel problem bedevilled the medical lexicographers as they sorted through what terminology from the past remained viable. Some tried to weed it out, while others were content for it to remain.

A significant point is that the schoolmen did not distinguish between term and art as Chambers does. Lexicographers more generally, Chambers claims, had been insufficiently discriminating in understanding what they were doing. While the hard-words tradition continued in English lexicography, and the resultant dictionaries targeted specific markets for publishers, little was likely to change,[8] Latin-English-Latin dictionaries and Vernacular-English-Vernacular dictionaries remaining tied to educational ends at various levels of both achievement and marketing, with similar results, despite their greater sophistication. For Chambers, lexicography was driven by a multitude of principles which remained largely undeclared and not thought through. Articulating these principles would help to purge dictionaries of their disorderliness and lexical excesses.[9]

Chambers could hardly have made such remarks without the development of the lexical dictionary, rather than dictionaries of translation equivalents, but he also played an important role in expressing this emerging view so succinctly.[10] What was coming to be the standard view of monolingual dictionaries, however, would find it hard to penetrate the structure of the medical dictionary while this remained a Latin-Greek-English compilation based on translation equivalents, a situation which persisted right through the eighteenth century and beyond. What would distinguish medical dictionaries in general was their encyclopaedic component, since their linguistic elements often constituted little more than a glossary.

THE Dictionary ... supposes the Advances and Discoveries made, and comes to explain or relate 'em. The Dictionarist, like an Historian, comes after the Affair; and gives a Description of what pass'd ... The Dictionary of an Art, is the proper History of such Art: the Dictionary of a Language, the History of that Language ... The Dictionarist is not supposed to have any hand in the Things he relates; he is no more concerned to make the Improvements, or establish the Significations, than the Historian to atchieve the Transactions he relates (1728: xxii)

---

8 For insightful discussion of the nature of the hard-words tradition in early modern English lexicography, see Lancashire 2007.
9 For an extended study of Chambers on definition, see Bocast 2016.
10 It is both interesting and indicative that translations of medical dictionaries such as that by Steven Blancard were not included in Emmerson's 1965 list of translations of medical classics.

Chambers' address to the King explains the magnitude of the task, which is "An Attempt towards a Survey of the Republick of Learning ... We have here the Boundary that circumscribes our present Prospect; and separates the known, from the unknown Parts of the Intelligible World" (Dedication) as understood at the present, a boundary which Chambers sees as being pushed far back into "the other Hemisphere" in the future under the King's patronage. He optimistically adds that "Former Lexicographers have not attempted any thing like Structure in their Works; nor seem to have been aware that a Dictionary was in some measure capable of the Advantages of a continued Discourse" (1728: i). Thus Chambers saw his task as imposing order and coherence on what he obtained from previous dictionaries, since his purpose "was as different from theirs, as a System from a Cento" (1728: i).[11]

The lexical dictionary is a compilation of discrete, small, textual components inter-related, if at all, by linguistic connexions, and consistently formatted, but it is not primarily a systematic narrative about the lexicon. Chambers wrote in introducing his *Cyclopædia* to the world in 1728 that:

> IT may even be said, that if the System be an Improvement upon the Dictionary; the Dictionary is some Advantage to the System; and that this is perhaps the only Way wherein the whole Circle or Body of Knowledge can be deliver'd (1728 Preface: i)

He sees a system as the web or chain of logical deductions and conclusions which go to make up a science. Chambers argues that all the minutiae must be "swallowed up in the Whole" (1728 Preface: i) rather than be allowed to dominate it, as would be the case in a purely alphabetical arrangement. Each minor point, he argues, should assist the imagination of the reader to envisage the whole, and vice-versa. Thus the use of systems and alphabetisation both offer advantages which Chambers wishes to exploit. This somewhat undervalues the extent to which a lexical dictionary reveals various linguistic systems, such as collocation and governance, but this was not Chambers' purpose, and any interconnected discourse is left to such prefaces and epistles as there may be.

Chambers is also very aware that most words have multiple meanings, and that lexemes with single meanings are rare. He is also aware of complex ideas and collocations: "The great Readiness and Propensity of the Mind to combine, and bundle up its Ideas, and thus pay or receive 'em in Parcels, has left us very few simple ones; I mean, very few Names which denote only one Idea" (1728: xviii). Chambers offers several definitions of a term, one being "a Word which denotes an Assemblage, or System of Ideas, relating to some one Point, which the Mind artfully complicates, or associates together, for the conveniency of its own Operations" (1728: xix). Terms allow us to order, contextualize, and communicate knowledge more easily.

---

11 A cento being a patchwork, something composed of scraps, a work composed of quotations.

Chambers also offers a justification for the collection methods employed by lexicographers. The bee image was a commonplace for this activity. Erasmus makes use of it in his *De copia*:

And so the student, like the industrious bee, will fly about through all the authors' gardens and will light on every small flower of rhetoric, everywhere collecting some honey that he may carry off to his own hive. Since there is such a great abundance of subjects in these, a complete gleaning is not possible, and he will be sure to select the most important and adapt them to the pattern of his work. (Erasmus 2005: 90)

It is also appealed to both verbally and visually in another dictionary, John Baret's *An aluearie or triple dictionarie in Englishe, Latin and French* ('the beehive'), first published in 1574. Denham, the publisher, supplied a fine title-page illustrating the beehive and depicting bees issuing from the central beehive to forage over a page liberally spread with trees and flowers. This image thus represents the dictionary as the beehive and its collectors and compilers, who were Baret's students, mentioned in the preface, as the bees. The preface to the reader describes his students, sent about their task of gathering words for translation, who soon created a mass of material. His title thus represents "a great volume, which (for the apt similitude betweene the good scholers and diligent Bees in gathering their wax and hony into their Hiue) I called then their Alvearie" (Baret 1574: To the reader). The frame surrounding the hive is surmounted by the heraldic image of two lions holding a wheat-sheaf, representing a fruitful harvest.[12]

More interestingly, Chambers is unrepentant in asserting that the foraging lexicographer commits no offence, despite appearances to the contrary:

NONE of our Predecessors can blame us for the use we have made of them; since it is their own Practice. It is a kind of Privilege attached to the Office of Lexicographer; if not by any formal Grant, yet by Connivance at least. We have already assumed the Bee for our device; and who ever brought an Action of Trover or Trespass against that avowed Free-booter ... 'TIS idle to pretend any thing of Property in things of This nature (1728: xxi)

Here Chambers also rather artfully exploits the notion of the grant of a privilege which bestowed copyright on an author as a form of property. The collection process he employs is not merely allowable, but by its very nature represents a legitimizing patent for such authorial activity. If it is free-booting, it is done for the public good. The bee image was a commonplace for this activity. Erasmus makes use of it in his *De copia*.

And so the student, like the industrious bee, will fly about through all the authors' gardens and will light on every small flower of rhetoric, everywhere collecting some honey that he may carry off to his own hive. Since there is such a great abundance of subjects in these, a complete

---

12 See Carruthers 1990: 38–9 for the bee image.

gleaning is not possible, and he will be sure to select the most important and adapt them to the pattern of his work. (Erasmus 2005: 90)"

1.3 Digests of learning

Great stress was put on the utility of compilations of knowledge in the eighteenth century, particularly in the form of encyclopaedias and dictionaries of the arts and sciences. These were seen as providing a convenient digest and a guide to knowledge, and as obviating the acquisition of a prohibitively large number of books on particular subjects. The implications of this notion are obvious enough, and provide an insight into what a compiler does, indeed, what he or she must do. To provide a replacement for a library of books, you must extract the essentials from precisely those books.

While the work of the French *philosophes* is widely recognised, we should also note that Ephraim Chambers' *Cyclopaedia* was a seminal influence on Diderot and d'Alambert in creating the *Encyclopédie* and that the medical dictionary of Robert James was also important. Diderot had undertaken translations of both these works in the 1740s. What the *Encyclopédie* editors sought was a demonstration of "the Order, Succession, and Connection of all the Parts of human Knowledge" (Alambert 1752: 2).[13]

The preface to the surgeon Thomas Wallis's *The farrier's and horseman's complete dictionary* of 1759 provides a useful comment on the nature and utility of dictionaries conceived as encyclopaedic as well as lexical: "This indeed is the great use of all Dictionaries, that they serve instead of many systems, and institutes; and prevent the trouble of turning over, upon every occasion, the various writers upon the subject" (Wallis 1759: iii); in short, a time-saving convenience.

Further, dictionaries can be shown to have been of genuine use, imposing linguistic order, communicating and prescribing; even facilitating the spread of new knowledge. An example is provided by James Keir in introducing his chemical dictionary:

> Mr. Macquer, certainly one of the most eminent chemists of his time in that kingdom, acknowledged that my notes to the translation of his Dictionary first excited his attention to the discoveries which had been made in England on the elastic fluids (Keir 1789 Preface: iv)[14]

The compilers of *A new and complete dictionary of arts and sciences* by "a society of gentlemen" of 1754 made little distinction between a dictionary and an encyclopaedia, especially in praising their own efforts:

---

13 See Alambert 1752: 116–122 for an extended discussion of Chambers.
14 For James Keir, see Smith 2013.

A performance of this kind being a digest of the body of learning, or, rather, of general knowledge, is thought capable of being made universally useful and instructive … It is father[sic] advanced, that, besides preventing, in some measure, the necessity and expense of a multitude of books, which too frequently retard rather than promote, and bewilder rather than guide in the pursuit of knowledge, there is no form or method of writing so advantageously disposed to propagate knowledge … or that can be made to comprehend so great a part of the circle of learning, and so well answer the purposes of a library, as a dictionary of this nature. (II: s.v. *dictionary*)

They then take up Chambers' argument about the compilers of dictionaries of the arts and sciences being exempt from accusations of theft: "their quality as dictionarists, or collectors, give them a title to everything that may suit their purpose, without rendering them liable to the imputation of plagiarism" (1754: s.v. *dictionary*). This distinction is however implied, since they perfectly well understand that "the caprice of authors, in coining a multiplicity of names for the same object, has subjected lexicographers to the cruel and almost endless task of explaining the various terms they have used for one and the same thing" (1754 I: iv). The answer they propose is to cross-reference consistently, both to synonyms and to subjects and their sub-divisions. They see the encyclopaedia as a work digesting and explaining the compass of human knowledge "in the form of dictionaries" (1754: s.v. *cyclopaedia*).

Despite their increasingly frequent publication, not a great deal has been written about the use to which medical dictionaries are put. Lamenting the fact that no new dictionary has appeared since Motherby, the editor of the *Edinburgh Medical and Physical dictionary* of 1807 writes that despite new discoveries and terms and new systems, "the student and the practitioner have been left to trace these subjects through innumerable volumes, for want of that indispensable article in a Medical Library, a Dictionary, in which they might be found, in a narrow compass" (ii). Expedition in dealing with the next patient is presumably a driving force here.

1.4 Dictionaries of botany and chemistry

While botanical nomenclature is of great interest and was of immediate relevance to medicine in the sixteenth and early seventeenth centuries, the considerable changes brought about by Tournefort and Ray meant that botanical lexicography and dictionaries had largely passed beyond the ambit of the medical dictionary by the late seventeenth century. This process had begun in England with the herbal by William Turner in the middle of the sixteenth century. The process was accelerated during the Linnaean reforms.[15] Works such as that by Linné and his student, Johannes Elmgren (1740–1794), the *Termini botanici* of 1762, were known in England; indeed a translation of this had been undertaken by Erasmus Darwin and saw the light of day in his

---

15 See also works such as Pulteney 1781 and 1790.

translation of Linné's *A system of vegetables* 1783 (see King-Hele 1981: 116–117). Since botany was firmly established as a discipline in its own right, and botanical works had long since ceased to be primarily lists of medical simples, botanical dictionaries are beyond the scope of the present work. There is much more interest in what botanical simples are included in medical dictionaries than in what botanical dictionaries say about them. Herbals, becoming in general a humbler and more popular genre, remained in use.

Botanical taxonomy and classification was central to the discipline in a way that did not apply to medicine and its various branches, so that making dictionaries was less significant to medicine, in which taxonomy was not an end in itself, whereas taxonomies, which share some features with dictionaries, were a fundamental objective of botany. The various disagreements of the early modern botanists were not over their intrinsic value but over how they were to be structured. Although botanical medicine did continue to thrive into the nineteenth century, attracting such advocates as John Skelton and I. A. Coffin (see Harrison 1987: 198–215; Brown, P. S. 1987), it was increasingly beyond the pale of mainstream medical practice. If there was a link remaining with medicine, it was through chemistry: "histories of the chemical analysis of many plants and of some animals ... might lead to a knowledge of medicinal or other qualities" (Keir 1771: iv). While Motherby's preface mentions the advances in chemistry as a contribution to the remarkable progress in medicine, it ignores botany (Motherby 1791: 5).

Dictionaries of chemistry, even though chemistry evolved rapidly as an independent discipline towards the end of the eighteenth century, remain of sufficient relevance to medicine to merit some comment and examination here. Their continued relevance through the eighteenth century is to some degree a function of the debates of the seventeenth century over the importance of this approach to medicine, instigated by Paracelsus, and given further impetus by Van Helmont and others. In England, iatrochemistry was supported by the renowned physician Thomas Willis, the scientist Robert Boyle, and the political polemicist turned medico Marchamont Nedham, among others.[16] The establishment of a Society of Chemical Physicians about 1664 was of serious concern to the medical establishment represented by the RCP, and a pamphlet war over this issue erupted just before the outbreak of the plague in 1665 (Cook 1986: 145–162).

Many of the substances listed in chemical dictionaries are familiar from medical dictionaries. The *Lexicon chymicum* by William Johnson (fl. 1652–1678), a Latin dictionary, was published in 1652 and reprinted in 1657 and 1660. Johnson lists both classes of medicaments as well as specifics such as *confortativa, diaphoreticum, diuretica, laudanum, mumia, odorifera, repercussiva, vomitivum,* and so on. Some names of diseases, such as *myopiasis, hemorrhoides,* and *icteritia rubea,* which he defines as "est

---

16 For Nedham's espousal of this cause, see Cook 1986: 145–146, 153–154.

Erysipelas", are also included. Johnson's dictionary does not contain linguistic information. The growth in scientific and medical interest in acids and alkalis is also
shown by comparing the entry in Johnson for the latter: "Alcali, dicitur sal omne quod
extrahitur è cineribus, vel calce cujusque materiæ per lixivium elixatum, proprium
omnibus rebus, liquidæ & solidæ" (8) ('Alcali is the name given to every salt which is
extracted from ashes, or from the substance produced by burning or roasting any material, drawn out by means of lye; it can be used of liquids or solids' with the massive
multi-page entries in James's and Motherby's medical dictionaries.[17] Johnson's entry
is from Gerardus Dorneus, (1584) *Dictionarium Theophrasti Paracelsi* Francoforti, 14.
Showing the tight interdependence of these various dictionaries, the original Latin
edition of Blancard (1679) has very nearly the same as Johnson: "Alcali, dicitur sal
omne, quod extrahitur è cineribus, vel calce cujusdam materiæ per lixivium elixatum,
proprium omnibus rebus, liquidæ & solidæ," while adding a suggested derivation.

To provide some further context, it is also worth noting the publication of Georg
Heinrich Behr's *Lexicon physico-chemico-medicum reale* on the continent in 1738.
Medical practice benefitted from progress in chemistry, particularly so towards the
end of the eighteenth century, connexions sometimes being made directly between
new chemical knowledge and experimental medical practice, as when Thomas Bed-
does proposed a Pneumatic Medical Institute in the 1790s, which opened in 1799. The
purpose was to test the possible medical benefits of the various "airs" then recently
discovered (see Schofield 1963: 373–377: also 179).

1.5 Medical dictionaries

Medical dictionaries in this period are best understood as special cases, either of the
encyclopaedia tradition so ably dealt with by Richard Yeo (2001: esp. 17–19), or as
special cases of lexical dictionaries, ranging as they do between these extremes. Robert James stands at the encyclopaedic end, attempting to comprehend all medical
knowledge into his massive work, and producing, not a successor to and expansion
of Quincy and Blancard, but in effect a greatly magnified and extended version of the
medical section of the encyclopaedist John Harris, whose *Lexicon technicum* first appeared in 1704. At the other, Quincy and Barrow in their various rather different ways
lean more towards the lexical dictionary, to some degree even extending the long-
established English notion of the dictionary of hard words. Barrow, despite the fact
that he relied heavily on James, comes into the category of the pared-down, largely
linguistic dictionary, as does the *Prosodia chirurgica* of 1729 ascribed to Benedict Duddell. Yeo draws attention to the relation between dictionaries of hard words and

---

17 Johnson's entry is from Gerardus Dorneus, (1584) *Dictionarium Theophrasti Paracelsi* Francoforti,
14.

encyclopaedias in that much of the vocabulary of the former belonged to the various technologies and sciences of the day (its "terms of art") (2001: 19–21), but such dictionaries also included words of neoclassical origin whose listing was intended to increase literacy, and to raise the status of those of modest education and modest claims to politeness and learning. As the title-page of Cawdrey's *Table alphabeticall* famously (or infamously) declares, it is a work

> conteyning ... the true writing, and vnderstanding of hard vsuall English wordes, borrowed from the Hebrew, Greeke, Latine, or French. &c. With the interpretation thereof by plaine English words, gathered for the benefit & helpe of Ladies, Gentlewomen, or any other vnskilfull persons. Wherby they may the more easilie and better vnderstand many hard English wordes ... and also be made able to vse the same aptly themselues. (1604: tp.)

This was a claim to be repeated by a number of Cawdrey's successors, and represented a form of dictionary still predominant by the end of the seventeenth century despite the gradually increasing sophistication of the monolingual dictionaries generally. In the eighteenth century, both J. K. (John Kersey) and John Wesley could still describe their works as dictionaries of hard words.

Yeo claims that the "wheel had come full circle" with the appearance of encyclopaedic entries in Dyche and Pardon's *New general English dictionary* of 1735 (Yeo 2001: 21), but such entries had already appeared sporadically in the early monolinguals, a case in point being the lengthy botanical entries in *An English expositor* by John Bullokar (c.1574–1641) published in 1616.[18] Blount's *Glossographia* (1656) also contains a number of encyclopaedic entries.

Yeo writes of the philosopher and encyclopaedist Pierre Bayle (1647–1706) that:

> Bayle established a defence of dictionary makers and their role in the Republic of Letters. In the preface to the Dictionnaire he cited and answered some prevalent negative perceptions ... 'of all the employments ... that can be had in the Common-wealth of Learning, there is none so contemptible as that of Compilers.' Bayle then quoted Scaliger, who observed that while compilers might be the 'drudges of learned men', they were nonetheless useful. In doing so, Bayle established a set piece for later dictionary makers of different kinds, such as Chambers and Johnson (2001: 44)

Dictionaries and encyclopaedias were compiled primarily to accumulate, codify, and disseminate knowledge. Both disseminate knowledge in their disparate ways, a process accompanying the huge increase of magazines in England in the early eighteenth century offering information on what was new and what to read. Titles included *The literary magazine*, *The London magazine*, *The daily post*, *The London gazette* and many others of all stripes, vending news, gossip, and useful knowledge to whoever could

---

18 The source (or sources) of these, the longest entries in the *Expositor*, has still not been identified to my knowledge.

pay or had access through such venues as coffee-houses. This period saw the commercialisation of knowledge, along with the emergence of the practice of publication by subscription list (Yeo: 46–58).

Yeo explains that the response in England to the growth of scientific knowledge was not to track and incorporate so much as to offer "selective coverage, a refusal to invade the territory of the historical dictionary and a decision not to replicate the detailed treatments of specialist dictionaries, be they philosophical, chemical, medical, or commercial." They "sought to condense and reduce knowledge ... to essentials in order to summarise the state of knowledge, accomplishing this in a methodical manner" (60). Yeo's attention to the role of the tradition of the commonplace book provides some helpful insights. Scientific dictionaries, he writes, like commonplace books, "sought to contain knowledge in the sense of reducing and managing it, not for the purpose of combining it into ever more copious forms" (106). The purpose was to bring the essentials of a subject together in one place to obviate the necessity of reading the ever-expanding numbers of works available (see Yeo: 110).

The process of ascertaining medical terminology was also important in this period, especially since it appears to have been rather unstable. Situations like the definition of *carpentaria*, which appears in Motherby 1775 and elsewhere is hardly satisfactory: "It is the name of an herb, but so variously spoken of, that it is impossible to say what herb it is." While this is an extreme example, entries which contain a comment that some other writer or lexicographer claims that the word means something other than the definition given are common enough. An example in Motherby is *epispasmos* "In Hippocrates, according to some it is inspiration; but others say it is a more quick inspiration than is usual." The ambiguity of this definition, which does not clarify whether the doubt is that of Hippocrates or of others mentioned by Hippocrates may simply reflect the basic underlying uncertainty about the term.

1.6 The titles of these works

The titles of medical dictionaries throughout this period represent a revealing semantic succession. Leaving Boorde aside, the next two use 'physical' in its fundamental sense of pertaining to medicine and medical practice. Since the first certainly and the second probably predates the influence of Newtonian physics on medicine, the next stage is represented by Quincy's *Lexicon physico-medicum*, a particularly pointed collocation suggesting that this work adopts a Newtonian stance towards medical practice. The next, James's *A medicinal dictionary*, uses *medicinal* in preference to a sense of *physical* which was available to him but in decline during the eighteenth century. James probably thought the word too deeply ambiguous to use in 1743. *Medicinal* had retained its primary sense of 'having healing properties' for centuries, further indicating that the *physical* in the titles of the earlier two suggest no more than 'medical'. Motherby uses the neutral *medical* in his title, but adverts in the sub-title to the notion of the dictionary as a storehouse of information by calling it a "general repository". The term *physical* meant simply 'medical', even this late, as we see in various catalogues advertising sales of 'physical' books (see Molini 1765), and in the title of Robertson's *A physical journal*, 1777. This means that we cannot necessarily impute a Newtonian medical sense to titles of medical dictionaries in the late seventeenth and early eighteenth centuries; John Quincy's title may be the only genuine exception.

1.7 The target audience for medical dictionaries

Who read and made use of these dictionaries is not easy to determine. This study has identified a number of copies of such works in sale catalogues, especially in the eighteenth century, but ownership does not necessarily suggest use. A medical dictionary lay at the intersection between the practitioner, the publisher, the compiler, and the user, and was thus a compromise in almost every sense. Professional and commercial interests both interwove and clashed. The user was as likely to be the patient as the practitioner. The author/compiler may well be beholden to the publisher, and may even have been a contract employee. The purchaser may be a professional, a patient, an interested amateur, or even simply be assembling a personal library. The profession concerned may not necessarily be medical, but may be the clergy, to take an example. Clergymen often practised medicine as part of their parish responsibilities, an example being the Reverend John Ward of Stratford, Warwickshire, in the mid seventeeth century (Ward 1839).

Generally speaking, medical dictionaries also crossed descriptive boundaries. The notion of a 'popular' publication has been considered by Fissell (2007: 110), who rightly finds it unsatisfactory, but then has to concede that her preferred alternative, 'vernacular', is also problematic. This is especially so in discussing these works from a linguistic point of view, which of course was not part of Fissell's declared remit once 'not in Latin' is excluded. 'Popular' awkwardly straddles the perspectives of the purchaser and the publisher/bookseller, while 'vernacular' is even more slippery as a concept once language and its manifold complexities (English, other vernaculars, various acts of translation, Latin, barbarous and apothecaries' Latin, Greek, and Arabic) are included in the equation. It seems that physicians had to know the Latin of the apothecaries in order to write their prescriptions, thus justifying the appearance of such terms in medical dictionaries; as Matthew Bramble writes to Dr Lewis in *Humphry Clinker*: "Heaven knows, I have often seen your hand-writing with disgust— I mean, when it appeared in abbreviations of apothecary's Latin" (Smollett 1771 III: 244). Conversely, the apothecary needed to interpret what the physician who used the more classical forms meant. As the teacher and essayist Vicesimus Knox asks:

How can the apothecary succeed without Latin? The physician's prescriptions are in Latin. The apothecary has recourse to his dictionary, and gives a tolerable guess by knowing something of the technical terms; but a guess is a poor dependence, when life and health are concerned (Knox 1789 1: 58)

For the present purposes, it seems better simply to let each dictionary speak for itself rather than apply labels to them.

As always, social concerns and distinctions could be important. A hint about the social considerations applying to medical practice occurs in a letter by Erasmus Darwin to his friend James Watt (20 Nov. 1789; King-Hele 1981: 196). Darwin tells Watt that he means to publish something about steam-engines, and that he will draw his information from two well-known encyclopaedias: "The historical part, as far as relates to the Marquis of Worcester, Capt. Savery, Messrs. Newcomen and Cawley, I think to abstract from Harris's Lexicon and Chambars's [sic] Dictionary", a matter about which he probably knew a great deal already given his involvement with the development of these engines. He then solicits something from Watt about his own improvements, again a matter on which Darwin was well-informed, telling Watt that if he does not wish to supply this information that he (Darwin) will do it himself: "2 or 3 quarto pages, and to consist of such facts, as may be rather agreable; I mean, gentlemanlike facts, not abstruse calculations, only fit for philosophers." Hence, Darwin means to produce a "gentlemanlike" piece by using dictionaries and encyclopaedias, implying that this epithet is appropriately applied to such works, but not to more technical publications. One immediately thinks of the many calculations inserted into John Quincy's dictionary, which was nevertheless the most popular of the eighteenth century. These, as we shall see, had been edited out by the time this letter was written. What, then, is actually implied by "gentlemanlike", and does it characterize medical dictionaries in general? Is the suggestion that a dictionary, even of medicine, was a gentlemanly acquisition for a library where a more specialised book was not? Does this explain the frequent appearance of medical dictionaries in the libraries of divines and the leisured class? Are such things as abstruse calculations beneath the notice of gentleman, or were gentlemen thought unable to cope with them? Austen's Elizabeth Bennet may have found this less perplexing than we do.

Darwin reveals another aspect of social distinction in commenting to his son Robert in 1790 that at "card assemblies—I think at Lichfield surgeons are not admitted as they are here;—but they are to dancing assemblies", and "Journeymen Apothecaries have not greater wages than many servants; and in this state they not only lose time, but are in a manner lowered in the estimation of the world, and less likely to succeed afterwards" (206; December 17, 1790). Robert had apparently asked his father for a recommendation for a friend who must have been an apothecary. Darwin's response is typically mischievous in tone, but it does elucidate some of the conventions and restrictions of the time on these medical professions and hence on a potential market for medical books. Such barriers might also be felt keenly by those who compiled and published dictionaries, as John Quincy obviously did.

It is easy to underestimate the role of the printing houses in the dissemination of knowledge and in particular the development of medical dictionaries. It has been pointed out that scientific progress before the nineteenth century was largely beyond the control of the state, the universities (and through them the church), and industry (see Bazerman 2011), which left a freedom to the presses which it is difficult to imagine now. The circle of enthusiasts, inventors, early industrialists and experimenters centring on Erasmus Darwin illustrates the point (see King-Hele 1981). "The printing houses proliferating across Europe no longer came under a single religious jurisdiction and therefore could not be uniformly censored or controlled" (Bazerman 2011: 27). Needless to say, the knowledge encapsulated in the printed text had value both as intellectual property and cultural capital as well as a market value.

1.8 Medical works with dictionary-like characteristics

Medical works frequently organised their content into broad alphabetical headings, but did not constitute dictionaries or glossaries, since they have descriptions of their head-words rather than definitions, lack linguistic information, and are centred on recognition and cure of the diseases. The great majority of the medical terms they contain do not appear as lemmas. Perhaps a better generic term for such a work might be either directory or compendium. An example is John Smith's *A compleat practice of physick* of (1656) which is organised under comprehensive headings. Some entries have definitions ("strangury, is wherein the water is made by drops with pain"), but many do not, merely describing causes, cures, and so on. ("HEAD-ACH. The cause is either a bare distemper, and then there is no heavinesse of the head...Or, Matter, from the common and proper signs". Sub-headings such as "The cause", "The cure", "The differences", "Signs diagnostick", and so on are in italics. Occasionally there is a gloss, as in "The Dropsie called Ascites. Is a tumor of the Abdomen, Scrotum, Thighs, Feet, from a watery humour". Alphabetisation in this work is loose at best. Two others are A. T.'s *Rich storehouse, or, treasurie for the diseased* of 1607, and the main part of *The skilful physician* of 1656, but these lack even the descriptive part of the entries, concentrating on cures and confecting medicines. A further broadly alphabetical example is R. T.'s 1657 translation of John Sadler's *Enchiridion medicum*.

The *a capite ad calcem* arrangement, standard in medieval medical textbooks known as practica (Wear 1998 11: 119, 126–127), gradually disappeared, to be replaced through the seventeenth century in books of general medical advice by straightforward alphabetical ordering. This generally meant a smaller number of longer entries. Philip Barrough's extensive manual of 1583 had used the head-to-foot layout. This arrangement certainly does persist, however, as shown by Lazare Rivière's work published in English in 1655 as *The practice of physick*, translated by Nicholas Culpeper,

Abdiah Cole, William Rowland, and an unnamed physician, and its partial use in the book on surgery by Felix Würtz, Abraham Fox's translation of which appeared in 1656.[19] Leonhard Fuchs had seen cleansing medical terminology of its barbaric medieval accretions as part of his remit in producing a practica in 1539 (Wear 1998 II: 12–123). It seems likely however that the head-to-foot arrangement ultimately became increasingly irrelevant and simplistic with the great efflorescence medical books and treatises coming off the presses in the seventeenth and eighteenth centuries, all offering an ever-increasing range of competing theories, descriptions of diseases, and terminology. A more comprehensive and sophisticated vademecum was required and the medical dictionary was designed to answer this need.

A partial answer was provided by the translation of Théophile Bonet's alphabetical listing of diseases, Englished as *A guide to the practical physician* of 1684. Alphabetisation is really the only obviously lexicographical feature of this work, since it lacks almost all linguistic data, and concentrates on long articles on aetiology, descriptions and treatments, with their own tables of contents. Some glossing is provided as under *arthritis*: "Arthritis, Podagra[,] or, the running Gout, and Gout." The "Arthritis, Podagra" then appears in the ruled running head on the verso, and the "running Gout and Gout" in the running head on the recto. In shorter entries, the headword and gloss appear on both the verso and recto, as in "Raucedo, or *Hoarsness*". This work, whose translator is identified only as "one of the Colledge of Physicians", is however, essentially a rather bulky vademecum, and has not been discussed below.

Some other works have been excluded from the present account, despite having at least some dictionary-like characteristics. Two such are Charles Alston's *Medicamentorum simplicium triplex* of 1752 based on the plants in the Edinburgh physic garden and intended for the use of students, and his *Index plantarum, præcipue officinalium* of 1740, an index of variant names of the simples. Another is Thomas Martyn's *The language of botany*, 1793. Martyn's is not a medical dictionary in any obvious sense, being essentially a list of the descriptive words of botany, not a catalogue of plants. Martyn is inclined to add a gloss as well, for the unlearned, as he points out in the preface (xxiii). Despite containing glosses, either in Latin or English, and Martyn's expressed concern in the preface about the proper language to use in botany, it contains no information about the medical uses of plants, and is thus beyond the scope of the present study. Martyn attempts an accommodation between Latin usage and that of "our sterling English" (xi–xii), while also being concerned to establish a consistent Linnaean terminology.

Another is the *Index materiæ medicæ: or, A catalogue of simple medicines that are fit to be used in the practice of physick and surgery* by the Scots anatomist, botanist,

---

19 On this traditional means of description, see DeMaitre 2013.

and man-midwife James Douglas (1675–1742), which appeared in 1724. This is an extended series of lists including officinal names, names in both Greek and English, as well as which part of the simple is to be used where it is a plant, and how if it is a mineral, arranged in parallel columns across the openings. In lexicographical terms it most resembles a three-language glossary accompanied by some brief descriptive material, representing a potentially valuable source of head-words for a medical dictionary. Further lists comprise *mineralogia*, *zoologia* and *phytologia*. A subsidiary list ("Medicamenta Simplicia, secundum Virtutes digesta") contains alphabetical entries under generic head-words, such as *absorbentia*, *emollentia*, and *vulneraria*, with the relevant simples as sub-entries but without glosses and descriptive material.

1.9 Some forerunners: Earlier printed medical dictionaries

Continental printed medical dictionaries preceded the English ones by many years. The earliest printed one is *Synonyma medicinae seu clavis sanationis* by Simone de Corda (Simon Genuensis 1250–?) first published in Ferrara about 1471–1472 (Rhodes in Besson 1990: 32), an edition which survives only in fragments. An edition was then produced by Zarothus in Milan 1473 (see Hajdu 2005). The next dictionary was Jacobus De Dondis's *Aggregator Paduanus de medicinis*, a work originally completed by 1355 (Drake 2003: 1842).

The year 1564 was a red-letter year for medical dictionaries. The first important humanist work published in this year was the dictionary by the immensely learned publisher, Henri Estienne (1531–1598), *Dictionarium medicum, vel, expositiones vocum medicinalium*, printed in Geneva by Huldrich Fugger, a work which influenced the re-introduction of Greek terminology into the tradition of medical lexicography. This is essentially a dictionary in Greek with Latin translations and a scholarly apparatus, based on ten of the most important Greek medical writers. Estienne begins the dedication to the eminent physician Philibert Saracenus "En tibi, mi Philiberte, ueterem nouum librum" ('Just look, my Philibert, a new old book for you'), capturing the fact that the ancient Greek sources of the work, Hippocrates, Aretæus, Galen, and so on, will be revivified in the present work. Konrad Gesner provided some notes for this work as well. Jean de Gorris (Gorraeus, 1505–1577), whose medical dictionary appeared in the same year, was at the forefront of the humanist attempt to reconstruct medical knowledge in the sixteenth century and to cleanse it of what were seen as the corruptions of the Middle Ages. It was also an effort to reinstate the Hippocratic tradition as the original source of medical wisdom, and to sideline Avicenna and his followers.

> Schon die Auswahl der Werke, denen sich Gorris zuwandte, kennzeichnet ihn als einen Vertreter jener Medizin, die seit dem 16. Jahrhundert gegenüber der lange vorherrschenden, zunächst auf der Grundlage der arabischen Werke in der Scholastik zunehmend ausdifferenzierten und systematisierten galenisch-aristotelischen Medizin immer mehr an Eigengewicht gewann: des

Hippokratismus. Nicht mehr Avicenna, wie Generationen von Ärzten der vorangehenden Zeit, sondern Hippokrates war ihm wie seinen Mitstreitern der »omnium medicorum princeps» (Stolberg n.d.)[20]

Greek, the less-known language in medicine, was also to be brought into a proper relation to Latin, the lingua franca of scholarship in Europe. In this respect, Gorris followed the lead of lexicographers such as the humanist theologian Simon Gryner (Grynaeus, 1493–1541), paralleling the monumental efforts of Henri Estienne in Greek and Latin scholarship. The overlap in these works is suggested by the fact Estienne had no medical training, and was essentially a classical scholar. The work was reissued in 1578 and 1601, and was re-edited by his son, Jean de Gorris the Younger, and published in 1622.

References to Gorris in England are infrequent, but they do appear regularly throughout the seventeenth century. The earliest occur in translations from the French of Jacques Guillemeau's *A worthy treatise of the eyes* (1587: 170–171) and Michel Marescot's *A true discourse, vpon the matter of Martha Brossier of Romorantin pretended to be possessed by a deuill* (1599: 28). Both appeal to his definitional authority; in the first for his distinction between a web in the eye and a cataract,[21] and in the second on a case of possession by a devil. John Gerard also makes reference to Gorris, citing his translation of verses by Nicander on the advisability of avoiding the poisonous yew-tree (1597: 1188).

Right at the end of the sixteenth century, a dictionary appeared which was to prove the most enduring of the period, that by Bartolomeo Castelli. First published in 1598, this work was widely published throughout Europe and acquired elements of other languages along the way, although it began its life as a Latin-only dictionary with a sprinkling of Greek glosses, unlike those of de Gorris and Estienne. The 1682 Jena edition incorporates Arabic, Hebrew, French, and Italian, as well as the original Latin. Editions came off the presses in Rotterdam, Venice, Geneva, Naples, Leipzig, Padua, Toulouse, and Nuremberg, among others, almost to the end of the eighteenth century.

Some comment needs to be made on the early printed herbals, such as Macer's herbal and Banckes's as well as those by William Turner, Lyte's translation of

---

20 The selection of the works to which Gorris turned already characterizes him as a representative of that Hippocratic form of medicine which, since the 16th century, was differentiated from the long-prevailing and systematized Galenic-Aristotelian medicine, first on the basis of the Arabic works in scholasticism, increasingly overcame the dead weight. No longer Avicenna, as for generations of doctors of the previous period, but Hippocrates, who was like his comrades-in-arms in the "omnium medicorum princeps".

21 A marginal note reads "as Gorraeus sayth it foloweth not that they are like. For the cataract is a collection and an heape of other humors, then of those vvhiche are naturally in the eye, flovving vnto it from some o|ther place: but glaucoma is properlye vsed when the Cristaline humor is dry and thicke".

Dodoens, and John Gerarde. Turner's *Libellus de re herbaria*, 1538,[22] should also be regarded as a dictionary in several important respects, such as alphabetisation and the inclusion of glosses and linguistic data. Both Banckes and Macer lack any introduction or preface, and the compilers of both feel the need to explain the alphabet; Macer by introducing each letter as it occurs, and Banckes by reminding the reader that the index begins with A.

Macer's herbal is medical in purpose, alphabetised, and contains glosses of the entry-heads, such as "Aperium is an herbe clepyd Cherfoyle, or Cheruyle." What is rather surprising is that the centred entry-head does not necessarily determine the alphabetisation, which follows the main subject of the opening paragraph of the entry. The work began with the assumption that the English word would head the entry; hence "Cherfoyle, Cheruyle", the main entry head, is alphabetised by *aperium*. Entries typically describe the herb very briefly and then proceed to the main matter, which is its medicinal virtues and uses. Similarly, *wormwode* is the entry-head for *absynthium*, and *smallache* for *apium*. This practice is abandoned after the entry for *agrimony* (*agrimonia*) however, the entry-head and the main subject agreeing by and large from there on. Thus we find "millefolium maior or yarow" under *myllefolium maior*, not *yarow*. Latinization is still not consistent, however, since there are still some entries in which the Latin name does not appear at all, including those for *rosemarye* (*rosmarinus*) and *townecresses*.

Banckes's herbal, the earlier, is more consistently organised, the entry-heads generally being Latin with the English gloss, if any, embedded in the first sentence of the body text. The entry-head also determines the alphabetisation. There are also some English entry-heads, including *cole-wortes*, and *morell* or *nyghte shadowe*.

Turner's *Libellus* is a multilingual glossary, with most entries containing three and some four languages. Turner uses Latin for the entry-heads, Greek, and English in most entries, as well as German on occasion. He also distinguishes at times between Latin as the "lingua officinis" and 'barbarous' Latin, the Latin of the Middle Ages. Regional usage is also sometimes identified, as under *cyanus*, where he points out that *blewblaw* or *blew bottel* is Northumbrian usage.

While herbals continued to be published throughout our period, a number of large and significant ones preceded our earliest dictionary. The reasons for commenting on herbals are made absolutely clear by Nicholas Culpeper in the preface to his *The English physician, or, an astrologo-physical discourse of the vulgar herbs of this nation* 1652: "a man reading Gerards or Parkinsons Herbal for the Cure of a Disease, he may as like as not, light upon an Herb that is not here to be had" (To the Reader). In other words, herbals were certainly still rummaged through for cures in the seventeenth century. A further complaint by Culpeper is that neither of these two herbalists ever gave a reason for writing what they did; again, the use of a herbal simply as a

---

22 See Rydén et al. 1999; McConchie 2011b for further discussion of this text.

reference work in the most general sense did not justify its existence. Providing useful medical information was the fundamental rationale of herbals for Culpeper.

The English physician has few of the features of a dictionary proper except for alphabetical order; it otherwise lacks synonymy, glosses, etymology, and definitions in the lexical sense, concentrating entirely on English herbs which are readily available, and their immediate uses in medicine. Culpeper, true to his agenda of making medical practice available to ordinary people, pointedly avoids Latin binomials and other borrowed names. Despite this, it is still a contribution to the growing tradition of alphabetical lists in medical works. Its single-minded concentration on the English language is also a precedent for John Quincy in the early eighteenth century.

John Gerard's *The herball or generall historie of plantes* of 1597 was one of the large herbals of the early modern period, along with that by William Turner published between 1550 and 1562. Gerard was a surgeon, and managed both the London garden of William Cecil, Lord Burghley, in the Strand, and his own garden in Holborn. The *Herball's* first edition was provided with a lavishly floral title-border, and a new one was supplied for the 1633 edition. Based on the herbal by Rembert Dodoens, the work is profusely illustrated, incorporating re-used blocks from Tabernæmontanus's *Eicones plantarum* (Frankfurt, 1590). Gerard's work was judiciously added to and revised by Thomas Johnson in the 1633 edition, since Gerard had relied heavily on the work of others and the first edition was by no means free of error. The 1598 edition contains an index and a glossary. The latter has head-words in English and glosses in either an English equivalent, a variant of the head-word, or the Latin gloss.

1.10 Dictionaries incorporating medical material

Some other works need to be mentioned as being medical to some degree and in often using alphabetical ordering, but declaring, say, a cookbook medical rather than not is an arbitrary decision. The appearance of medical advice and instructions is not surprising, since housekeepers were expected to keep a supply of remedies on hand for everyday medical problems and to know how to use them. Preparing these was simply another kitchen task. Fissell, who described these as "the only really ambiguous category", determined that about twenty-five percent of medical material was her cut-off point in identifying a medical book among these works (2007: 111), but rather than make such a decision here, it seems simpler to discuss one or two as proxies for the rest. William Salmon's *The family-dictionary* appeared in the last years of the seventeenth century, and is a cento whose content is divided between cookery and family medicine, equally the responsibility of the woman in charge of a household. The medicaments should be easily prepared and inexpensive, and the ingredients should be readily available (1705 Preface). The alphabetical list contains recipes, simples, and descriptions of diseases along with food, so that *apopleptick water* is followed by the ways to restore *appetite*, and this by the recipe for *apple cream*.

John Nott's *The cook's and confectioner's dictionary* of 1723 contains its share of medical recipes; under *almond*, we get the recipes for various healthful concoctions, such as Dr Blacksmith's and Dr Atkin's almond milk; the latter useful to cleanse the kidneys. Both are largely confected from familiar simples. We also find recipes such as the Lady Spotwood's stomach-water, as well as nostrums to cure bad breath, remove pimples, and remove scurf under the entry for *water*. Aqua mirabilis and other useful concoctions can also be found. On the other hand, this compilation has no linguistic information, and is only dictionary-like in being alphabetised. Hannah Glasse's *The art of cookery* of 1747 incorporates two remedies for the bite of a mad dog at the end, as well one against the plague, and advice on keeping clear of bugs. The author protests that she will not "meddle in the physical Way" any more than these (To the reader: ii).

Despite his concentration on other areas, such as mathematics and heraldry, John Harris offered quite a few terms in anatomy, and made specific mention of medicine, pharmacy, and anatomy, as well as the dictionaries by Castelli and Blancard in his proposal for the *Lexicon technicum* in 1702, although his use of Castelli was limited as it turned out. Yeo claims that specialist lexicons were available in anatomy and other medical topics, but this claim does not seem right (Yeo 63). There were treatises and some glossaries, but few lexicons.

Perhaps the only one of these works which concerns us immediately is the translation of Chomel's *Dictionaire oeconomique*, englished as *The family dictionary* (1725). Chomel had had immediate experience of practical medicine, as well as consulting medical works. The preface informs the reader that he had served as the superintendent of "the great Hospital at Lyons", and that, among other assistance, he had the help and advice of a work by Dr Antony Mizaud, a Paris physician, on the care of gardens and the ways to prepare medicines from them. In Lyons, Chomel was able "to observe Variety of Diseases, to consult the Nature of them, and to learn the Remedies that were used against them" (Preface).

Members of his immediate family had also been physicians. The work thus contains "great Variety of Recipes for the preserving of Health as well in Mankind as in Cattle and other Creatures" (Preface). The dictionary contains not merely botanical entries, however, but also outright medical ones such as *contusion, convulsion, deafness, flux* (which has several sub-heads), *hæmoirhagy* [sic], *philectena, rheumatism, ulcer,* and *uvula.* The head-words are conspicuously in English form.

1.11 Manuscript dictionaries

Manuscript dictionaries and manuscripts with dictionary material did not cease with the introduction of printing.[23] These continued to be compiled, used, and added to, as witnessed by the manuscript owned by the alchemist, astrologer, and medical practitioner Simon Forman (1552–1611), dated by him February 2, 1574 (King's College Cambridge MS 16). This work by Johan Cockys has copious notes and additions by Forman in the margins, as well as additions, mainly from Andrew Boorde, on interleaved pages.[24] These interleavings contain runs of entries for the most part in alphabetical order, suggesting that they were written up in an orderly way before being inserted.[25] The implication is not that Forman was a medical lexicographer as such but that he added to a manuscript medical dictionary in a principled way which preserved lexicographical features such as derivations (sometimes) and alphabetical order (largely), that he used it as a dictionary, which might therefore have lent itself to publication as a dictionary.[26] Elsewhere, the Wellcome Library's MS 408/6, apart from recipes in both English and Latin, contains a glossary in Latin and English in fols. 71–75.

The manuscript medical text tradition in the late middle ages and into the early modern period has been extensively surveyed over recent years.[27] Recent research has indicated that manuscript compilations were significant in the supply, exchange, and dissemination of medical knowledge, especially since the initial locus of medical treatment was the family home (Leong and Pennell 2007: 133–134), and that the advent of printing by no means put paid to this lively tradition.[28] Indeed, the introduction of printing, which was consciously conservative and popularising, may have affected scientific work negatively (Voigts 1989: 350–351). Such collections of remedies and treatment procedures might well have had partial or complete indexing and alphabetisation in order to rationalise the content and render it more accessible. The tradition of keeping manuscript collections of medical information obviously continued through the period; Robert James has a rather disparaging entry for *receptarii medici*, of whom he remarks "Physicians who collect or write vast Loads of Prescriptions, to the great Detriment of their Patients, are thus called by way of Reproach," but such practices are known to have produced at least two of the dictionaries surveyed in this book, and possibly more may have been compiled this way. A great

---

23 For early modern manuscript lexicography, see Lancashire 2004.
24 For Forman, see Kassell 2013.
25 One of the exceptions is *cutis*, which appears in a run of the letter D.
26 For more on this, see Jones, P. M. 2011: 40.
27 See Taavitsainen et al., 2011: 9–11 for a brief account; Jones, Peter Murray 2011: 36; Norri, Juhani 2016.
28 See Voigts 1989 for an extended survey of late medieval manuscripts in science and medicine. For an early modern example kept by Valentyne Bourne of Norwich, see Fay 2015: 50–52.

many more never made it to the print shop—domestic compilations, often the work of women, but were put to practical use by the compilers throughout the period (see Furdell 2002: 96–98).

1.12 The present book

The arrangement of this book is chronological, but with a few exceptions. The chapter on glossaries comes before that on Nicholas Culpeper and the *Physical dictionary* simply because glossaries are all the medical lexicography that is published in Britain between Boorde and Culpeper, and that they continued to appear across the whole period. Since the eighteenth-century ones added little to what had already appeared, there seemed no justification for an additional chapter on them. Surgical dictionaries are lumped together in a single chapter because they are modest enough in size to justify this. The Latin dictionaries by Thomas Burnet and John Cruso, although different in many ways, appeared relatively close together in time, and are put together in their own chapter. The chronology of the book stops short of William Turton's *A medical glossary* of 1797.

It has also been essential in preparing this book to research and reconstruct the lives of most of our medical lexicographers. No dictionary is free of bias, and will tend to reflect the preconceptions of its creator, especially in an age not yet subject to the internal licensing and copyright arrangements within international publishing houses which tend to homogenise and standardise dictionary content. Just as R. J. J. Martin found it necessary in his article to explain John Freind's history of medicine in terms of this famous physician's life and career, so knowing about the lexicographers of medicine will shed light on their reasons for publishing such works (Martin 1988), although for the present purposes biographical material has been limited to that which has immediate relevance to a dictionary.[29]

---

29 It is hoped that books on the life and works of Drs John Quincy and Robert James based on much material which does not appear here will be published in due course.

2 Andrew Boorde (1490?–1549) and *The breuiary of helthe* 1547

Andrew Boorde's *The breuiary of helthe for all maner of syckenesses and diseases the whiche may be in man, or woman doth folowe, expressynge the obscure termes of Greke, Araby, Latyn, and Barbary in to Englysh concerning phisicke and chierurgye* was printed by William Middleton in July 1547. Some details of Boorde's life and career are known and generally agreed upon. He went to Oxford and was first admitted into the Carthusian order, but left about 1528 and went abroad to study medicine. Boorde travelled widely through Europe during the 1530s, even visiting the Holy Land and living for a while in Montpellier as he himself tells us (see Fletcher 2002; Furdell 2004). Although it has not been recognised as such, Boorde's *Breuiary* is arguably the first printed English medical dictionary—it certainly is so on a fairly strict understanding of what a dictionary is, despite having been seen simply as a vademecum for the poor and unlearned. This account is not wrong, but the work is clearly more than that and is a medical dictionary in a strong sense. Earlier views, such as those of the surgeon John Aikin are rather censorious (1780: 52–60), accusing Boorde of being coarse and trifling. Thomas Warton, whose account of Boorde is much more scholarly, takes him rather more seriously (1774 III: 70–78), arguing that a reputation for levity does not preclude being serious as well. It may be as well to recall, as Wear put it, that Boorde's *Breuiary* was in English, which was "the sine qua non of a popular medical book" (1998 IX: 22), a stark contrast to the works by Estienne, Foës (Foesius) and Gorris, not to say an outright affront.

2.1 Boorde's posthumous reputation

Boorde's medical reputation has been somewhat obscured by his being identified, probably quite incorrectly, as the original 'Merry Andrew' (see Guthrie 1943: 507), and being associated with joke-books such as *Scoggin's jests* and the early tale of the *Mylner of Abyngton*.[30] Other considerations may have conspired to assist Boorde's eventual but later association with Merry Andrew. He is a consistent and serious advocate for mirth as salutary. He addresses one of his dedicatees, the Duke of Norfolk, thus:

> the dyuers tymes in my wrytynges I do wryte wordes of myrth/ truely it is for no other intency-on/ but to make your grace mery for myrth is one of the chefest thynges of Physicke the whiche doth aduertyse euery men to be mery, and to beware of pencyfulnes (*Regiment*: Aiii^r)

---

30 *Scoggin's jests* was still being reprinted as Boorde's at the end of the eighteenth century.

https://doi.org/10.1515/9783110639186-002

a warning he repeats in many other places. A realistic assessment of Boorde's contribution to medical lexicography must however discount the association with Merry Andrew.

2.2 Boorde's works

An account of Boorde's works is by no means straightforward, the loss of some of them complicating it still further.[31] There is little point in exploring all the ins and outs of his publications and the various attributions here, but for our purposes it is significant that three of his major works were printing simultaneously about 1547: *The pryncyples of astronamye* and *The introduction of knowledge* at Robert Copland's printing house, and the *Breuiary* at William Middleton's. These and the *Breuiary* appear to form an interconnected series. Not all were to appear in that year. Copland was also printing a prognostication in the same year, which seems not to have survived, but is mentioned in passing in his preface to the *Pryncyples*, along with the association between the other two works:

> wher I haue ometted & lefft out mani matters aprtayng to this boke latt them loke in a book namyd the Introduction of knowleg a boke of my makyng the which ys aprintyng at old Robert Coplands the eldist printer of Ingland the which doth print thes yere mi pronosticacions. (The Preface)

In the same work, he likewise mentions *The introduction of knowledge*

> Who so euer wolde haue a forder noticion of the sygnes and the planetes & of theyr influence or constellacyon. let thē look in a book that is now a pryntyng at Robert cooplondes namyd the Introductyon of knowleg. And he that wyll haue the knowleg of, all maner of sycknesses & dysesys let them looke in the breuary of helth whiche is pryntyd at Wyllyam Mydyltons in flet stret. (Ciii^v)

It seems that he saw these works as interrelated, as was *The introduction of knowledge* (1555), there being a number of cross-references, such as the allusion to a particular fact in the *Breuiary* at cap. 261, *Os*:[32]

> Euery man the which hath all his whole lymmes hathe .ii.c.xlviii. bones as it doth more playnly appere in my Anothomy in the Introduction of knowlege whiche hath bene longe a pryntynge for lacke of money and paper, and it is in pryntyng wt pictures at Robert Copland prynter.

---

31 For a lengthy discussion of the various editions and datings of Boorde's works, see the introduction to Furnivall 1870. This includes some account of his lost works on 23-27.

32 Each numbered entry in the *Breuiary* is called a 'capitle', but is in fact a separate lemma. I will refer to these as chapters in this section, but use the abbreviation 'cap.' in references to them.

Boorde's frustration with the delays in publication is apparent, and Copland's position appears to have been parlous (Erler 2008). This may also account for the fact that the promised anatomy does not appear in the book. The hold-up may not in fact have been at Copland's establishment, since Boorde may be implying that it had been delayed elsewhere, and is now in press at Copland's printing-shop at the sign of the Rose Garland. The financial and supply difficulties alluded to here suggest that the publication of this work was delayed by a number of years, finally appearing under the imprimatur of William Copland, the successor and quite likely the son of Robert (Tedder 2004: 2008). The ESTC says of the *Introduction*: "Printer's name and address from colophon; publication date conjectured by STC", but it is tempting to assume from the inter-references that this work might also be from 1547 or not very much later. Boorde suffered the misfortune of both his publishers dying in 1547—Middleton in June (Erler 2008), and Copland presumably after the publication of the *Breuiary* on the fifteenth of July 1547. Copland's exiguity may partly explain the long delay in producing the *Introduction* some years after Boorde's own death in 1549. What Boorde seems to have had in mind was a set of inter-referenced introductions and a dictionary-like handbook in the vernacular for the use of the ordinary and unlearned Englishman.

Boorde's short *The boke for to lerne a man to be wyse in buyldyng of his howse for the helth of body* of about 1550 is proof, if it was needed, of the eclectic approach Boorde took to medicine and medical writing. Boorde argues that the situation and construction of a house as well as the air in the immediate vicinity had potential effects on health (Fay 2015: 39–41). This work also contains advice for daily living, including "myrth and reioysing doth strength a mānes lyfe, and doth expell syckenes" (Ciii[r]).

Boorde clearly intended that several of his works should be inter-referencing and should form a medical whole. He comments in *A compendyous regyment or a dyetary of helth* (1542), printed by Robert Wyer, that "If any man therfore wolde haue remedy for any syckenes or dyseases, let hym loke in a boke of my makynge, named ye Brevyare of helth" (Preface: Aii[v]). It seems then that the *Breuiary* appeared in an earlier edition than 1547, and Guthrie has suggested that they were companion volumes (1943: 507), which seems to be Boorde's implication; this in spite of the disparity in dates of printing. Boorde says that the *Introduction of knowledge*, also mentioned at the same spot, is being printed next to St Dunstan's church within Temple Bar (Aii[v]); that is, by Middleton. This work begins with the matter of the *Boke for to learne* verbatim, but continues with a number of additional chapters, beginning with Chapter nine on "replecyon or surfetynge" (Eii[v]). These latter chapters are to do with diet, the qualities of various foods, and the kinds of diets which are appropriate in coping with various ailments. It also seems that there is a version of the *Dyetary* without this material, apparently produced fraudulently under Thomas Linacre's name, not Boorde's (see ESTC; Thornton 1947, 1948).

The introduction of knowledge (1555?) is an account of a wide range of countries and languages, presumably reflecting Boorde's travels, either wholly or partly. A general impression of first-hand knowledge is often apparent. The book must have been published earlier than this edition, apparently the earliest now known, since Barnes alludes to it in 1541? in his attack on Boorde's work on beards, as does Boorde himself in the *Regyment*. The dedication is addressed to "the ryght honorable and gracyous lady Mary, doughter of our soverayne Lorde kyng Henry the .viii.", and signed from Montpellier on the third of May 1542.[33] Boorde also calls it "thys first booke", which presents somewhat of a problem. Is this his first book of all, or the first in the series he was writing in Montpellier? If the first of all, then it must precede the lost book on beards of 1541. Further, if the work had first been published in 1555, it would have had to be addressed to Mary as queen.

A short book which, although primarily an astrological handbook, mainly emphasises the medical implications and directions for the timing of such things as blood-letting and administering medicines is *The pryncyples of astronamye* (1547?). In a retraction, he mentions with just a hint of false modesty the circumstances of composing this work: "Now to conclud I desier euere mā to tak this lytil wark for a past time, for I dyd wrett & make this bok. in. iiii dayes and wretten with one old pene and with out mendyng" (*Pryncyples*: Dv[v]).

2.3   *The breuiary of helthe*

The *Breuiary* was written in the early 1540s while Boorde was in Montpellier, but was only published after his return to England. This work followed hard on the heels of Sir Thomas Elyot's Salernitan manual for the preservation of health, *The castell of helthe* (1539?),[34] but went much further in being original rather than a compilation of other works. It has not thus far been seen for the ground-breaking work it is. Previous accounts of the work are revealing, mainly for what they do not mention. Frederick Furnivall summarised it as simply "an alphabetical list of diseases, by their Latin names, with their remedies, and the way of treating them", as well as indicating that there are some other 'subjects' which are not obviously medical, such as the neglect of fasting (Extrauagantes fol. iiii[v]-v[r]). Furnivall also dismisses the work as a matter for a "Medical Antiquarian Society ... to reprint" (1870: 22). Guthrie saw it as a 'handbook' consisting of a large number of short chapters alphabetically arranged, without ever seeing it as a dictionary by another name and, like so many earlier commentators on medical works, treats it strictly as a source of med-

---

33 Williams 1962 lists only seven such dedications to Mary before her accession to the throne.
34 This is an ESTC date. There is also a version dated 1537. The date 1534 is used for the first appearance of the title-border in which it appears (McKerrow and Ferguson 1932, no. 30), and Elyot's work has sometimes been mistakenly been attributed to this year.

ical information, curiosities in particular. Its essentially lexicographical structure is quite overlooked. Guthrie is however happy to praise Boorde's medical common sense and forward-looking approach (1943: 509). Craig Muldrew describes it as "a self-help book of remedies and preventatives" (2011: 35), while Elizabeth Lane Furdell calls it a "paean to sensible living as a way of preserving vitality" (2002: 31). These accounts of the work, while revealing something of the characteristics of the *Breuiary*, do not come to grips with its real nature as the earliest attempt at a published medical dictionary in English, exhibiting all the main features one would expect to find in such a work.

There is rather more to the *Breuiary* than these comments would suggest; like *The introduction of knowledge*, it is also a richly linguistic work which merits further attention as an exercise in medical lexicography. The cross-references between the *Dyetary* and the *Breuiary* suggest that they were seen as interdependent works (Furnivall 1870: 21–22); indeed they may possibly have been conceived as part of a larger whole, along with his *Astronamye*, which was never fully realised, as we have already seen. He certainly seems to have been working on these books simultaneously in Montpellier. If John Bale (*Scriptores*, ed. 2) is referring to the *Breuiary* when he mentions Boorde's "Promptuarium physices", as Furnivall suggests (1870: 33), then this may mean that Bale understood very well the reference nature of the work, a promptuarium being a repository or storehouse, a place where things are kept ready for use.

Boorde's *Breuiary* proved to be popular and enduring. The work was reissued in 1552, 1557, 1575, 1587, and 1598, and still turns up in the sale catalogues for the libraries of a number of physicians and surgeons into the eighteenth century (Sir Richard Jebb, John Woodward, and others). The work was thus widely sold and presumably used, despite Aikin's description of it as "a very trifling and weak performance, extremely coarse in language, and injudicious in matter" (1780: 55). It is hard to find justification in the text for Aikin's abhorrence, despite the very occasional lapse in the expected decorum, such as the note on belching and farting for relief under *timpanitis*, cap. 345, albeit probably sound advice. In general, Boorde's tone is sober, serious, and indeed pious, exhorting the reader to avoid vices and to honour God. The text itself is quite often interlaced with advice about virtues and vices as well as reproducing familiar Tudor moral imperatives, as under *luxus* (intemperance), which should be avoided, since "where there is no order there is horror" and "al the kindes of sensualtie the which can neuer be subdewed wtout the recognision & knowlege of a mannes selfe what he is, of him selfe, what god is." A further example occurs under *febris*, as Boorde chides the young in a rather pointed afterthought: "Amonge al the feuers I had almost forgoten the feuer lurden with the which many yong men, yonge women, maydens and other yonge persons be sore infected nowe a dayes" (cap. 151 *febris*). OED defines this as "the disease of laziness".

2.4 English and foreign

Boorde seems at pains to stress his Englishness on his title-page; the juxtaposition of "Doctour" and "an englysh man" seems anything but coincidental. Indeed it is rather provocative since he is an Englishman aggressively insisting on using English for a medical text. The sense one often gets that it contains some significant autobiographical material is intriguing. The *Breuiary* also offers the occasional comment about Boorde's many foreign peregrinations, as in cap. 61, in which we are effectively told that he has been in Greece:

> Caro is the latyn worde. In greke it is named Sarx, but I dyd learne amonges the grekes Creas, as thus to saye, geue me some flesshe. In greke they saye Dos so moo creas, this is no true greke although it be the comon speche in greke.

In the 'Extrauagantes' (Giii^r *vrynes*), he informs us that "The phisicions in Grece & in Constantinople doth determine that a reed vrine doth signifie adustion of coler".

A substantive linguistic question is raised under cap. 118 *spyytynge of blode*: "*Emoptoica passio* be the latyn wordes. In greke it is named *Hæmoptoicon pathos* or *Phthisis*. And the true latyn worde is named *Tabes*."[35] *Tabes* appears to be the regular Latin term for wasting away. Identifying the 'true' or 'proper' term was a persistent difficulty for early modern medical terminology. What precisely is meant by 'true' here is intriguing. Boorde uses this descriptor a number of times in such contexts, including his mention of the "trewe latyns" in cap. 278, *phrenitis*, whose usage follows Greek, as well as in cap. 376, *vvlua*, where he instructs the reader to look for remedies under "the proper names" of the words. There is no explanation of what this expression means here, but this advice can only be helpful if what is meant is the alphabetised head-words rather than the chapter headings. Another mention occurs in the Introduction, where Boorde discusses Welsh: "I do not wryte true Welshe I do write it that euery man may rede it and vnderstand it without any teachynge." (Ci^v). In all of this, the sense seems to vary between 'formal' and 'official', perhaps under the more general sense of conforming to an acceptable or recognised standard or form (see OED sense 4). It is hard to see it as meaning 'classical' in reference to Latin, given the extensive post-classical medical writings Boorde must have known. 'Not barbarous' may be sufficient to cover it in some cases.

There is also a suggestion that while in Italy he had acquired some Italian, as in 'Extrauagantes' cap. 16 *excoriacio* "in Italion it is named *Malum Mule*." We do know that he was in Rome, possibly more than once, and for an extended period. We hear that he had lived there, and we also hear of an exorcism which he personally witnessed. A very long description of this ensues, in which, as narrator, he becomes a bystander at the event. In 'Extrauagantes' cap. 11 *demoniacus*: "The fyrste tyme that

---

35 I have used italics where Boorde actually has small capitals.

I dyd dwell in Rome there was a gentle woman of Germany, the whiche was possessed of deuyls". This woman had been brought to Rome to have the devils exorcised. The exorcism takes place at the obelisk in the precinct of St. Peter's, apparently the traditional place for such rites.[36] The response she gives to the priest's interrogation so appals Boorde that he leaves for fear of being possessed himself. "I considerynge this, and weke of fayth & aferde crossed my selfe & durste nat to here & se no more suche matters for it was to stupendiouse and aboue all reason".[37] There is also a long report in which he mentions other things and places, and is extremely critical of the corruption and vice in Rome. He also alludes to medical practices which apparently differ from those in England in cap. 317 *scrophule*: "For this matter in Rome and moundpyller is vsed incisions." There is also a reference to the same treatment in Montpellier under *timpanitis*, cap. 345.

At the same time, he admits both his own shortcomings and those of his material:

> I haue redde De Ostocopo,[38] but it is so longe agone that I haue forgotten what it is. And whan I dyd make this boke I was there that I had no Auctours nor Doctours to helpe me, but only by my practyce. (Extrauagantes' cap. 49 *oscedo*)

As far as is known, Boorde's is the first original printed medical work written in English, Elyot's being a translation, so that any models he might have used would probably have been in Latin. The sometimes conversational and at times hesitant tone he uses is entirely understandable in these circumstances. In cap. 341 *tenismos*, he concedes that "I am nat so good a grecion to declare, discusse, or defyne as some auctours doth wryte in th[is] matter for as many doth saye that *Tenasmon* is a dyffyle thynge for a man to make his egestiō or seege".

Even his illnesses are sometimes mentioned, as in cap. 50 *cacecia*, a condition of poor or insufficient nutrition which Boorde defines as slack or poor digestion: "I was in this infyrmyte, and by great trauell I dyd make my selfe whole more by labour than by phisicke in receptes of medecines." His remedy is moderation, not drinking either late or before eating, and hard labour. Perhaps this is an oblique allusion to the story of his aversion to beards as a result of a night of hard drinking in Montpellier (see Barnes 1541?: Aiiijʳ), but calls for moderation in life-style were the norm.

---

36 Described by Boorde as "a pyllar of white marble grated rounde aboute with Yron".
37 He is also appalled by "saynt peters church downe in ruyne & vtterly decayed and nothyng set by" as well as the "beggers, & baudes, hores and theues" haunting the place. He visits other places in Rome, such as the house of the Celestines and the Charterhouse, in which he finds disorder, and sees "Lechery & boogery, decyt and vsury in euery corner & place" in Rome. See also Foster 2008: 31-34.
38 It is not clear what Boorde is referring to here, but see Adams 1995: 304-305, s.v. *ostocopus*.

Another important point to recall is Boorde's acknowledgement of the difficulty of adumbrating the medical lexicon in full. Under the remedy for cholera, having given directions as to what to use, he comments that "I nor no man els can nat in theyr maternall tonge expresse the whole termes of phisicke" (cap. 79 *colera*).

2.5 The title

The title of the work raises some pertinent questions. The OED etymology shows that it is ultimately from "Latin breviārium 'summary, abridgement', from the neuter of breviārius 'A brief statement, summary, epitome." The word is listed as obsolete. In Boorde's day, however, it was a neologism in English, and a widely used term in Latin. Boorde seems to have been original in using breviary in his title, an Anglicisation of a Latin word which had a lengthy and exclusive association with religious texts in the sense of an abridgement or compendium of the canonical office. The next known use of the English word in a secular context from that period is in Nicholas Haward's translation of Eutropius published in 1564, and it does not appear in a secular title in English again until Humphrey Llwyd's *The breuiary of Britayne* of 1573. A sense a little more closely related to Boorde's is provided by Abraham Fleming's preface to the reader in John Caius's *Of Englishe dogges*, a work Fleming describes as a "breuiary or short treatise of such dogges as were ingendred within the borders of England" (Aiij^v). The word is also used by George Baker to describe a work by Arnold de Villa Nova in his translation of Konrad Gesner, entitled *The newe iewell of health* (1576).[39] Finally, Philip Barrough describes the glossary in his *The methode of phisicke* of 1583 as "a breuiarie or abridgement of phisicke" (*vj^v).

Since Boorde uses the word in a context of many references to the various short compilations of the Latin canonical order so often printed in the early sixteenth century, he explains in the preface that

> for as much as euery mã now a dayes is desirous to rede brefe and compendiouse matters. I therefore … pretend to satysfy mens minds … namynge this boke …The Breuyary of Healthe and where that I am very brefe in shewyng brefe medcines for one sicknes (Bij^v),

explicitly stressing the notion of brevity and implicitly detaching the term from its familiar religious sense, but perhaps recalling the breviary as a compendious text intended for regular use, containing in short form what it is necessary for the laity to know and observe. This is certainly a claim he makes for this medical work, offering the reader just enough knowledge to cope without supplanting the expertise of the

---

39 He describes a cure "borrowed out of the Breuiarie of *Arnoldus de villa noua* in the Chapter of the palsie."

professionals. Given the lack of such medical works in readily available printed form, Boorde may also have hoped to see his established as an enduring and traditional text. If this is so, it is all the more significant that he should do so in English rather than Latin.

The long title of the *Breuiary* is also revealing in a number of ways. First, it stresses the idea of the obscurity of the terminology covered by the work. There is also a very marked declaration of Boorde's Englishness as well as his profession, which is particularly striking in an age when medical works in English were the exception rather than the rule, and when the innumerable editions of the medical classics were mostly from the continent. The dominating English author-physician of the age, Thomas Linacre, translated Galen from Greek into Latin, but not into English, and was widely published on the continent, both in Paris and Lyon, but especially in Leipzig (see McConchie 2012; see also Helmstaedter 2005). The choice of languages employed in the *Breuiary*, "Greke, Araby, Latyn, and Barbary", is also declared in the title, and is thus given as much prominence as the medical content of the work. This draws immediate attention to its role as a polylingual glossary. It is also significant that these 'obscure' terms are to be translated into English.

The title-page itself uses a wood-cut border which appeared on subsequent editions of the *Breuiary* in 1552, 1557 and 1561. There was no particular reason to use this border, since it has no imagery or symbolism relevant to medicine, but it had already been used for three of Thomas Linacre's editions and translations of works by Galen and one of Linacre's *Rudimenta grammatices* by Richard Pynson in the 1520s (McKerrow and Ferguson 1932, no. 7), giving it some general association with both medicine and learning.

2.6   The preface

The work is introduced by an unusually long, painstaking five-part preface in which Boorde undertakes to address both readers and users of the book. The first part is addressed to doctors, urging them first to master the requisite knowledge, and only then put it into practice; the second to surgeons, who are encouraged become learned and have a steady hand as well as to consult a physician where necessary; the third is to patients, who ought to absolve their sins, make their wills, and do what the doctor or surgeon directs; the fourth is to the readers, Boorde informing them that he will explain the hard words; finally, "The Apendex to all the premysses folowethe" (Bii^v), being a general injunction to obtain spiritual remedy, live moderately and remain without sin. God has provided physical remedies as well as spiritual. Although he does not mention that the work was a new departure in English medical writing, it certainly is that.

Like the title, the preface to the work gives considerable time to the linguistic aspects of the *Breuiary*, adumbrated under the section addressed specifically to the readers.

> Gentyl reders, I haue takē some paine in makynge this boke, to do sycke mē pleasure and whole men profyte, that sicke men may recuperate their helthe and whole men may preserue thē selfe from sickenes (with goddes helpe) as well in phisicke as in Chierurgy. But for as muche as olde auncient, and autentyke auctours or doctours of phisicke in theyr bokes doth wryte many obscure termes, geuinge also to many and diuers infyrmites darke and hard names diffycyl to vnderstand some and most of al beynge greke wordes, some & fewe beynge Araby wordes, some beyng Latyn wordes, and some beyng Barbaruse words, Ther fore I haue trāslated all such obscure wordes and names in to englyshe, that euery man openly and apartly may vnderstande them. Furthermore all the aforesaide names of the sayd infyrmites be set togyther in order accordynge to the letters of the Alphabete, or the A B C. So yt as many names as doth begyn with A be set togither and so forth al other letters as they be in order. (Preface: Biᵛ)

His first declared intention is thus to make the terms of medicine plain and easy to understand, and to do so without concealment ('apartly') in the best interest of the poor and the unlearned.[40] His reasons for being brief, somewhat contradictorily, are that first, he will conceal as much of the art of medicine as is necessary to preserve the integrity of the science; second, he wants to prevent the incompetent from being encouraged to practise. Boorde also discusses the fact that he has left Latin terms in their nominative case rather than match them to the appropriate case in English, a concession to his unlearned readers intended to simplify their task. Despite the risk of criticism from learned circles, he points out in introducing the 'Extrauagantes' that "I do nat wryte these bokes for lerned men but for symple and vnlerned men that they may haue some knowlege to ease them selfe in theyr diseses and infyrmytes" (The Preface: Aiᵛ).

Whether Boorde achieved the aim of reaching out to the poor is probably now beyond our knowing. It seems, however, that despite Paul Slack's claim in his deservedly widely-cited article that such works could hardly do so (1979: 237), Boorde seems to have believed his assertion. That such claims in the prefaces of medical works were "calculated advertisements rather than statements of fact" (Slack 1979: 237) is not untrue, but it is not the entire truth either. That illiterate people could not read is not necessarily a barrier, since they could still be read to, and the knowledge Boorde offered could make its way through the social ranks and medical hierarchy by trickle-down diffusion. People who were educated, such as the clergy and women in charge of better-off households, saw it as their responsibility to pass on knowledge to others as well as to heal where they could (see Shapiro 2018). The books themselves may not have been in the homes of the poor, but their influence could be felt nonetheless. Slack cites instances of the discussion of medical

---

40 See OED *apertly*, sense 1.

knowledge between friends and neighbours (1979: 260). Another barrier to diffusion is the technical terminology used by the professionals, but that is precisely what the *Breuiary* is designed to overcome. Boorde is not merely producing a text in English as a matrix text, but is consistently offering glosses for the obscure terms used within it. Not all were prepared to do this even much later, retaining the medical terminology as the last professional bastion.

Boorde also makes large claims for the content of the book:

> Also there is no sicknes in man or woman the which may be frō the crowne of the heede to the sole of the foote but you shal fynde it in this boke, as well the sickenesses the whiche doth pertayne to Chierurgy as to phisicke, and what the sicknes is, and howe it doth come and medecines for the sefe same. (Preface: Bii[r])

Perhaps this should be seen in the light of the point he makes elsewhere that no one is able to compile all the terms of medical knowledge in a single volume. Since there was some agreement at the time that the diseases adumbrated by Hippocrates and Galen were all that there were, this suggests that the knowledge of the terminology was in fact much less fixed than that of the ailments themselves.

Turning more specifically to what the *Breuiary* actually contains, a study of the 455 head-words shows Boorde's comments on the languages he uses are not wholly borne out by his text. He remarks that among the obscure terms the majority are Greek, some are Arabic, some Latin, and some barbarous (Bi[v]), but the great majority of the head-words (62 percent) are in fact Latin, while the Greek component is much less at 29.5 percent.[41] The separate listing of barbarous terms, which amounts to variants of familiar medical terms, indicates that Boorde is thinking not strictly in terms of languages, but of linguistic usage within the medical profession. Barbarous usage presumably identifies terms used by the apothecaries. This term can also be found outside the medical profession however, being more used in the context of religion, history, politics, and law than in medical works by the early eighteenth century. The division between the various language categories is Latin 285, Greek 134, Arabic 17, Barbarous 11; nil, that is, no language attribution 6, and Physicke 2.

---

41 I have strictly followed Boorde's own ascriptions here, and made no adjustments for him possibly being incorrect.

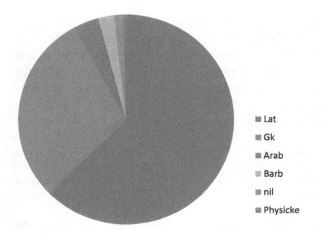

- Lat
- Gk
- Arab
- Barb
- nil
- Physicke

Fig. 1: Language attributions in *The breuiary of helthe*: Latin, Greek. Arabic, Barbarous, no attribution, and Physicke in percentages

Boorde now makes his claim in the title to 'express' the foreign terms in English more explicitly, claiming that they will be translated; in other words, glossed. These terms will also be put into alphabetical order, he suggests, although the order adopted is not entirely strict in the modern sense, being A- order and, rather inconsistently, AB- order.

2.7 The structure of the *Breuiary*

The work consists of two parts, the *Breuiary* itself, and what he calls the 'Extrauagantes', the 'extravagants', which sounds like a collection of afterthoughts or material found while the *Breuiary* itself was in progress but could not be changed. However, the fact that there are many references in the *Breuiary* to words in the 'Extrauagantes' gives the lie to this presumption. Perhaps it represents a change of mind about what should be included, but it can hardly have been composed later. The use of this term in the early- to mid-sixteenth century would suggest that what is in this section is 'stray'; either beyond the canon of medicine, or overlooked.

The chapter total is 383 in the *Breuiary*, seventy-three in the 'Extrauagantes' and a further three in the small additions section, ending the *Breuiary* alphabetically with *zimie*, although the large number of cross-references to terms within entries and some insertions of 'minor' lemmas (see *blohosos*, under Al-; *dia, diuramator*[sic], etc.) suggests that the total number of medical terms in the work is much higher. It is further increased by the fact that some entries contain terms for parts, as under *oculus*, where we find *rhetina, secundina, sclerosis, tela arena, vnca, cronea*[sic], and *conjunctiva*, as well as some compound English terms for complaints of the eye, such as *goggle-eyed* and *dim-sighted*. Of these, *retina, secundina* (*secundina pellis* being a different medical phenomenon), and *tela arena* are unrecorded elsewhere, *sclirosis* [sic] is listed and cross-referenced to *febris de trachea*, while *conjunctiva* and *cornea* are appropriately cross-referenced. These additional terms are usually indicated in the text by the use of italics. A manicule or a fleuron also introduces a variable number of sub-lemmas at the end of many entries, such as *anathomia* and *apepsia* at the end of cap. 26 *aptæ*. This distinction into main entry head-words and entry text, while obscuring the presence of many other terms, has been done on the assumption that this is Boorde's fundamental category distinction, and that more generally in the process of transferring lexicographical data from one medical dictionary to another, this is a point of fracture or discontinuity.

Each chapter is arranged under a heading which includes an English term or description, presumably when a single term was not available, but this is not the alphabetical head-word for the entry. The chapter heading seems to include the best-known term, often English rather than Latin, Greek, or Arabic and sometimes a word, sometimes an explanatory phrase. This head-word introduces the next section, and is indicated by a drop capital and the Roman font, the text itself being in black-letter. This heading is also indented, in a smaller type-face, and is prefixed by the early modern pilcrow, or a capitulum, which serves the same function as a manicule. Alphabetisation is governed by the head-word, almost never in English, Boorde indicating the source language in most cases. Alphabetisation is generally adhered to after the initial letter, but there are many exceptions, such as the sequences *cornix–chimosis–ciphac–cherade* and *expergifactio–exanthemata*.

The glosses follow, usually in the order Greek, Latin, and English, with variations such as Arabic, Latin, and English, depending on the derivation. The entry for *epilepsia* is an especially complex one, the remedy section of this chapter also containing some English versions of Latin terms used elsewhere, e.g., *oyle of philosophers*. The glossary part is sometimes accompanied by a definition, and then a section headed "The cause of this impediment/these impediments/infyrmyte" or something similar. The last section, also separately headed, usually contains a remedy for the complaint, and sometimes several, as under *capillus* (hair). This is sometimes followed by a set of cross-references and/or a few extra terms not given full entry status. This last represents a useful and consistent means of cross-referencing. An example of one sub-entry which is not a cross-reference but relates to the main lemma occurs at the end of *fistula*: "*Fistula cimbalaris* is a pype in the throte ye whiche doth meliorate a mannes voyce or breste" but might have been incorporated into the text of the main entry, while one which is entirely separate from the main lemma is "*Chilis* is the name of a vayne the which dothe sprynge out of the lyuer," which falls between *cornix* and *chimosis* (Iiiiᵛ).

Italics are used for the terms other than English, but these may occur in the text in black-letter as under *coriza*, where *eliborus albus* is in black-letter; likewise *emptoica passio*: "let the pacient be let blode in a vayne named sophena, and thā abstract a lytle blode out of cephalica," where *sophena* and *cephalica* are in black-letter. English terms are seemingly never in italics, although long-established borrowings such as *morbus* and *mithridatum* are, and established anglicisations such as *sarcocol* and *iliac passion* may appear in black-letter.

There are some exceptions to the structure adumbrated above. The entry for *febris* stands out since it has several chapters of its own, and there are further types and terms which are not given full chapter status, especially at the end, such as *febris homothena, febris augmastica* and *febris epamastica*.[42] Among the many other sub-lemmas, some are treated as for main lemmas in that they appear with translations, synonyms and a gloss, as in *lacerti*. A few other entries have their own chapters, although not nearly so many as *febris*; *melancholia* and *nares* have two chapters. *Morbus* is treated somewhat the same, the various diseases under this head being given two separate chapters; *morbus regius* and *morbus gallicus*. In between these are *morbus caducus, morbus comicialis*, and *morbus arquatus* as sub-lemmas. Interestingly, there are sub-lemmas which have the full linguistic range of glosses, and even a manicule at the beginning of the entry as well as a marginal note.

Anomalous chapters occur, such as cap. 316, for which there is no actual head-word. This chapter is headed "The .316. Capitle doth shewe of many infyrmytes names which shalbe found, in theyr capytles." What is listed here is simply the terms *scabies, scirrhus, scarificacio, scliros, sebel* and *semiapoplexia*, each preceded by a manicule and with their cross-references; in other words, a list just like those so often appended to the end of main entries. The number can also be paralleled elsewhere, although infrequently, so that it hard to see why Boorde has deviated from his usual practice. Among other entries, *salsum flegma* is followed by five sub-entries with manicules, but no entries with five sub-lemmas occur between *cephalargia* and *salsum flegma*, the largest number in this section being four between *emoptoica* and *ephialtes*, and there are some examples of three. After *algarab* and *catarrhos*, however, there are no less than six, and five occur after *alboras* and *asthma*. Since the marginal glosses usually provide the English rather than Latin or Greek, the entry for *herpes* has "tetter" as its marginal gloss, *sirones* has "wormes", and so on. *Madness* in the 'Extrauagantes' lists four Latin terms without stipulating one as the main entry.

Boorde's choice of word to head the alphabetical entry needs some consideration. Given that most are Latin and many are Greek, but there are also Arabic and barbarous head-words, he presumably does not rely primarily on a preferred language. The chapter headings themselves and the marginal glosses are largely in English as we have seen. My assumption has been that there is an underlying principle of using the 'best-known' term, but this is a very slippery concept. Best-known to whom and by whom? One would certainly expect a compiler such as Boorde, with

---

42 For the detail invested in the classification of fevers, see Slack 1979: 268.

his aggressively positive attitude to the use of the vernacular to do this. Boorde does not use the barbarous term simply where there is no alternative; thus under *siatica passio* [sic], a head-word described as barbarous, he has given the English terms in the chapter heading "a goute named Sciatica", *sciatica* being in black-letter, and then informs the reader that it is known as *dolor scie* in Latin and *ischias* in Greke. We also hear that 'some' call it "*Coxendrix* or *Coxendricis morbus*." Likewise, *quinancia*, the preferred barbarous head-word, has equivalents in Latin *angina*, and Greek *synanchi*. Since the English term given here is the familiar term *squyncey*,[43] the choice of the barbarous gloss to head the entry seems very marked. The alphabetical head-word *anastropha* is also designated as barbarous, and is followed in order by the Greek and English terms. The chapter heading for this is "casting vp of a mans meate," and it is also glossed simply as "a vomiting" in the definitional section. *Catharacta* is another leading barbarous word, as are *coriza*; *grossities, gurta, limphaticarom*, and *nureticus*, the last four in the 'Extrauagantes'. The method seems to be to lead the chapter with the English term, follow with the alphabetised head-word, then Latin, Greek and Arabic, in no particular order, where applicable, and then round off this section with a repetition of the English term. Any of these languages may include further glosses as well. It is difficult to determine whether there is a principle in play here. If Boorde is choosing the most familiar word to head the alphabetised sections, how would we know except by taking for granted what we hope to show? It might be more informative in this respect to analyse his choices than to attempt to reconstruct what might have been familiar to him from present-day historical dictionaries and corpora. Another possibility is that he is simply taking over material from his source(s), possibly a manuscript, but this would contradict his claim that he has had no models to follow. A check of the *Synonyma medicinae seu clavis sanationis* of Simon Genuensis (1473), a possible source, only located a scattering of corresponding head-words *acrochordones/acrocordines, alboras/albaras, algarab, amigdale, anasarca, animus, antrax/anthrax, bulimos, cacecia/cachecea, xrophthalmia*[sic]/*xerotalmia, zerma/zerna*, etc.), insufficient to suggest that this was in fact a source for Boorde. Perhaps more telling is the large number of obvious head-words in Simon that Boorde does not use.

2.8 Barbarous words

Although barbarous Latin is often mentioned in other medical works, Boorde uses "barbarous" alone, rather than barbarous Latin, so that variants of Greek and Arabic may also be barbarous for him. In fact, words he lists as barbarous are either from Latin, such as *catharacta, gutta, quinancia*, or Greek, as in *argemata*. A few are uni-

---

43 See OED quinsy/squinsy.

dentified so far, such as *tarphati*.[44] Thus it is not entirely clear what he means, although he may simply be referring to the usages of apothecaries irrespective of derivation. In all, fifty-two barbarous terms are mentioned aside from the head-word occurrences. The great majority are essentially spelling variants of the head-word, although there are some inconsistencies within this such as the ending '-us' for '-os'. In a few cases, the terms are unrelated, and in one case, *lichena*, it serves for no less than three different head-words, including lichen itself. The other unrelated terms are *impetigo* and *zerma*.[45]

Making only a brief assessment of the source language as stated in the OED and ignoring mediation through languages such as French shows that *acroconides*, *anastropha*, *asma*, and *cremastres* are directly from Greek. The great majority are from Greek via Latin in some way or another, and just one, *mirac*, is from Arabic through Latin. The majority are from Greek through some form of Latin, although I have not noted whether this is classical, post-classical, late Latin, etc. and a few are directly from Latin, such as *emigrania*, *quinancia*, and *ungula*. The point is that when Boorde uses 'barbarous/barbary', he does not necessarily mean barbarous Latin only. There is of course no guarantee that Boorde would agree with the OED's etymologies.

There are many suggestions that Boorde is reflecting uncertainty and variation in medical terminology. One of the more intriguing comments appears under *febris hectica*, where he writes that "*Febris hectica* is the greke worde. The latynes doth name it *Hectica passio*. The barbarous persons with some latyntst[sic] dothe name it *Febris Etica*, In englysh it is named the feuer Etycke, or the Etycke passion". It seems here that Boorde means to suggest some overlap between the usages of the apothecaries ("barbarous") and the learned ("latynysts"). Since the word hectic derives from the Greek ἑκτικός, Boorde attributes *hectica* to the Greeks, and *etica* to those using barbarous terminology. Further overlap between the classical and barbarous usages is suggested by the entry in cap. 172 "*Haemorrhoides* is ye greke word. In olde tyme the latyns dyd vse this barbarous worde named *Emoroides*," as well as cap. 371 "*Vndimia* is the latyn worde. And some doth say it is a barbarous worde," which indicates a degree of doubt about the status of this term.

There is also some overlap both in what the 'Latins' are called ("latyns"/"latenists"), as well as which term is used by whom. Cap. 278 *phrenitis* suggests that "the barbarus worde is named *Frenisis*. The trewe latyns doth vse the terme after the grecions." Who are the "true latyns"? The truly learned? Classical writers who wrote in Latin? The lexical discussion can become quite complex, as in cap. 54 of the 'Extrauagantes':

---

44 Used by Mesue 1549: f. 14ʳ.
45 For allusions to the usages of medical practitioners in Elyot, see Stein 2014: 281-2.

Pvlmonia is the latyn word ...there be .ii. kyndes, the one ... is named *Pulmonia* or *Pipulmonia*, and some doth name it *Peripneumonia* the other dothe cleue to the rybbes, and is named *Pluritis*, or *Peripulmonia*, of[sic] *Plurea*, or *Pluritis*, or *Pluris*, or *Pluresia* al is one thing, saue that some wordes be barbarous wordes.

Examples of multiple choices of terminology include: "Some doctours do name this infyrmyte Ruonia. And some do name it *Gutta rubia* and *Gutta rosea*" (cap. 48 *buriga*). In this case, the variation is between doctors themselves, not between doctors and, say, apothecaries. Barbarous words may also be productive, as suggested by cap. 343 *thetanos* "The barbarous worde is named *Tetanus*, out of the whiche is vsurped a worde named *Tetanisi*"; that is, those who suffer from tetanus. Boorde also has some mixed derivations; under *aschachilos* he gives this as the Greek word, but then says that the word *asca* in Arabic means corruption and that *chilos* is Greek. Usage is also called into question, as in the very hesitant "*Porrigo* or *Porre* or *Furfures* some latenist[sic] dothe vse these termes."[46] The list upon which this discussion is based accepts the first attribution of language in the entry, not any subsequent mixed etymology, as under *aschachilos*.

Some entries are also signalled by a marginal note or heading, generally the larger ones, but there are exceptions. Boorde is happy to correct perceived errors, as under 381 *Ydroforbia* "I haue sene & redde that the barbarous worde is named *Euforbium* the whiche is false, for *Euforbium* is a gumme. ... *Hidroforbia* in englyshe is abhorringe of water as I lerned in the partes of grece". Suggestions about etymologies occasionally appear, as in Ex. cap. 29:

Hyostianum is a kinde of frantycknes, and it doth take the name of a greke word named *Hiostianus*, the whiche in englyshe is named Henbane, for who so euer doth eat of Henbane or an herbe named Dwale shal fal into a frantycknesse or a fantasticall minde.

2.9 Duplicates

Four terms appear in both the *Breuiary* and the 'Extrauagantes': *caros*, *lepus marinus*, *pulse* and *tortura*. Three of these involve homonymy or polysemy. The duplicates *caros–caros* are merely homonyms; lethargy in the *Breuiary* and crapula (hangover) in the 'Extrauagantes'. Similarly, *lepus marinus* has been cross-referenced from the *Breuiary* because it has two different possible meanings: "some dothe name this sicknes a wateryshe skabbe that ronneth abrode and some doth take it for a kynde of vometynge, loke in the capytle named *Lepus marinus* in the 'Extrauagantes' in the end of this boke." The exception is *pulse*, which is the arterial pulse in the *Breuiary*, but in the 'Extrauagantes' the same meaning is given a far a

---

46 This has been recorded as Latin in my list nonetheless.

longer account, again cross-referenced from the *Breuiary*: "they be named pulses because they be euer knockynge and laboryng [sic] For this matter loke in the *Extrauagantes* & in the capitle named *Arterie* & in the capitle named *Vene*."

2.10 Glosses and definitions

There is a tendency for the English gloss to be a definition rather than a gloss, whether there is an English word or not, as under *empima*, etc. An example of one which is both in effect is *excrementa*: "*Excrementa* is the latyn worde. In englyshe it is these thynges the which be digested and expulsed, and there be excrementes of the egestion, of vrine". Sub-divisions with their own terms sometimes appear, as in *exitura*. The lexicographical tradition in Boorde's day did not often recognise what we would call definition, since dictionaries were by definition bilingual or polylingual, so that the significance of Boorde's work for lexicography cannot be overestimated (see McConchie and Curzan 2011).

Glosses are sometimes embedded comfortably enough in the English text as an explicit explanation, as in cap. 45 *bocium* "In englyshe it is a swellynge the which doth grow in the throte and in the necke ... naturall bocions comonly chyldren hath". Examples of the gloss fully implicit in the text also occur, as in cap. 77 *coitus*, the remedy part of which mentions "Medecines for a man the whiche can nat do the acte of matrimony thorowe impotence" and "Medecines to helpe a man or a woman to haue chyldrene" and "Medecines to kepe a man or a woman lowe of corage". The deficiency of the native lexicon is also commented upon in cap. 79 *colera*. Under the remedy, after directions as to what to use, Boorde remarks that "this must be done of a potycary the which hath ye practyce of al suche matters, for I nor no man els can nat in theyr maternall tonge expresse the whole termes of phisicke."

2.11 The use of 'some'

Boorde, like many early modern lexicographers and those with terminology to explain, makes use of the indefinite 'some', presumably to express doubt over the proprieties of usage. This usually introduces an alternative expression, but without the pejorative sense that 'barbarous' would involve. For instance, in cap. 88. *ilirica passio* (alphabetised head-word *cordapsis*), after the glosses we get "Some men dothe name this sicknes volnulus."[47] In the case of cap. 286 *polipus*, 'some' prefer a lengthy periphrasis: "And some doth name it *Excrecensia carnis in naso*", and in cap. 315 *siatica passio* we read "and some doth name this infyrmyte *Coxendrix* or

---

47 This should obviously read 'voluulus' ('volvulus'), the 'n' being a turned letter.

Coxendricis morbus." Cap. 341 *tenismos* sets up 'some' under a further category with a separate form: "some dothe name it *Tenasmon*. The barbarus word is named *Tenesmus*. And the latenystes doth name it *Tenesmus*. And some latenystes doth name it *Gemitus*." In this case, it is left unclear whether the first 'some' is a sub-species of 'barbarus' or a separate category, while the second clearly applies to a sub-species of Latinist. Expressions of uncertainty in the work of Sir Thomas Elyot which are similar to those in Boorde have been pointed out (Stein 2014: 271–273).

2.12 Conclusion

Boorde is at pains in *A compendyous regyment or a dyetary of helth* to justify his plainness of speech (pointedly using a number of aureate terms to do so, as well as the then fashionable doublings), informing his lordship the dedicatee that "I ... haue not ornated and flourysshed it with eloquent speche and rethorycke termes, ye which in all wrytynges is vsed these modernall dayes" (The preface: Aii^v–iij^r). His decision not to consistently valorise Latin or Greek any further than as the usual alphabetised head-word for his entries is significant, as is his attention to both barbarous terms and English.

The introduction of knowledge points out that "The speche of Englande is a base speche to other noble speches, as Italion Castylion and Frenche, howbeit the speche of Englande of late dayes is amended" (Bij^r). Boorde thus embraces the problem of the perceived insufficiency of English, assertively declaring the language's right to be taken seriously. He also stands near the beginning of the trend towards the printing of medical works in English (Pahta 2011: 117), a natural if somewhat tardy response to the vernacularisation of both medicine in particular and science more generally in the late middle ages in England (see Voigts 1989). When Simon Forman later wished to expand his manuscript medical word-list, now King's College Cambridge MS 16, he turned to Andrew Boorde for much of the additional material, and Boorde's work was reprinted a number of times. Boorde thus has a legitimate place as a pioneer in medical lexicography, adapting the dictionary format to English use.

3 Medical glossaries

Glossaries, which are by definition less than stand-alone dictionaries, occur in some printed medical works of the period we are concerned with as a supplement to a particular text and an aid to the reader.[48] By and large they are relatively straightforward lexicographically, usually including simply a head-word and a gloss or definition. Ian Lancashire pointed out in 2002 that glossaries (and indeed many dictionaries) in this period translated words rather than defining them, a practice apparent throughout the medical glossaries. This translation work adds particular point to Lancashire's view, given that exactly what a glossary does by way of either defining or rendering equivalences is not very clear. No one criterion for what constitutes a glossary is absolute, but they include limited scope, both as appended to a specific work and to a specific subject, alphabetisation, both translational and explanatory equivalence, lexical definition, and a relative lack of encyclopaedic content, Essentially, the medical glossaries are alphabetical, while other familiar characteristics of dictionaries are only sporadically present. Alphabetisation is also used now and then by works which could not otherwise be classified as either dictionaries or glossaries, medical reference works usually preferring some conventional professional categorization, such as the head-to-foot description of the body familiar from late medieval manuscripts. This appears in such works as the translation of Christof Wirsung's *The general practise of physicke* (1598) and the list of anatomical terms in Randle Holme's *The academy of armory* (1688), or the classification proceeds by such means as type of remedy, disease or symptom, and so on.

Compilations such as the list of simples appearing in the 1618 London pharmacopœia lack both glosses and definitions, and are only alphabetical within large categories like *ligna*, *animalia*, and *cortices*. Pharmacopœias retain this structural characteristic throughout our period, and thus cannot be considered as genuinely lexicographical in nature, although they do provide lists of potential head-words, albeit separated into categories (see RCP 1632), but since they are primarily organised topically, acquiring a word-list from an existing dictionary is more convenient for the would-be lexicographer.[49]

John Tanner's *The hidden treasures of the art of physick* of 1659 provides a fairly typical example of a medical glossary. Almost any sample page, taking in this case the opening page of the letter S, shows variation between translational equivalence (loosely, glossing) as with *situation*, *sediment* and *sincere*, and explanatory equivalence, as in *saphæna* or *scarification*. The latter shades off into encyclopaedic content

---

48 Most of the sixteenth-century glossaries mentioned here are described in Schäfer 1989.
49 For an account of the Arabic origins of much of the traditional content and terminology of early pharmacopoeias as well as a useful survey of the earlier works on pharmacy, see Hueget-Termes (2008).

https://doi.org/10.1515/9783110639186-003

and, in this glossary, classification is modified by the fact that the head-words are seen as English.[50] We are not dealing here strictly with bilingual lexicography, but with specialist terminology heavily dependent on its Greek and Latin sources, much of which has been long-established in English but little altered in form from the source language.

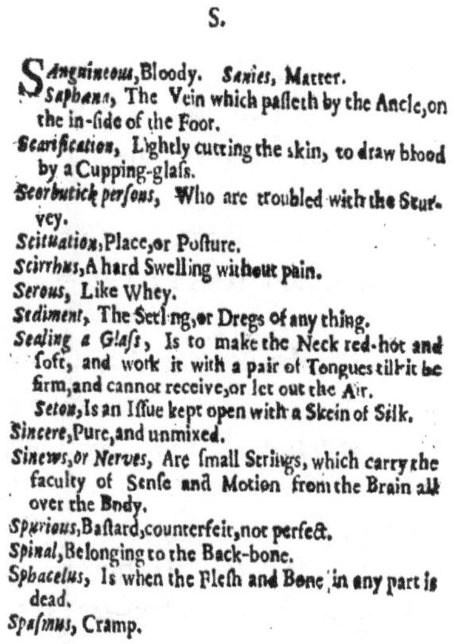

S.

Sanguineous, Bloody. Sanies, Matter.
Saphana, The Vein which passeth by the Ancle, on the in-side of the Foot.
Scarification, Lightly cutting the skin, to draw blood by a Cupping-glass.
Scorbutick persons, Who are troubled with the Scurvey.
Scituation, Place, or Posture.
Scirrhus, A hard Swelling without pain.
Serous, Like Whey.
Sediment, The Setling, or Dregs of any thing.
Sealing a Glass, Is to make the Neck red-hot and soft, and work it with a pair of Tongues till it be firm, and cannot receive, or let out the Air.
Seton, Is an Issue kept open with a Skein of Silk.
Sincere, Pure, and unmixed.
Sinews, or Nerves, Are small Strings, which carry the faculty of Sense and Motion from the Brain all over the Body.
Spurious, Bastard, counterfeit, not perfect.
Spinal, Belonging to the Back-bone.
Sphacelus, Is when the Flesh and Bone in any part is dead.
Spasmus, Cramp.

Fig. 2: A page of the glossary from John Tanner's *The hidden treasures of the art of physick*

An obvious question about the various glossaries is whether they provided material for dictionaries, or influenced them in some other way. The majority are too small to have a perceptible effect, and it seems that the massive collection accumulated by Randle Holme was not only rather ad hoc, but also more an end-point than a beginning. There is little to suggest that lexicographers used the material in pharmacopœias in this way either. Glossaries tend to be either general or specialised in nature, always allowing for the fact that 'hard words' are a specialism in themselves. I will merely survey some of the more significant glossaries chronologically in this chapter and point out general trends.

---

50 For discussion of the nature of translation equivalence in its various forms, see Adamska-Salaciak 2016: 148–154.

3.1 Traheron's translation of Vigo

A translation of a work by the Italian Giovanni da Vigo (1450?–1525) appeared in 1543. Bartholomew Traheron (c.1510–1558?), the translator, appended a list of what he called "The interpretation of straunge wordes, vsed in the translation of Vigon" (Zz^r), making this perhaps the earliest of such printed glossaries in printed English medical books. Traheron, keeper of the King's Library from 1549–1553, is not known to have produced any other medical works or to have practised medicine.

Vigo's *Chirurgerye* proved durable, being republished in 1550? (by both Wyer and Whitchurch), 1552?, 1555?, 1571, 1562, 1564, and 1586 (see ESTC). The work is little discussed by modern scholars, however, except for the question of the use of the vernacular in medical writings (see Williams 2011: 58–59). Both Thomas Elyot and Robert Recorde had felt it necessary to mount explicit and spirited defences of the use of English in their medical publications. Traheron's translation and extensive glossary must also have helped to elevate the vernacular. [51]

Traheron's glossary contains 420 head-words, including those treated formally as sub-lemmas, that is, without the head-word centred on a separate line and repeated at the commencement of the entry text. These are not all that frequent, amounting to nine in all, three of these at the beginning of the letters A, C, and O. Traheron's count makes it only slightly short of the total of Boorde's *Breuiary* (457), although the average entry in Boorde is rather longer than those in Traheron, as would be expected in a fully-fledged medical dictionary rather than a glossary. Traheron's entries are certainly richer than in most glossaries, however.

The entire work is printed in black-letter, a significant departure from the usual distinction between this and italic, with centred head-words and a repetition at the start of the main entry. Sometimes however the last word of the previous entry takes up the left side of the line with the centred head-word. Letters are handsomely introduced by historiated drop-capitals. There are some sub-lemmas with uncentred head-words, rather as in Boorde, including *excrescences* and *exciccation*, which are usually just given a gloss rather than a fuller and more explanatory entry.

Quite a lot of doubt about the meanings of words is expressed in this glossary. Under *acetositas citri*, we find Traheron first telling us what he has done and then patiently declaring his doubts about it, as well as introducing the familiar quandary of what to do about the usage of apothecaries:

> I dyd translate it ones or twyse, the soure iuce of an orenge; howebeit the apothecaries make this syrup wt the iuce of a citron (as they haue shewed me)[sic] Natheles Fuchsius techeth that they ben both of lyke vertue and effect. And Io. Agricola sayth yt citrō signifyeth an orenge, and also

---

51 For Traheron, see Trueman 2004.

a limō. And bycause this name is doutfull, I leue it to thy iudgemēt, good reader, whether thou wylt (when thou fyndest the ryndes of a cytron, or ye iuce) vnderstand an orēge or a pome citrō.

Lexical meaning and species significations are not clearly distinguished here; the apothecaries have demonstrated something which does not fully reflect Traheron's translation, and he regards the claims of German physician and botanist Leonhard Fuchs (1501–1566) about the medical benefits as equivalent to that of Agricola about the identification of the actual fruit.[52] His solution is to abandon final judgement to the reader, having set out the somewhat conflicting accounts. A modern dictionary reader would expect full disambiguation between what the correct translation is and what to use to confect the remedy. The entry for *acorus*, while shorter and more straightforward, is equally problematic. Traheron offers the reader the identifications of Otto Brunfels (1488–1534), Mainard (probably Ioannes Mainardus Ferrariensis), and what we often find in the early glossaries and dictionaries, the attribution to what the indefinite 'some' call it: "Some take it for galingale."

Considerable doubt about translation strategy appears in *aqua gariofilata*:

> Aqua gariofilata is the water of cloues: as it appeareth in the fourthe boke of abridgementes. Howbeit, by cause gariofilata is commenly taken for ieloflours, for that, that they haue the odour of cloues called gariophili I thynke I dyd translate it ones, the water of iellyflours. Here ye shal note that though gariofillata be commenlye taken for ielofloures, yet other well lerned men thinke it to be Auēs, and so perchaunce I haue translated it sometymes.

It seems here that Traheron is hedging his bets and translating it both ways at various times. *Centorie the greater* again provokes a list of alternatives. Likewise *centrum galli*, *consolida the greater*, *memithe*, *minium*, and *mumia*. He also hedges over the identity of *lanciola*: "Vigo sayeth that Lanciola is hote and drye in the fourth degre, & therfore I thinke that he meaneth speareworte Lāciolata signifieth the lesse plantaine."

There are often attempts at derivation, as under *aematites*, which is given a Greek derivation from 'Hema'; others include *apium risus*, *bechichie*, *chilis*, *diaphinicon*, *epithema*, *eupatorium*, *gumme elemi*, *maturatiue*, *omphacine*, *obthalmia*, *parotides*, *philomum*, *psillium*, *pyretrum*, *sarcoeides*, *sclerotike*, *serpillum*, *sticados*, *storax*, *suppositorium*, *tenasmos*, *terra sigillata*, and *trociskes*.

Barbarous words are often noted: "the barbarous auctors vse alcohol, or (as I fynde it sometymes wryten) alcofoll"; likewise *collyrie*, *os laude*, *pustles*, *rasceta*, *saphatum*, *sclerotike*, *sirsen*, *undimia*, and others. Those who use such terms are identified as authors, and at least once as doctors (under *rasceta*). An explanation of the difference in usage occurs under *obthalmia*: "Ophthalmos in greke, sygnifyeth an eye. The barbarouse writters leue out the aspiration or lettres h h, and turne P, into B;" thus it seems clear that the head-word here is the barbarous form. The language of

---

52 Possibly Georgius Agricola (Georg Pawer, 1494–1555).

apothecaries is noted under *coloquintida, infusion, ireos* ("the Apothecaries vse the genitiue case for the nominatiue"), *malabathrum, miuam, paucedinis,* and *trociskes,* and a herb known only to the apothecaries, *ermoline*: "Ermolinus is an herbe, wherof I haue founde nothing wryttē. Howbe it ye apothecaries affirme that they haue it." *Palea marina* he claims is a term of which he has read nothing, but may signify a marine product "whyche they thynke to be spuma maris, that is ye fome of the saye." He declares his uncertainty about what Vigo meant by the term *chaff of the sea*. Latin, Greek and other glosses are sometimes given as well.

Under *bozomus*, Traheron claims that "This worde Bozomus is found in no good auctour, that euer I chaunced to see. Bromus in greke signifieth the corne which we call Otes, let the reader iudge, whether Vigon vse bozomus, for bromus", while under *pericranium*, Traheron comments that he feels obliged to add to Vigo since, he claims, Vigo is obscure on the anatomy of the head. This becomes a very lengthy addition as Traheron extends it to other principal organs as well—the heart, liver, and stomach—supplying some information on each of them. Some extra terminology is provided in these entries as well. *Pyretrum* involves a lengthy language discussion. All in all, this glossary is far more sophisticated than many appearing much later. Two English authorities are mentioned: William Turner under *aristologia* who, Traheron relates, "shewed me that he founde thys herbe in Italye", which tells us something about the fact that they knew each other as well as Turner's peregrinations in Europe. The entry for *chamepiteos* refers to Robert Recorde, whose own glossary in *The urinal of physick* is a very modest series of lists of diseases and simples between pages 62 and 65 (see Schäfer 1989: I). A gross error occurs under *cancrena*, where we find the complete entry for *gangrena*, not where it should be, a mistake still not corrected by the 1571 edition.

An obvious question is the relation between Traheron's glossary and Boorde's dictionary.

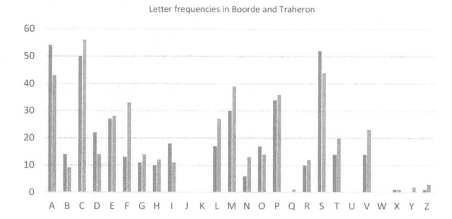

Fig. 3: Letter frequencies in Boorde (red) and Traheron (blue)

In short, none is apparent; although the distribution of letters is similar as the figure shows, they only share a paltry 33 of the 830 words in all; that is, 3.9%. Even allowing for the fact that Boorde's list is general and Traheron's is putatively specialist, this is a remarkable lack of overlap. These terms are (Traheron's spelling): *acorus, agaricke, amygdale, anthrax, arthetica, cancrena, catarrhus, cataracte, emunctories, epiglottis, epilepsia, eschare, estiomenos, exiture, fauus, formica, glandules, herisipelas, herpes, impetigo, incision, inflation, lethargus, macule, nuke, obthalmia, panaritium, scotomia, scrophules, spasme, tenasmos, varices, uuea,* and *vuula.* Traheron prefers an English form in many of these cases, perhaps in deference to his assumed readership of surgeons.

3.2 Other sixteenth- and early seventeenth-century glossaries

Both Thomas Elyot and Robert Recorde had felt it necessary to mount explicit and spirited defences of the use of English in their medical publications in the mid-sixteenth century. Traheron's translation and extensive glossary must also have helped to promote the vernacular. The main reason for its being called a glossary is being appended to a larger work rather than a lack of dictionary-like features. In other respects, it is formally very similar to Boorde's *Breuiary*.

The translation of Pope John XXI by Humphrey Lloyd, *The treasurie of healthe*, published in about 1550, incorporates a list of weights used by physicians and "the interpretacyon" of the names of the compound medicines as well as containing an unalphabetised list of medicines and simples (fii^v–gii^r). The list of compound medicines include descriptions of them (their "exposicyon" as the title-page declares);

these are in effect definitions, but there is little sense that these lists are an exercise in lexicography. The epistle to the reader indicates that the descriptions may be Lloyd's own additions. William Bullein's 1562 glossary, forming part of the dialogue between Sickness and Health (I.ii^v–I.iii^v) and not alphabetical, seems to depend substantially on that in Lloyd or to share a common source, since forty-six percent are matches, sometimes verbatim.

John Hall writes in the Epistle Dedicatorie to his translation of Lanfranc of Milan (1565) that an anatomy has been appended, and

> a table of the interpretation, as well of all maner of strange wordes, as also of all maner of simples, by any occasion treated of in this profitable worke: By me collected, according to myne owne experience and the meaning of good authors, as well ye aunciētes as the new writers (¶i^v)

A dedicatory letter by William Cunningham confirms that these words are so strange that their difficulty will exacerbate the problems confronting students, and describes this table as "expositive":

> But for because briefe treatises want not obscuritie, especially to the yonger studentes: Iohn Halle hath made an expositiue table, setting plainly out as well the perfect natures of those simple medicines mentioned of Lanfranke, as also of all the termes belonging to the arte. (*1^r)

Cunningham also stresses the purpose of the translation as being to benefit students of surgery, returning to this notion several times. There is also a subtle difference in that while Hall alludes to the meaning of the words, Cunningham mentions only the "perfect natures" of the substances themselves, suggesting that he does not consider the linguistic problem of definition that Hall does as translator. At this period, there was no very clear distinction made between glossing and genus-species definition, this latter then being largely unrecognised in lexicography.[53]

The expositive table is introduced with a good deal of fanfare, indicating that it forms a more significant part of this publication than merely an additional and perfunctory list. It begins with a new title-page, and with new pagination on Ai^r, although it does revert to the original pagination after the preliminaries. Hall adds two more categories of potential user to the information about the table already cited on the first title-page, claiming that it is "Very commodious to the vse of all professors of the medicinall Arte, and especiallye to the Apothecaries that are desirous of perfecte knowledge in simples." Since, Hall argues, England produces most of the drugs needed, he will supply a list to augment Lanfranc's text. Examples of such lists in medical texts have been less easy to find than his remark that providing these is a

---

53 See comment on the forward-looking practices of Christopher Langton at the same period in McConchie and Curzan 2011.

common practice may suggest, however, and Hall's list represents a relatively new departure.

The long proem is followed by a letter from Hall's brother Thomas, whose praises are equally for the surgery, the expositive table, and the anatomy, as the three mainstays of this work. He lauds both the surgery and

> hys exposityue table therof, whiche he hathe gathered and adioyned therto. And lastly ... his Anatomy in the end: bothe the whyche, he hathe (at my sute partly) decked with the Greeke, as wel as the Latin names, of symples, diseases, members .&c. as the purpose of teachinge the yoūger sorte gaue occasion (Niii^r)

The list itself consists of entries with centred head-words, as in Traheron, attractively set out and easy to navigate. As usual, the head-words are in Roman italic with the entry text in black-letter. Many entries contain Greek and Latin glosses where appropriate as well as English explanations, and comment on derivations is by no means unusual. Now and then a term with an unmarked gloss is simply incorporated into the text, as in "*Aqua*. Water is of temperament cold, contrarye to fier".

It is perhaps important to note that in spite of the 266 main headings in the table, Hall's index contains far more terms than this. Still more terms are either explained in the table entries, in the main text of the translation, or are not explained at all. Quite a lot of English terms which do not appear as head-words in the expositive table turn up in the index (*matter, southernwood, turnep*, and so on), but there are also similarly unlisted foreign terms, including *gymnocrithon, linospermum, mastix*, and *trithales*, all of which might well have found a place in a table of obscure terms. The reason for their exclusion can only be surmised. The head-word total for Hall and Traheron combined is 621. There are 44 words shared between Hall and Traheron but not Boorde (7.0%), more than between Boorde and Traheron, but still not a large percentage.[54] There are only six shared between all three.[55]

The physician Philip Barrough produced his *The methode of phisicke* in 1583. Barrough outlines his intentions in the preface:

---

[54] These are accidents, aematites, aloes, anotamie, antimonium, aposteme, baucia, baurach, bdelium, bolearmenie, cassia, cicers, crassula, euphorbium, exiture, galbane, gariofilata, gentian, hermodactyle, laudanum, manna, maturatiue, mumia, mundificatiue, olibanum, opoponax, orobus, parietaria, phlegmon, pruna, restauration, sanguis draconis, scammonie, scarification, serapine, spodium, storax, tamarindi, terra sigillata, turbith, titia, ulcers, undimia, and vngula (Traheron's spelling used in this list).

[55] That is, *acorus, anthrax, cancrena, formica* and *glandules*, the entries for which show no relation; *herpes*, in which entry part of one sentence only is shared between Hall and Traheron (Traheron's spelling in this list).

> I haue (good Reader) for thy benefit, collected out of sundrie authors, as it vvere a breuiarie or abridgement of physicke, and togeather vvith those deductions, I have interlaced experimentes of mine ovvne, vvhich by long vse and practice I haue obserued to be true.

This lengthy work contains only one modest formal glossary, an unalphabetised ten-item list of weights placed immediately after the table of contents. There are however a couple of other points to be noted. The table of contents is alphabetical rather than being listed in page order, as one might expect. The alphabetisation is broadly speaking by key word; thus "Of flowing of Menstruis" appears under M, but "Of the Dropsie Anasarcha" is under D, not A. "Paines in the teeth and ears" are under P, as is "Of Panting of the hart," but pain in the stomach is under S, so that the choice of headword is not necessarily consistent where a noun plus noun or a noun and deverbal are available in the same heading. There is considerable discussion of medical terms and their equivalents in other languages throughout Barrough's text, especially the extended discussion of terminology mentioned by McConchie (1997: 67–72). There are also elements of lexicographical practice throughout the text, some chapters being introduced by a discussion of the synonyms and variants of a term; hence the section on the iliac passion ("Of Iliaca passio") begins with the sub-heading "de ileo", and the text begins "The Iliaca passio, is a disease causinge most grieuous & deadly paine in the small guttes. The Latines do call this disease, voluulus & convoluulus. The barbarous do call it Iliaca passio" (103). It is also noteworthy that Barrough choses to head this entry with the 'barbarous' term, possibly because it is the most familiar, as we saw in Boorde. A lengthy example occurs in the very first entry of the book, which deals with headaches, supplying Latin, Greek, and barbarous glosses, and a number of terms for the various types of headache. A briefer example is Chapter 46 (138) which is headed "Of difficultie of pissing" and subtitled "de difficvltate vrinæ". This is followed by the gloss *disvria* which opens the running text. Not all entries contain such material, however. A more characteristic arrangement is an English title, a Latin subtitle, and no further linguistic information in the running text. The entry for *sciatica* (III Chapter 65; 162) has an even more elaborated set of glosses and related terms, including the derivation *ischaidi* for those who suffer from this complaint. Thus although Barrough's is not a lexicographical work, he does use a number of familiar dictionary elements throughout, and the text is rich with medical terminology.

John Gerard's *The herball or generall historie of plantes* contains a list of popular plant names (Schäfer 1989 I: 43), which is mainly of simplex entries but does have a number of glossarial ones, such as that headed "Whickentree, that is wilde ashe." This does not precisely reflect what is in the entry, since the heading reads "The wilde Ash otherwise called Quickbeam, or Quicken tree", illustrating the way in which an index could be made to supplement what is in the text itself, even inadvertently, and the extent to which an index might take on some of the characteristics of a glossary.

Gerard's indices also list Latin, barbarous and Arabic terms separately.[56] As with any other sixteenth-century herbal, the medicinal qualities of the plants are an essential part, and are again separately indexed. The temperatures and virtues of the plants appear at the end of each entry where relevant as well as some recipes and uses for particular diseases. By the time that English medical dictionaries had begun to appear with any regularity, this medicinal function of herbals was disappearing, and with it the relevance of herbals to medical lexicography. Gerard's last list, "A Supplement or Appendix vnto the generall Table, and to the Table of English names: gathered out of ancient written and printed Copies, and from the mouthes of plaine and simple Countrie people" deserves comment as being partly vernacular terminology derived from oral sources. This may show in forms such as "Croneberries, *vaccinia palustria*", which form is recorded by the OED as a rare variant of *cranberry*. Some of the glosses in this list are the Latin binomials, while others are English variants or alternatives, as in "Crow leeke is *Hyacinthus Anglicus*" or "Groundwill is Groundswell" and "Herbe Peter is Cowslip," and "*Stonnord* is stonecrop", *stonnord* being recorded as a variant of *stonehore* in the OED.

Jacob Mosan's translation of the *Artzneybuch* by Christof Wirsung (1500–1571) was published in 1598 and again in 1605 and 1617. The continental version of Wirsung published in 1597 has two registers, one of German terms and the other of Latin. In Mosan's translation, there are three 'tables': the first of diseases and medications in English, the second of simples in English with Latin and Greek glosses, and the third of "all the Latine, Greeke, and other strange names of all Simples, especially of those which are mentioned in this Booke". The first is, as expected, a simple index of subject headings and the corresponding page numbers. The second and third tables, however constitute a brief two-way dictionary. The preamble to the second explains that

> This second Index contayneth all the Simples that are specified in this Worke, as Rootes, Herbs, Flowers, Fruits, Plants, Iuices, Gums, Woods, Stones, Barks, Metals, Minerals, and Earths: Also all the parts of Beasts, and of the body of man, that are or may be vsed in Physicke. (Eee4ʳ)

This list has English head-words and Greek, Latin, and Arabic glosses as well as lengthy definitions. Several other categories are presented as linguistic in this work, including the terminology of apothecaries, the barbarous, herbarists, simplicists, and the ubiquitous 'some' terms, as in "and some do call it". Many entries contain large numbers of glosses, especially Latin. Text and head-words are in black-letter, and glosses in roman italic.

The third index is Latin-English, the preamble in this case being much more detailed and explicit:

---

56 The use of the 'barbarous' category was by no means confined to medical works; see Adam Littleton's dictionaries (1677, 1703).

> This third and Latine Index, contayneth all the Latine, Greeke, and other strange names of all
> Simples, especially of those which are mentioned in this Booke, as Rootes, Herbs, Floures,
> Fruits, Plants, Iuices, Gummes, Woods, Stones, Barks, Metals, Minerals, Earths, Deere, and
> whatsoeuer else is vsed in Physick: Also all mixed and compounded Medicines, as Electuaries,
> Confectures, Syrupes, Iuleps, Conserues, Cakes, Pils, Salues, Oyles, Potions, and distilled wa-
> ters, with their names, not only as they are called by the auncient Greeke and Latine Physitions,
> but also as they are now named amongst the common Physitions and Apothecaries: In like sort
> also all inward and outward parts and members of the body, with all the diseases that euery one
> of them is subiect vnto. (Hhh3ᵛ)

This table is much simpler than the second, containing head-words and glosses. While most entries are short and simple, some occasionally contain further information, as under *cardamom*, which gives quite a lot of information about variant names, types of cardamon, and advice for purchase; or information about the plant, as under *hyacinthus*, and so on. Although called an index, it is in fact a glossary, since it has glosses and sometimes variants, and alternative names and some short definitions, but does not have page references. It looks as if it ought to complement the second index, as in a two-way dictionary, but it does so only sporadically, since many head-words have no English equivalent.

A quite aberrant glossary appears in M. A.'s translation of the *Artzneybuch* of Oswald Gabelkhover (1539–1616) in 1598; aberrant in the sense that it looks more like a list of errata, is ordered by page number, not alphabetically, and is laid out as a block of running text, not as a list in columns.[57] Hence it is primarily a finding-list of Latinate hard words as the reader encounters them, as the heading makes explicit:

> The expositione of such wordes which are in this Booke deriued of the Latines, vvhich for the
> common, and vulger people is made, because they should the better vnderstande the meaning
> of the harde vvordes [395]

as well as explaining how it is to be used as a memory bank for the reader whenever this might be required: "Therfore I vvill explaine one vvorde, and so forth may you reade (gentle Reader) vvhersoeuer that vvorde shall shevv it selfe agayne in other places of this sayed Booke." It is however phrased as one would expect a list of errata: "Puluerisated, reade beaten, p. 1." and so on. In these respects, it is the oddest of the medical glossaries. Not all the terms listed are in fact Latinate, since they include *snipperinges*, for which OED suggests a German cognate. A number are very infrequent, including *cibaries*, *foraminated*, *insparge*, and *floscle*.[58] Some, such as *insparge*, appear in only one other work, most often Tomlinson's *Medical dispensary*

---

57 For more on this glossary, see Lancashire 2007: 113–115.
58 *Perfricate(d)*, as in "Perfricated, read rubbed, p. 15" is still unrecorded in OED, as an adjective, as is *contund*; both *ientation* and *periclitation* are also unrecorded.

(1657), and Cawdrey's *Table alphabeticall* (1604), as in the case of *pluiviatile*. *Effodicate* is a nonce-word.

This glossary is fascinating for another reason. The OED has used the text of Gabelkhover, but not the glossary. Using the glossary only, a modest 113 items, however, to check against the OED, produces no less than thirty-nine absolute first citations (35 percent), as well as eighteen (fourteen percent) which have three citations or less. There are also six unrecorded words: *curvefy, desude, ientation, periclitation, præterlapsed* and *resude*. In twelve of these cases, *fastidiousnes, combure, pulverisated, corroded, cibaries, frigify, inoculated, minutlye, puluiscle, pluuiatile, snipperinges*, and *viuificent*, the OED also cites Cawdrey's *Table alphabeticall*. Adding the words actually in Cawdrey but not cited in the OED, 25 (22 percent) are not recorded at all, a small enough figure to suggest that Cawdrey might have relied directly on M. A.'s glossary for some of his vocabulary.[59] The omissions are *ana, carnositie, cenation, circumvolve, contund, crughe,*[60] *debile, desude, diurnally* (but *diurnal* is present), *effodicated, elevation, eradicated, exsiccated, fervour, illiquifacted, imbecile, incend, liquefy, lixivy, meliorization, permutated, polus, resudate, supranominated, ternally reduplicated*, and *tumour*. If Cawdrey did not use the glossary, it is hard to explain the presence of related forms like *ebullient* and *ebulliated*, the very odd term *snipperinges*, or the large percentage of terms with few enough citations to suggest their rarity. Not that all this has been said and done—the lexical resources of the fifteenth to eighteenth centuries are still under-researched, and some apparently extremely infrequent items in Gabelkhover may yet prove to have had a larger life.[61]

The standard and complexity of glossaries declines from about the end of the sixteenth century, during which glossaries were much more dictionary-like and even somewhat encyclopaedic, as is attested by Gervase Markham's glossary in his *Cheape and good husbandry* of 1614. This is designated as simply a hard-word glossary, but much of it consists of familiar medical terms, almost all of them herbal. Although many might indeed have puzzled the reader, it is hard to imagine that a term like *eyebright*, described vacuously as "an hearbe growing in euery meadow" by Markham, would have been unfamiliar. *Chiues, lettice, house-leeke, hearbe-Robert*, and *yarrow*, among others, come into the same category. If the description of eyebright offered here was intended to assist the reader in recognising this plant, it would obviously fail to do so. In terms of the purpose outlined in the preface to the reader, however, which explains that common herbs are available to effect cures of animal diseases, this description might help a reader who already knows eyebright to recognise that it has medicinal value, clearly valuable information. Some definitions are

---

59 Lancashire (2007: 114) has already noted the first citations in A. M.'s Gabelkhover.
60 Glossed as "coughe", but what M. A. intends here is far from clear.
61 For useful general comments on this, and on the particular illustrative case of *chimaericalness*, see Considine 2014: 31.

more helpful than this, and some offer alternative names. *Knot-grass* is described in some detail, but the average description is quite insufficient for positive identification. *Stubwort* seems typical—"an hearbe which growes in wooddy places and is called wood-*Sorrell*." Seventeenth-century glossaries often consist of an elementary word-list with glosses of either one or two words.

A rather different glossary occurs on pages 312–328 of John Woodall's *The surgions mate* of 1617. This is strictly an alphabetical list of symbols ('characters' as distinguishing marks or signs, as he calls them). While Tyrkkö correctly points out that "[it] is in fact much more than a simple gallery of alchemical symbols" (2018: 276), it is also true that it is primarily and essentially a list of these symbols. There is also a short preliminary listing of the seven planets, again with their 'characters'. The arrangement is a head-word in large type, followed by the symbol (usually in two forms), then the English gloss, which often suffices for a definition, and sometimes the characteristics and use of the substance in question. Woodall frequently moves straight to the use, as in *lapis prunella*, which is "good against the toothache" among other conditions. In some few cases, an alchemical equivalent is offered, as in *chalibs* "*Steele* The most valiant Sonne of Mars, it openeth obstructions, and stayeth the fluxes, &c." Iron ("or Steele") also appears in the list of planets under Mars.[62] Many other medical things are mentioned throughout the text, including surgical instruments such as *speculum ani*, *terebellum*, and *spatula*, although they are usually not described, but simples and remedies such as *mel saponis*, *tragacanthum*, *mumia* and *sulphur* and their uses are described. "Chymicall verses" outlining principles for the young practitioner, or 'artists' as he calls them, and using although not necessarily explaining a number of terms then appear. As the verses explain:

In terms of Art which diuers are,
instructed he must bee,
Amalgamate, alcolizate,
and cohobate must he. (333)

And so on alphabetically. This is followed by a third glossary of a more traditional kind. This list unusually consists mainly of processes, such as *cohobation*, *ferrumination*, *levigation*, *purgation*, *torrefaction*, and a few general terms for generic medicinal substances such as *lotion* and *quinta essentia*. This list, Woodall explains, provides definitions of the terms in the verses.

Lazare Rivière's *The universal body of physick* (1657) contains a short 'dictionary' of hard words at the end, presumably added by the translator, William Carr, and consisting of only three and a half pages. Despite its title, it is in fact a small glossary of hard words consisting of head-word plus glosses or definitions. William Carr is described as "Practitioner in physick" on the title-page, but little is known about him.

---

62 For a fuller discussion of Woodall and his glossary, see Tyrkkö 2018.

Various glossaries were published in 1655–1657, but these are dealt with in more detail in Chapter four since they provoke the publication of a stand-alone medical dictionary in 1657.

John Tanner (c.1636–1715) published his *The hidden treasures of the art of physick* in 1659, a work to which he appended an example of the many short and straightforward seventeenth-century glossaries. This work is addressed to those who cannot afford to consult with a physician. This glossary is by no means sophisticated, Tanner writing that it is intended to explain "the Terms of Art and other Words, which are not in the reach of Vulgar Capacities" ([545]). While there are Latin terms in his word-list, a great many are anglicised; thus we find *astringents* rather than *adstringentia*, *symptomes* rather than *symptomata*, and so on. Other familiar terms such as *scirrhus*, *hypogastrium*, and *pus* are, as one would expect, given no obvious anglicised equivalent.

His work, he declares, is also for penurious students and those who are not able to manage large volumes before first gaining an acquaintance with the subject through a compendium, thus holding out the prospect of a quick and easy introduction. Such people will also be able to inform the physician better about the symptoms, not leaving him merely to "joggle in the Piss-pot" (To the Reader). There is a strong suggestion that his work has emerged from experience and possibly a commonplace book, arising as it does from "my wandering Meditations ... [and] my Daily Collections" (To the Reader). This work was reissued in 1667 and 1672.

Not only is there a tendency to simpler glossaries at this later period, there are also more instances of monolingual glossaries with English head-words, such as that in Robert Johnson's *Enchiridion medicum* of 1684. This is a short glossary of hard words, amounting to a mere six and a half pages and 248 words. Most are in English and are quite straightforward, such as *antidote, amulet, apoplexy, cartilage, ducts, dysentery, medicinal, Neapolitan disease, pest, puncture, tumour*, and *unguent*, which suggests the intended readership for this work; indeed the impression is that Johnson understood very few as being anything other than English, exceptions being *aetites, chylus, hydrocephalos*, and *spina dorsi*. The preface, predictably enough, mentions that students formed a part of the target audience. A number of the various medical compendia, enchiridions, handbooks and guides published frequently in the latter seventeenth century contain lists, sometimes topical, sometimes alphabetised, but not strictly intended as glossaries.

3.3 Randle Holme

The most remarkable, surprising, and least-known medical glossary, however, appeared in 1688. A considerable number of terms appear in the various lists and the text of *The academy of armory* by Randle Holme (1627–1699), the third of that name in a family of genealogists and heraldic painters in Chester. Holme, while writing a handbook of heraldry, seems to have been unable to resist the temptation to include everything he knew or could find out about a subject alongside the potential heraldic charges that pertained immediately to his craft. The title-page declares that this work is useful for "all such as desire any Knowledge in Arts and Sciences." The work contains such divers and abstruse matters as the ways of curling hair and both the kinds of periwigs and terms used in their making (II: 463–464), shoes and their parts (III: 14), coins (III: 25–37), terms used by mowers and haymakers (III: 72–73), monastic officers (III: 177), instruments of torture (III: 310–312), and a description of the ark of the covenant (III: 463), to mention only a few, loosely combined into a narrative about heraldry.

While his work is a handbook of arms and heraldry on the face of it, it is in another sense a remarkable encyclopaedia, arranged rather like a nomenclator. Three books were published in 1688, but there were insufficient funds for the rest. The part which remained in manuscript was eventually published by the Roxburghe club in 1905. An example of the kind of specialist lexical study elicited by this work is Dyer's 2007 article on Holme's list of brewing terminology and the use that might be made of it in blazons and cognisances.[63]

The original work contains roughly 3900 medical terms, depending on how they are counted, arranged in seven alphabetical lists. The first list is in bk. II, 379–393; 398; 401–402; 403–406, these being terms for the parts of the body. The second, also in bk II, is a brief list of the vital and natural faculties of the body on page 414. These are followed by a third, on the human anatomy, in bk. II, xvii, 416–427). Short lists of humours and complexions are incorporated into this one. The fourth list, on diseases, is in bk. II, vxii, 427–436, while the fifth, a loosely alphabetical one covering terms of art used by anatomists, is in bk II, 439–450. The latter ends with a list of further reading, including a reference to the English edition of Blancard of 1684. The sixth list, surgeons' instruments, which is copiously illustrated, is in bk. III, xi, 420–438. The list of surgical instruments may be from the translation of Johannes Scultetus (1595–1645) *The chyrurgeons store-house* of 1674, also an illustrated work. There is also a short list of these in Thomas Johnson's translation of the works of Paré, 1634, 1113, which is illustrated. The seventh and last list, bk III, xii, 438–447, is of the names of medicines. At the end of this list, Holme mentions that "ALL which variety of Phisical names may be reduced into English termes, under these three heads; thereby to avoyd a multitude of unheard off[sic] words, which rather confound then giue Instructions." His three heads are "Inward Medicines to Comfort", "Medicines to Purge" and "Outward Medicines". Further sub-heads are provided, such as *Infusions*, *Purges* and *Salves*. There are lists of medicines, surgical instruments, and of other "practical

---

63 See also the homepage of the Stone Roofing Association at http://www.stoneroof.org.uk. For some notions of the activities and interest of the Holme family, see Tittler and Thakray 2008; for Holme's pictorial resources, see Alcock and Cox 2000.

terms", as he calls them. There is also a list of many terms relating to diseases and anatomy in Book II, Ch. xvii. These begin with "bones in the head" on II 416 and run through to II 450. Definitions are usually provided, as are glosses in many cases. Entries are usually short.

A glossary of terms for instruments used by physicians, surgeons and apothecaries, methods of preparing oils and waters, medicines, as well as "other practical terms used by Phisicians, Chyrurgions, and Apothecaries" (III: 442), begins on III 420 and ends on III 447. A further short list of surgeon's instruments occurs on III 398–399, an account which is likely to be derived from Scultetus. In all, it contains many hundreds of terms, mainly in English but many in Latin, and some given Latin equivalents, such as "the retort ... in Latine it is called *Retorta*" (III: 424), or "The second is the *Spatula Linguae*, or a Tongue Spatula" (III: 426). Multiple alternatives are sometimes offered, as under tent: "Of the learned it is termed *Tarpia*, *Tenta*, or *Turunda*, and *Turundula*" (III: 434). Some terms also occur repeatedly throughout the text,[64] and there are many combining forms, such as *goose-bill pincers* (III: 434) and *three-toothed levitor* (III: 436). Not all the terms in the first section, which is not alphabetical, are strictly medical.

The present word count is mostly confined to head-words, words marked as variants or glosses of head-words, and words marked in running-text sections dealing with medicine which are usually in black-letter, and sometimes italics. The underlying assumption is that if Holme intended them to be understood as medical terms, he marked them accordingly. This means that many glosses in English incorporated into definitions are excluded, but it is difficult to decide what should be in a specialist list of medical terms, especially English terms. *Cornea* clearly should be, but should *eye* be included as well? It will suffice for the present purpose to note the possibility of exclusions and remark that the size of the list is almost certainly understated here. Even given these caveats, it is a remarkable assemblage of medical terms. A further problem is that they are scattered about the work in several sections.[65] There are also a few medical terms scattered throughout the rest of the text, some of which could add a little to the total.

The relation between Holme (RH) and Blancard (BL) deserves further detailed research, especially given that Blancard was such a recent work for Holme, but a preliminary survey shows that it was used and how. *Anthysterica* (Bk. III: 439) is a fairly close fit.

---

64 Duplicates have been removed from the count, but this may also have removed a small number of genuine homonyms.
65 No attempt has been made to read the entire text for terms outside these lists for this study, however.

> RH med: against fits of the mother
> BL *Anthysterica* are Medicines good against the Fits of the *Mother*.

Apochylisma is a new English form, and a synonym is added.

> RH Apochylism, or Apothermus, or Robub, is a boiling of any juice with sugar & honey to a thick substance or hard.
> Bl *Apochylisma*, called *Succago*, *Robub*, and *Rob*, is the boiling and thickning of any juice with Sugar and Honey, into a kind of a hard consistence.

Catharticum shows drastic reduction. RH III 439 offers "Catharticum, medicines to purge the Stomach, and the gut" perhaps reducing this by about two-thirds to what one might normally expect in a medical dictionary under this head-word.

The term *nascalia* is clearly dependent on Blancard, but shows editing.

> RH III 441 little globular bodies, to put into the neck of the Matrix to cure a Disease. See Pessarium.
> BL Nascalia, are litle globular Bodies, which are put in the neck of the Matrix, made of the same substance as Pessaria. See Pessaria.

Sacculi shows heavy deletion and a changed head-word.

> RH III 441 Sacculi Medicinales, is a Bag quilted with several simples compounded and beaten together, put in and applied to the places grieved.
> BL Sacculi Medicinales, are when several Simples, according to the Nature of the Disease, are compounded and beaten together, and tied up in a little Bag, to be applied to the part affected. The Bag is to be sewed or quilted down in several places, that the Ingredients run not altogether in a Lump.

A possible example of eye-skip occurs under *acopum*, which Holme renders as "Acopium, a medicine applied by fomentation, is compounded of wearming and molifiying things", where "wearming" appears to conflate 'weariness' and 'warming' in Bl:

> a medicine which applied by fomentation, allays the sence of weariness, contracted by a too violent motion of the body, compounded of warming and mollifying ingredients.

3.4 Eighteenth-century glossaries

Another glossary was produced in the early eighteenth century by Daniel Turner in his *The art of surgery*, vol. II, 1722, to which he appended an extensive "Tabula Ætiologica", as he explains,

> Giving an Account of some hard Words contained in the foregoing Sections, with their Derivations both from the Greek and Latin; for the Benefit of such who are less conversant or acquainted with those Languages, here explain'd, and Alphabetically digested.

Turner lists 544 lemmas in all.[66] He obviously prefers to use an English lemma where he can; hence *ablactation*, not *ablactatio*, *mithridate* not *mithridatum*, *repulsion* not *repulsio*, and so forth. Lemmas which can be anglicised usually are, although not consistently, exceptions including *diaphoretica*, *mundificantia*, *narcotica*, and *temperamentum*. Others which are conventionally not in anglicised form are not, including *ancryoides*, *enarthrosis*, *pericranium*, *phægadena*, etc. Turner's etymologies are often from verbs to nouns as in "*Comminution*, ex *comminuor*, to break or shiver to Pieces" or "*Dislocation*, à *disloco*, to put out of Place". He prefers definitions to mere glosses. While short of being outright encyclopaedic, these are relatively full. There seems no obvious reason for some of the terms in this list, including *diary* in the journal sense only, *ludicrous*, *mathematist*, *paradox*, *pusillanimity*, *system*, and *vehiculum*. Curiously, and perhaps indicating a particular source, the definition of *nonnaturalia* is mostly in Latin.

Interestingly, he uses 'ex' not 'from' in giving the etymologies. Not all lemmas have etymologies but do include a gloss; e.g., "*Scrobiculum Cordis*, the Pit of the Stomach, called of some the Heart-Pit; the Word *Scrobiculum* standing for a little Pit or Furrow." Sometimes he simply proceeds to the definition, as in "*Sutura*, the first of the Species of Articulation, under *Synarthrosis*, belonging to the Bones of the *Cranium*". This list is certainly not a list of aetiologies, however, so that the sense in which he uses this word is unclear.

The anonymous *The ladies dispensatory* (1739) contains a very short, but revealing glossary consisting of a mere 41 lemmas. The natural assumption would be that this represents those terms in the text that the intended readership might not be familiar with. The declared audience is women who can read English, and no other language, and the purpose is to understand and treat specifically female complaints while allowing the reader to maintain her feminine discretion, so that she can cope without "discovering her condition" (tp.).

A first question is thus whether the items listed do actually appear in the text. A preliminary search suggests that some do not, including *cacochymic*, *callus*, *discutient*, *emaciate*, *friction*, *lymphaticks*, *rarefaction*, *scirrhosity* (but *scirrhous* appears several times), and *sutures*.[67] Some appear only once, such as *feculent*, or infrequently, such as *restringent* (138, 199). Another point is that the terms in the glossary are not necessarily those preferred in the text, so that *hæmorrhoids*, for instance, is in the index and is glossed and defined on page 128 of the text, but the term "piles" is generally preferred.

It is also noteworthy that terms like *aperitive*, *lochia*, *prolapsion sphincter* (147), *tumefaction* (150), *seminal effluvium* (175) and *sanious* (156) are not in the glossary. At

---

66 For further analysis of Turner, see Chapter eight on surgical dictionaries.
67 A complete search may locate some of these, given that that searching on ECCO is a bit hit-or-miss. It is easier to locate a term than to guarantee that it does not appear at all.

the same time, *lochia* is named and described on page 286 and *prolapsion* is glossed in the text on pages 184 and 143, so that there are instances where an in-text explanation is offered. Further instances of a word not in the glossary is *rectum*, glossed as "great Gut or Rectum" on page 146 and again as "Rectum or Fundament" on page 148, as well as "Diascordium, or Syrup of Quinces" on page 137. These points suggest that perhaps the glossary was at least partly derived from another source than the text. A further hint that the source of the glossary may not be the text itself is that we find *hystericks* in the glossary but the word is always spelt "hysteric" in the text and the index and is always an attributive adjective, not a noun. The same applies to *lymphaticks/lymphatic* (221), but not to *plethoric*.

This may thus be a glossary from a different source. Another possibility is that there were separate compositors with different spelling conventions setting the text. but it will require a study of this publishing house's conventions at the time or a search for an original glossary to resolve this. It may be hard to establish the latter given the brevity of the glossary and the considerable number of potential sources available.

At the end of the eighteenth century, Buchan's *Domestic medicine* contains a glossary not so dissimilar in layout and function to Tanner's, nearly a century and a half earlier. The first edition of this work in 1769 did not have this glossary, which only appeared in the tenth edition (1788). Two American editions of the work appeared in New London and Philadelphia in 1795. both containing the glossary (see Guerra 1962). These are essentially the same, apart from the New London version's erroneous headword *mysentary* appearing correctly as *mesentery* in the Philadelphia edition and being entered as the first entry under M, not the last, and the entry for *exacerbation* being shorter in the New London edition. *Mysentery* appears in the 1788 edition, as does the short definition of *exacerbation*. One wonders why it took so long to make the correction to *mesentery*.

To conclude this chapter, mid-sixteenth-century glossaries have a format, typography, and depth comparable to that in the first printed dictionary, Boorde's *Breuiary*. By the mid-seventeenth century, they are becoming more simplified, and by the eighteenth they tend to have English head-words in preference to Latin or Greek, although there are sufficient exceptions in each century to suggest that it was not a principled decision to make this change but simply a reflection of trends in the actual use of the medical lexicon. Neither does there seem to be any conscious attempt to neologise in English. These later glossaries also tend to be restricted to the vocabulary of the work in which they appear. Allusions to the lexemes being hard words persist. Finally, there is a tendency, not at all surprising, for these glossaries to be confined to popular works and compendia rather than the more learned tomes. The mid to late eighteenth century has yielded little of further significance. While glossaries continue in such works as the late editions of Culpeper, and translations of the works of Astruc, the famous French surgeon, they are small, simple and straightforward.[68]

Another obvious feature of the history of medical glossaries is that they move from containing encyclopaedic material to abandoning it altogether, which medical dictionaries certainly do not. A primary consideration is that, by definition, a medical glossary is intended for the use of the unlearned, especially those without access to a physician, or to tyros, which becomes less true of medical dictionaries over time. While glossaries shrink, medical dictionaries grow and bifurcate. Robert James's massive three-volume medical dictionary appears almost contemporaneously in the mid–eighteenth century with John Barrow's minimal medical dictionary intended for students, the first genuine surgical dictionaries appear, and the slightly earlier dictionary by John Quincy promotes the vernacular aggressively. There are also sporadic glimpses of overlap between indices and glossaries. The texts to which glosses are appended also contain many terms which might well have found a place in a table of obscure terms, but do not. The reason for their non-inclusion can only be surmised, and might well be a subject for further research, especially since they may reflect contemporaneous views as to which words were familiar to a particular readership and which not.

---

68 My thanks to Teo Juvonen for a conducting a search for these.

4 The physical dictionaries of 1655–1678

The years 1655–1657 saw the appearance of two works entitled *A/The physical diction-ary*, as well as the publication of a stand-alone version of one of them, thus constitut-ing the first printed medical dictionary under this title in English. These years are the point at which medical glossaries and a medical dictionary are once again closely re-lated, although not for the reasons that applied in the sixteenth century. Given the titles, I will refer to these works as dictionaries in this chapter, but they are glossaries insofar as they are appended to other works.

4.1 Lazare Rivière's *The practice of physick* 1655

The first of these dictionaries was issued by Peter Cole in 1655, appended to a trans-lation of Lazare Rivière (1589–1655) under the title *The practice of physick* (hereafter PP) standing under the names of the physicians Nicholas Culpeper (1616–1654), Ab-diah Cole (fl. 1602–1664) and William Rowland. The first printing of Rivière in Eng-land is *Lazari Riverii consiliarii ... observationes medicæ & curationes insignes*, pub-lished in London by Miles Flesher in 1646. This is a non-lexicographical work, with merely an index at the end. Rivière's work was obviously well-received in England about the middle of the sixteenth century, and Nicholas Culpeper made more of him than most. The dictionary, supplied with its own title-page, forms the eighteenth and last chapter of the PP, but its separateness from this work is indicated by its being described on the cancel title-page thus: "With these Books is bound a *Physical Dic-tionary*", a formula repeated on the inner title-page (*The compleat practice of physick*), which also describes it as the eighteenth book. Although "bound with" might suggest that the dictionary was a separate production, the foliation is in fact continuous. Sig-nificantly, the title-page declares that it is of use in understanding not only the hard words in Rivière, but those in other works as well, since the implication of general use puts it potentially beyond the scope of a glossary. This dictionary only uses A- order, which makes look-ups less efficient.

Further explanation of the presence of the physical dictionary comes in the ad-dress by the printer to the reader.

> For the worthy sakes of which honorable Ladies and Gentlewomen in the first and chiefest place, and for the ease of all others unacquainted with the Greek and Latin Tongues, and consequently unable to understand divers terms of Art, and other words drawn from the said Tongues (which it was necessary to retain for brevity sake, and to avoid tedious Circumlocutions) I have caused a *Physical Dictionary* to be added at the end of these Books, explaining all such terms of Art aforesaid, as are used therein. (A2ʳ)

Several points are worth discussing here. First is the specific reference to use by lit-erate gentlewomen who, as managers of a household, were expected to administer

https://doi.org/10.1515/9783110639186-004

medical assistance as a matter of course, and indeed to prepare some of the medicaments. Second, the allusion to the unlearned reader is a standard trope in such works,
and predictably includes surgeons and apothecaries. Third, it is striking, looking
through the entries of these physical dictionaries, that they contain a number of terms
not obviously in medical use. In this case, these include *axiom, adverse, generating,
coincide, intercepted, intermediate, occult*, and *scituation*. The presence of such terms
suggests the recognition of a 'halo' lexicon, or medical metalexicon, which enables
the core medical lexicon by way of explanation, avoiding 'circumlocutions', as well
as reinforcing its status through the use of a further set of hard words.

Peter Cole also points out in the address to the reader that difficult terms are
glossed where they occur in the text (Aii^{r-v}), offering the example of *masticatory*, a
medicine meant to be chewed, *gargarism, empyema*, and others. Such in-text glossing
was a long-standing practice, by no means confined to medical texts, but occurring
across a broad range of genres. Thus on page 426, a remedy for a pregnant woman
suffering from 'womb-fits', that is, a difficult labour is: "It is also good to lay unto the
soals of her Feet, this Epispastick, or drawing Cataplasm, or Pultis". *Epispastick* is in
the dictionary. Some however are not, as with "External causes depend upon things
necessary and things contingent, the things not necessary are such as Physitians call
res non naturales, things not natural" (518). This term does not appear in the dictionary. Terms not included are relatively easy to find, as with *glaucoma*, explained rather
than glossed on page 66: "The chief Disease ... is called *Glaucoma* (or changing of the
Crystalline Humor into a fiery redness)" and *anacollemata*, described as "repelling
Medicines such as are vulgarly called *Anacollemata*, things to be applied to the fore-
head" (66–67). Others include "*Miasmaza*, or vapors infective" on page 170, and
mydryasis, page 74: "The Dilatation of the Pupilla ... is called in Greek a *Mydryasis*".

Culpeper was aware of the language problem surrounding the use of the vernacular from the outset of his career. His first edition of the translation of the London
dispensatory, *A physicall directory* of 1649, is prefaced by a list of eight terms which
he regards as important to know. As he puts it,

> Although I did what I could throughout the Book to express my self, in such a language as might
> be understood by al, and therefore avoided terms of art so much as might be, yet it could not
> sometimes be avoided but some words were quoted which stand in need of some explaining
> (Directions)

these terms being listed as *balneum marie, manica hippocratis, calcination, filta-
tion*[sic], *coagulation, natural vitall and animal spirits, infusion*, and *decoction*. He defines these terms, but does not offer such lexicographical elements as a derivation or
glosses. Neither does he offer them, bar two, in Latin form in the first place, which he
might well have done. Clearly the linguistic reference point for this is English rather
than Latin.

On the other hand, the list of weights and measures, such as *cochlearium* and
hemina, he offers in Latin, because "I know not well what English names to give

them" (Biiiᵛ). He also mentions measures such as the *handful* and the *pugil*, the latter known (according to OED) since the later sixteenth century, which he defines as "properly so much as you can take up with your thumb and two fingers".[69] This translation is provided with a considerable indexing and quasi-lexicographical apparatus. Further lists then follow, such as that of the compounds, without language comment, the list containing many Greek and Latin terms, in italics. In the third list, that of "vertues", there is again no language comment, and the head-words swap abruptly from Roman to italics part-way through, at the letter I. Towards the end of this work, Culpeper is also explicit in his commitment to English in the heading provided for the general index, describing it as "An exact alphabetical table to the English names in the catalogue of simples", the Latin head-words from the body of the London dispensatory being retained. The catalogue and the index thus constitute a nascent glossary taken together.

This physical dictionary itself is, frankly, rather messy. A number of head-words are needlessly repeated, and some occur not merely out of alphabetical order but in the wrong letter altogether, an instance being *iron-water*, which is in L. Why *livid* should occur a second time five entries later and with a slightly expanded definition is not obvious, although one possibility is that more than one person was working on the list and the duplication was not noticed while the final compilation was done, an oversight rendered easier by not having complete alphabetisation. One compiler perhaps added to the source definition while the other left it as was.

The user would also sometimes have struggled to find terms treated simply as synonyms, as distinct from variants. Thus *Capital opiate* forms part of the entry for *Cephalick ... opiate* and is not listed elsewhere, whereas *conjoyned matter* cross-references *conjunct cause* for a full definition. Some antonymous pairs are cross-referenced, but others are not. The entry

Intension and *Remission*: Increase and decrease, growing stronger or weaker

is not matched by a cross-reference for *remission*, although *remitted* is present, and *sulphurous and bituminous bathes* does not have a corresponding entry for *bituminous* (bathes).

Since medical lexicons are dominated by nominal forms, an obvious linguistic characteristic of the present list is the almost forty participial verb forms listed without a corresponding infinitive. Most are past participial adjectives, judging by the definitions. Examples include *affected, aromatized, contracted, couched, concocted, derived, diminished, dissipated, dissipating, depraved, embrochated, exasperated, extinguished, eventilated, going about, illustrated, impacted, producing, relaxing,*

---

69 Compare the definition in the *Physical dictionary* of 1657: "as much in quantity as may be taken up between the three fore fingers and the thumb."

recruted, stupefying, steeled, suppurated, suffocating, terminated, and *ulcerated.* The majority of those mentioned here do appear as verbs in the main text, the exceptions being *concocted, stupefying, steeled,* and *suffocating,* which appear only as participial adjectives. *Recruted* is given its correct spelling in the main text.

A few which are potentially polysemous have a definition seemingly restricted to the medical context, such as *expressed* ("squeezed out"), but more have definitions which are not unambiguously medical, such as *intercepted* ("stopped in the middle way"), *precipitated* ("thrown head-long, forcibly cast down"), and *repelled* ("driven away"), again suggesting the perceived importance of the halo lexicon.

Going about is one of the very few non-Latinate ones, not perspicuously defined as "by fits" in the main text on the subject of vertigo: "But those Vapors are sent up from evil humors, not continually without intermission, but by compass and going about, and at a distance, namely, as often as they are raised up by an external cause" (35). This appears to have been identified as a specialist sense in this definition, although the general sense of moving in a circular motion (s.v. OED *go about,* v. 1a) persisted at least into the eighteenth century.

Among the several re-issues of the PP dictionary, the issues of 1661 and 1668 show some degree of editorial attention.[70] The 1661 edition, also published by Peter Cole, is a new version of his 1655 physical dictionary, with a few corrections and changes, not always for the better. The entry for *essentially springing* has been entered twice in 1661, but the repetition of *laxe* in 1655 has been removed. Other duplication errors have been left in place, such as the repetition of *contracted.* A fresh typographical error is *centree* (1661) for *centre* (1655); likewise *defluxion* (1655) is replaced by *defluxtion* (1661) and *precede* (1655) by *percede* (1661). In the 1668 edition, the last two, along with a number of others like *defluxion/defluxtion, fluxive/fluxtive, intermediate/intermeditate, magistral/magistical* and *sphacelus/spacelus,* have been restored to the 1655 readings, possibly indicating that this edition was set from the 1655 text, not the supervening one. Against this interpretation, however two apparent errors in 1661, *pupula* for *pustula,* and *sphincther* for *sphincter* were not changed in 1668. *Paralysis* (1655), replaced by *paralisis* (1661), was not changed in 1668 either.

Among the minor changes which are not obviously errors are *axiome* (1661) for *axiom* (1655), *physical regiment* (1655) by *physicall regiment* (1661). There are also a few signs of editing independent of both 1655 and 1661 as in the change from *dilatation* to *dilation* with an unaltered definition. Probably as a matter of printing-house style, *coindicants* beomes *co-indicants* in 1668, and *tile tree* becomes *tile-tree.* Similarly, *distention* is rendered *distension* and *anticulate voyce* [sic] as *articulate voice* in 1668. There is also some variation between doubled letters as in *distillations* and *distilations.* The change from *vital functions* to *vital function* may indicate a perception that this term and some others are uncountables. In general, then, changes and

---

70 The last was in 1678, but I have not had access to this edition.

mistakes in 1661 are corrected in 1688, but otherwise few alterations are made. One final point is the placement of the antonymic doublet *systole* and *diastole*, which should appear under the head-word *systole* but in fact appears near the end of the letter O. This remains unchanged throughout.

4.2 Jean de Renou's *A medicinal dispensatory*

The translation of Jean de Renou's *A medicinal dispensatory* by Richard Tomlinson, the vehicle for the second physical dictionary, exists in no less than five versions of 1657, two of which actually incorporate the dictionary. The edition printed by John Streater and James Cottrell, which were to be sold by George Sawbridge, is the first to contain the dictionary (Wing R1037). "A physical dictionary" was added to the end of the edition to be sold by Sawbridge, but not to Streater's other editions of the same year, which were for sale by Henry Fletcher and Giles Calvert (Wing R1037A). There are two other impressions by the same printers in the same year, for sale by Francis Tyton and by Calvert and Fletcher (Wing R1037 and 1037C), but these do not incorporate the dictionary.

The declared purpose of the dictionary is anti-establishment: "It is intended for such Persons as spend their time and employment in studying Physick, and are acquainted with no other than their Mother tongue" (To all English Practitioners: Ai^r). The dictionary itself was clearly produced at the instigation of John Garfield, but his preface dances around the question of who actually wrote it. Garfield claims that "I hope for ... friendly Acceptance amongst you, having preserved this Dictionary for your Good," pointing out further on that he has sought expert advice on the meanings of the terms used by Tomlinson: "I have caused them to be Explained by Able Persons, well Acquainted with the Practice of Physick" (The Stationer to his countrymen).

A fourth impression was printed by G[ertrude] Dawson for Garfield, who was also the vendor. This impression was supplied with a new title-page proclaiming "*A physical dictionary or, an interpretation of such crabbed words and terms of art as are derived from the Greek or Latin, and used in* physick, anatomy, chirurgery and chymistry", despite the fact that most of the work is in fact Tomlinson's translation of Renou. Finally, it was issued in small format as a stand-alone (Wing 2143), now divorced from the Renou translation. Little is changed, the letter from the stationer to the reader still alluding to Tomlinson's translation.

While the question of the authorship of the *Physical dictionary* is still open,[71] Culpeper apparently has no qualms about claiming credit for translating if not the authorship of his own dictionary, having several explicit marginal notes in his

---

71 For an exhaustive account of the problem, see Tyrkkö 2009.

translation of Jean Prevost (1655) which refer to it as his 'physical dictionary' such as the marginal note on the expulsive faculty: "what that is, see my translation of *Riverius* Practice of Physick in the Physical Dictionary at the end of the aforesaid Book" (16). As Boorde had done, Culpeper here makes a number references to and between his own works. This inter-referentiality through marginalia is a very consciously constructed web guiding the reader through any possible difficulties. Culpeper fell short, however, of undertaking a full-scale, stand-alone dictionary, despite having plenty of material to hand, given that his *The English physician* of 1652 is an alphabetised encyclopaedic list. In other works, such as the *Directory for midwives*, Culpeper uses the marginalia both sparingly and more conventionally as a key guide to the contents and for source references. This, from *Medicaments for the poor*, the Prevost translation, seems to be a standard formulation for such notes: "What Emulsions are, see my Translation of *Riverius* in the Physical Dictionary at the end thereof" (42). Others are supplied for *diureticks* (59) and *gargarism* (73). This is also anticipated in 'The Printer to the Reader' in Prevost (1656): "If thou meetest with hard words that thou dost not well understand, look at the end of *Riverius* Practice in English, and most of them are there explained." A noticeable difference between the Culpeper and Garfield dictionaries is that Culpeper's is presented on the title-page as an appendage to the main text, placed low on the title-page and in small print, while Garfield's is increasingly highlighted in various issues.

The epistle to the Renou dictionary, which urges the necessity of a medical dictionary, addresses the unlearned reader, and is undersigned by fourteen surgeons, physicians, and apothecaries: George Starky, George Thornley, Thomas Herbert, John Rowland, John Hawkins, John Roane, John Baech, Philip Frith, Ralph Woodall, John Bryan, Anthony Rowe, John North, John Straw, and John Harry. Interestingly, the Sawbridge version uses the Streater title-pages; hence there is no mention of the *Physical dictionary*. There is then a preface by John Garfield, "the stationer to his covntrymen."

This dictionary occasionally has an italicised synonym after the main entry, in which case I listed it as forming part of the dictionary (see *catagma ossum*, where *fractura* is mentioned as well. There is a separate entry for *fracture*). If it is simply a variant of the main entry it is ignored. It also shows the fairly consistent and familiar use of the plural for count nouns in the entry-head. Further points are that it is much longer than the Culpeper physical dictionary, and much more accurately alphabetised.

4.3 Comparisons between Renou's and Culpeper's physical dictionaries

Opinions have varied as to whether there is any relation between the Renou glossary and the Culpeper physical dictionary. They appeared to Alston to be dependent on each other, but others have claimed that they are entirely independent (see Tyrkkö 2009: 178–179). My own limited study of the head-words shows that the PP dictionary (598 head-words in all) shares 224 head-words with Renou; that is, thirty-seven and a half percent of the PP entries also appear in Tomlinson/Renou, suggesting a relationship between them. Further evidence of this is the nature of the shared terms. While one would expect terms like *bolus, contusion, diacatholicon, mortification*, or *pugil* to be shared, being basic items in a seventeenth-century medical lexicon, others are surprising, especially some of the binomials. These include *carminating medicines, coction of humours, febris catarrhalis, habit of body, solution of continuity*, and *vaporous matter. Treble quality*, not an obviously medical term at all, also appears in both. There are also shared phrases such as *species retained in the mind* and *state of the/a disease*. No attempt is made to regularise language, in that those which are in Latin or Greek in the one are also in Latin or Greek in the other; likewise English spelling variations among these shared terms are also very few. The most striking change, *breathing vein/breathing of a vein* is apparently editorial, although perhaps in the circumstances should be regarded as a transcription error since it is a singleton example. Analysis shows a somewhat increasing dependence as we move through the alphabet, with more shared entries as a percentage, and less original ones. The change begins about the letter M, where the balance between the two is almost equal.

In compiling a list for this research, head-words only were considered for the most part, although occasionally there is an italicised synonym after the main entry. These alternative head-words were ignored for the present analysis, such as "*Matter*, or *Quittor*", simply listed as *matter*. Simply variants of the main entry were ignored. Others, such as *aspera arteria*, under *rough arterie*, is not listed separately, but many are cross-listed as head-words, as is *quittor*. Words in the definition text and italicised which are not obvious glosses also sometimes appear separately as head-words, so these were ignored as well. Further points are that this dictionary has far more head-words than the Culpeper physical dictionary, and is much more accurately alphabetised, although definitions tend to be shorter. The dictionary also shows the fairly consistent and familiar use of the plural for count nouns in the entry-head. Errors occur; for instance, *suppression* is listed twice, both instances being cross-references to *stoppage*. For *sinew*, we find "*Nerves*, Sinnewes" where the putative headword follows its gloss and is not italicised.

We turn now to the definitions. As with the Rivière physical dictionary, non-medical terms figure relatively largely. These include *adjacent, acquires, alacrity, appellations, bonity, castigation, diuturnity, investigate, miscellany, probable, profound, renovation, symbolical*, and *tact. Profound* occurs in seventeenth-century religious works often but only rarely in medical works, and *symbolical* is largely used in religious and philosophical works. *Bonity* is almost entirely confined to religious works in the seventeenth century, aside from the occurrences in the text of Renou's *Medical dispensatory*. Non-medical terms, again, have no obvious function in such a compilation, other than their representing words in a metalexicon which support the medical lexicon contextually. Although copiousness for its own sake is a possible motivation and one familiar in the lexicographical practice of the time, it seems unlikely here, especially in an appendix which must perforce be limited in size.

Verbal forms are prominent relatively speaking. Some 3rd-person singular verb forms, such as *attracteth, coruscateth, depurges, deturpates, emanates, emends, erugates, exacts, expletes, extrudes, extergeth, impinguates, indicates, inebriates, jugulates, liberates, minuates, projects, reficiates, represses, respondeth, sapors, stimulates,* and *suppeditates* appear. Another repeated verb pattern is the past tense/part participle without the infinitive, e.g., *coacted, contracted, dilated, infused, mutilated, obdulcorated, præcipitated, remitted, repelled,* and *suffocated.* These are more likely to be accompanied by a nominal form such as *infusion* or *suffocation.*

The stand-alone Wing 2143 changes to a two-column format, but is simply the other reset. Nevertheless, some small points of comparison emerge. We see that the erroneous *euntiates* for *enuntiates* has not been corrected, nor *fugacius* for *fugacious.* or *oesephagus* for *oesophagus.* Some corrections of 2143a in 2143 include *berillus* for *brillus, chologogon* for *cholagogon, dilacerate* for *dilacerat, pubes* for *pules, pulverization* for *pulverication,* and *refecilate* for *refocilate* (OED *refocillate*). Page D4^{v}-D5^{r} is duplicated in 2143, and is recopied in 2143a without any change (*coagmentation-colature*), while *dulco-acid* replaces *dulcoacid.*

4.4 Comparisons between Rivière 1655 and Renou 1657 (Wing 2143)

There are 1911 head-words between these two dictionaries. Determining the degree of relationship is often straightforward, as in

> Rivière 1655: *cardiogmos,* heart-burning.
> Renou 1657: *cardiogmos,* heart-burning.

but at other times it is fraught with difficulty. Both likewise gloss *carabe* with the single and obvious term *amber,* which is not surprising in itself, *carabe* appearing in a number of sixteenth and early seventeenth-century medical texts. A great majority of the verbatim entries are one-word glosses, and some show a trivial deletion or addition. Trivial change between entries is illustrated by *aromatized*:

> Rivière 1655: *aromatized,* Spiced, perfumed.
> Renou 1657: *Aromatized,* spiced, or perfumed.

and a different kind by *indicate*:

> Rivière 1655: *indicate,* declare, point out.
> Renou 1657: *indicate,* declare, point at.

An example of the complex way in which dependence between entries manifests itself may be illustrated is the definition of *aneurism* in these two dictionaries:

> Rivière 1655: *Aneurism*: a swelling caused by a dilatation of the Arterie's external coat, the internal being broken
> Renou 1657: *Aneurism*, a swelling caused by the breaking the internal coat of an Artery, the external being whole.

where the grammatical structure of the definitions matches quite closely, but the conceptual structure is focussed quite differently. A number of entries consist of the same core gloss, but with substantial material deleted in Tomlinson/Renou, as in

> Rivière 1655: *Atomes*: smal motes hardly visible, and that cannot admit of any division.
> Renou 1657: *Atomes*, motes.

While this is a simplification of the entry, it comes at the expense of significant definitional material. The next example removes two synonyms and makes a conflation:

> Riviere 1655: *Carus*; foulness, rottenness, corruption of a Bone.
> Renou 1657: *Carus*, rottenness of a bone.

Glandules shows a definition which is almost verbatim, and an expansion which adds little of substance:

> Rivière 1655: *Glandules*, kernels, such as are about the Throat, aad[sic] are called the Almonds of the Ears, and such as the Sweet-bread, &c.
> Renou 1657: *Glandules*, kernels such as are about the throat, and are called the Almonds of the ears, also the sweet-bread; and whatever is like to these is said to be of a Glandulous substance.

Under *cornea*, the Tomlinson/Renou version shortens that in Rivière somewhat:

> Rivière 1655: *Cornea*, a Coat of the Eye like the horn of a Lanthorn.
> Renou 1657: Cornea, the coat of the eye of a horny substance.

But *horny coat* was a familiar name for the cornea, so that the similarity here seems less significant than the lack of a reference to a lantern in assessing the degree of dependence. In the case of *efficient cause*, the first clause is verbatim, but is followed by an analogy; in Renou to the making of medicines by an apothecary, but in Rivière to the making of clothes by a tailor. Thus once again the entry is structurally similar but quite different in detail.

Among entries that are the same, the coincidence of single-term glosses are the least significant: the longer the definition the more significant the coincidence. The following chart shows the percentage per letter of entries which are either verbatim or with either insignificant changes or verbatim along with some addition or deletion. In interpreting this graph, it should be remembered that Q and W are outliers, since one of a mere five entries in Q is verbatim, but three of seven in W are, yielding an unrealistically high result compared with, say A, which contains six among 170. Even making this allowance, however, the trend is clearly upwards from N, suggesting increasing dependence between the two to parallel the increase noted above. An alternative reading is that there are two rises, one through each half of the alphabet. There is no obvious reason for the sharp decline at L-M, although one might conjecture that a break in the work occurred at this point and that these two letters were somehow overlooked. Nevertheless, these two dictionaries are independent for the most part, Tomlinson relying on Culpeper for only about 6.4% of his entries overall.

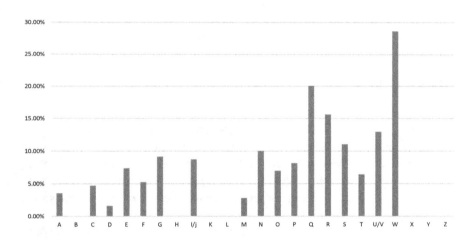

Fig. 4: Verbatim and near-verbatim entries per letter in Rivière and Renou

Garfield's sense of the commercial potential of the *Physical dictionary* itself has already been noted by Tyrkkö (2009: 174–175). This work did not however arise at a stroke, fully-fledged and free-standing, but took its course through various stages in the publishing industry of the time, as reflected in its various impressions, title-pages, publishers, and vendors. In fact, the Rivière physical dictionary had the longer publishing career despite never being issued as a stand-alone, lasting until the first medical dictionary to appear at once complete and independent in nature, the translation of Stephen Blancard in 1684. The appearance of this work must have rendered both the existing physical dictionaries irrelevant.

5 Latin medical dictionaries: Thomas Burnet and John Cruso

We turn now to discuss two works which were published in Latin, and do not necessarily exhibit all the characteristics of a medical dictionary. Medical handbooks and enchiridions had to strike a balance between a system and a form of order which made them accessible, whether to the professional reader or the unlearned general reader, a requirement which saw their authors exploit alphabetical order at least to some degree, as well as glossaries and indexes. This meant that a medical vademecum or enchiridion might certainly take on a number of the characteristics of a dictionary for the convenience of the user while never actually being intended as such by its compiler. I will discuss an example of such a work, as well as an outright dictionary whose matrix language is Latin, not English; common enough in the continental tradition, but only once undertaken by a Briton.

5.1 Thomas Burnet (1638?–1704)

The first of these, by the Scot Thomas Burnet, does meet most of the requirements, but is entirely in Latin and exerted influence elsewhere than Britain. Burnet, among the original members of the Royal College of Physicians of Edinburgh, serving as its president between 1696 and 1698 (Payne 2004), is not to be confused with his brother Gilbert Burnet, who became the Bishop of Salisbury, or with the Thomas Burnet who was the master of Charterhouse and author of the controversial *Telluris theoria sacra, or sacred theory of the earth* (1681).

The theses submitted by Burnet for his licence and his medical degree were published in 1659.[72] The medical school in Montpellier was known for its staunch Galenism (Furdell 2001: 186), a fact which is reflected in Burnet's published works, the best-known of which is the *Thesaurus medicinæ*, published in 1673. There are two versions of this first edition, one with a title-page indicating that the work was published in London, and the other indicating that it was to be sold (*prostant*) in Edinburgh.[73] The latter version also incorporates the London title-page on C4r, that is, immediately after the list of errata.

This work proved to be popular in continental Europe. Editions were published in Geneva by J. H. Widerhold in 1678, with additions by Daniel Puerari (1621–1692); it was translated into French in Lyon and published by Hilaire Baritel, 1691; in Geneva

---

72 *Currus iatrikus trumphalis* for his licence (1659a), and *Quæstiones quatuor cardinales pro suprema Apollinari daphne consequenda* (1659b) for his doctoral degree.
73 "Londini: excudebat G. R[awlins]. pro R. Boulter bibliopola Londinensi, & prostant apud R. Brown, J. Carnes & J. Mason, Bibliopolas Edinburgenses".

https://doi.org/10.1515/9783110639186-005

a second time, this edition by J. A. Chouët & D. Ritter in 1698. Puerari was a physician and professor of philosophy at the Academy of Geneva. A very early edition appeared in Venice, issued by Gasparis Storti in 1681, followed by re-issues in 1687 and 1694 by Storti and others. Venice also saw a later edition by Hieronymus Savioni in 1733. The *Thesaurus* was obviously directed at the medical profession, being entirely in Latin but, as a compendium, was probably specifically intended for students.

Burnet also wrote *Hippocrates contractus* (1685), a compendium of the works of Hippocrates, although the content is not exclusively Hippocratic. Like the *Thesaurus*, this work was well-received, editions continuing to appear well into the eighteenth century. Burnet also produced an abridgment of the *Thesaurus* in 1703. His *Hippocrates contractus*, possibly the last of the purely classical medical textbooks to survive, was still being published as late as 1743 by William Bowyer in London, an edition by Cornelius Haak in Leiden in 1752, and König in 1765 in Strasburg.

The *Thesaurus*, which is encyclopaedic, does not include herbs and other simples, being restricted to anatomy and diseases. The entries themselves certainly do include medicines, however, since there are a great many remedies included. The *Thesaurus* is not organised by conventional dictionary standards, but it is orderly and consistent. There is first a large subdivision into books which correspond to letters. The books predictably exclude K, Q, W, X, Y and Z, and naturally incorporate I with J and U with V; hence there are eighteen altogether, but the claim in the title that it is organised by alphabetical order is not strictly true since, while the highest level is by letter, this is followed by a numbered section, then by an alphabetical keyword, and finally by a numbered subsection again ordered by alphabetical keyword. Book ten, for example, begins at L ("Liber Decimus. De Affectibus à Litera L incipientibus"). The reader then encounters the first section, and under that the "Pro Labiorum pustulis, decorticatione & fissuris", where *labiorum* is the alphabetical keyword. Under the main heading, a division into a numbered 'subject' or section' is used, and the keyword alphabetisation then returns. Hence "Sectio undecima Pro Oculi tumore carneo/ Sectio duodecima Pro Oculi vulnere" (656). Thus alphabetical entries under superordinate but increasingly delimited subject headings alternate with numerical subdivisions. The arrangement also preserves things such as prepositions, as in "De Ægilope", *de* introducing sections in most cases, and *pro* introducing subsections, while ignoring them for alphabetical purposes. Clearly *de* is used for the introductory explanatory section while the *pro* subsections contain advice on treatment and remedies. Exceptions do occur but are orderly; for example, under H: "Sectio quarta/Pro Hæmorrhagia ex Vulnere". These occur when there is no corresponding subsection.

The page headlines, while they normally follow the section headings, may not entirely agree with either section or subsection heads; e.g., "De Hysterica Passione", a wording which does not occur under either the corresponding section or subsection headings, the appropriate section heading being "De Hysterico Affectu". Subsection headings are frequently repeated, "Pro Hæmorrhagia Narium" appearing as the heading for the first six subsections of section two of letter H, "De Hæmorrhagia

Narium". In short, finding material by the section and alphabetical ordering provided is rather limited. The index eliminates these repeats, although in other respects it simply reproduces the layout of the text headings. Thus a heading like "Pro Hydrope Ascite" does not generate a separate entry for *ascites* in the index.

This work by Thomas Burnet is the only English medical dictionary of this period to have a substantial publishing history outside the British Isles. It was in fact far more successful in Europe, despite the 1685 and 1703 Edinburgh editions, as the many editions in France, Switzerland, and particularly Italy show. A rather scholarly production, it clearly met a practical need. It must however be recalled that this is a dictionary only in a very loose sense. It does not have formal single-word lemmas, has an alphabetical structure which coexists with numbering, lacks linguistic information such as the derivations and glosses then found in medical dictionaries, and has little or no definitional material, except in the sectional entries. At the same time, medical dictionaries in the more conventional sense do include a great deal of the kind of material found in the *Thesaurus*, and it is a reference work.

5.2 John Cruso (?–1717?) *Medicamentorum Ευποριστον thesaurus* [1701]

Little is known of Cruso, who was it seems an apothecary since he is designated "pharmacop." on the title-page of his thesaurus, and who was obviously learned. He seems to be from Brecon.[74] His being an apothecary is also confirmed by the translator's preface in 1771, adding the fact that he was trained by Thomas Lee, who apparently supplied "the famous Dr. Bowles", that is, George Bowles (1604–1672) (Cruso 1771: ix).[75] Cruso's work itself has an odd history, being first published in Latin in 1701 and then no less than seventy years later in English, without making an intervening appearance.

The work itself, which is prefixed by a statement of the approval of the college signed by several members of the RCP and dedicated to the Brecon merchant and MP, Jeffrey Jeffreys, and Sir Charles Duncomb, is an alphabetical listing of diseases with the appropriate simples for their cure, also arranged in alphabetical order under the

---

74 An inventory for an apothecary of that name dated 1717 which may well be his is lodged in the National Library of Wales (BR/1717/5).

75 See Munk 1878 I, 332 s.n. Bowle. The only Dr Bowles I have been able to identify appears on page 63 of Robert Pierce's *Bath memoirs* of 1697, and then practised in Oundle. A Dr Bowles is also mentioned in John Ray's *Joannis Raii synopsis methodica stirpium Britannicarum* 1724, 205. This Bowles is mentioned by a few later eighteenth-century writers, and is associated with Ray. *The family guide to health; or, a general practice of physic: In a familiar way: containing the most approved methods of cure*, 1767, also mentions Bowles on p. 70 on the curative effects of mistletoe in a reference from Robert James, s.v. *viscum*.

main lemma, and incorporating glosses in English which are capitalised and in black-letter. Hence there are no definitions as such in English. To illustrate, *rachitis* (rickets) is followed by five potential treatments based on *agrimonia, calamintha, fragaria, hypericon* and *plantago*. Cruso's list arose as a result of his own botanising and for the purposes of keeping a record and a memory aid. In the original edition, Cruso offered a straightforward list of simples; "quandoquidem non pompose congestam, nec à longinquò petitam medicamentorum farraginem; sed simplicia, atq; ubiq; ferè nascentia, eximiis tamen virtutibus prædicta ostendit" (Lectori candido).[76] Included among the lengthy list of sources in the forematter are the Englishmen Samuel Dale, the controversialist and physician Marchamont Needham (Nedham), John Ray, Thomas Sydenham,Thomas Willis, and the surgeon Richard Wiseman.

There does not seem to be a work comparable to this. The main listing may contain sub-entries; hence *interna, putrida*, etc. appear under *Vulnera in Genere*, and the head-words are also sometimes generic enough to include entries which would normally be separate head-words, such as *achores, alopecia, capilli, furfur, tinea, ulcera* and *vulnera* under *capitis affectus externi*, these sub-entries being preceded by a longish rule to distinguish them. They also lack the drop-capital of the main head-word. The entries for the simples are in italics, with a brief English gloss in black-letter, the main text being in Roman. Entries generally include a reference to an authoritative source.

This work was translated and reissued many years later as *A treasure of easy medicines*. This later edition begins with a glossary of terms and a general index follows immediately, both lacking in the first. This edition thus compensates for the lack of the definitions in the first to some extent, although this by no means makes the work a dictionary in the full sense of the word. Copious additional notes have been added from various sources, including Robert James's dictionary and the influential *Gardener's dictionary* by Philip Miller, which first appeared in 1724 and went through many editions.

The translator of the 1771 edition does seem to be attempting to have it both ways in claiming that the work is of use to the learned and had been recommended by the RCP for younger physicians with access to herbs, but that it was also designed to assist the "poor patients destitute of advice" (Cruso 1771: vii). This reads more like publishing puff than anything else; an attempt to revive a forgotten work by a now rather antiquated appeal to the popular and the learned market. The Latin names have been retained, as this is more convenient for the physicians and other learned professionals, and a glossary and index provided for other readers (Cruso 1771: viii). With all this added labour and apparatus, the work is then offered as one of general use—its failure to run to another edition suggests that the general reader did not agree.

---

76 In the 1771 translation: "as it does not consist of a pompous or far-fetched collection of Medicines, but of Simples only, which grow every where, yet are endued with admirable Virtues" (vi).

6 Steven Blancard (1650–1704)

Steven Blancard was a Dutch physician and iatrochemist, as well as an entomologist who made some significant contributions to medical science, including his demonstration of the existence of a capillary system, and writing the first Dutch book on paediatrics.[77] He began work as an apothecary, but then practised medicine in Amsterdam after graduating from the University of Franeker. His *Lexicon medicum, græco-latinum*, a dictionary in Greek and Latin like its predecessor by Bartomoleo Castelli, appeared in 1679. As is often the case, Blancard is mentioned mainly for his non-lexicographical work as an anatomist and entomologist and, predictably, for a series of disconnected curiosities, including the that fact that he alludes to particular diseases in his works, such as bulimia (Margocsy 2009: 194–195; Stein and Laakso 1988). His dictionary has been credited with first use of the word psychology (Colman 2009: s.v. *psychology*).[78] He is also discussed in an article on the controversy over the rete mirabile (Pranghofer 2009), as well as for his advocacy of the benefits of drinking coffee (Poukens and Provoost 2011: 171), but not for the fact that he wrote a particularly enduring and influential medical dictionary.

6.1 The continental editions

The English translation of Blancard of 1684 was not long coming, the first continental edition having appeared only five years previously. Perhaps it was the newness of this work that appealed; after all, the famous and widely-reprinted medical dictionary by Bartolomeo Castelli, *Lexicon medicum graeco-latinum* (1598), had been on the market since the late sixteenth century. Blancard's popularity was by no means confined to England; in fact, it lasted longer on the continent. His dictionary was, among other editions, published in Jena in 1683 by Müller and in 1693 by Weimann, Leiden

---

77 Spellings such as Stephan/Stephen Blankaart, Blanckaert, Blancard, Blancart, Blancardus, and Blanchard occur. 'Blancard' is the preferred form in this work, since that is what was usually used in the seventeenth and eighteenth centuries in England, but he appears under 'Blankaart' in the ESTC.
78 Colman ascribes this word to Blankaart himself but, as it does not appear in the first English edition, it should thus be attributed to the anonymous English editor who addded new material to the second edition. Further, this editor attributes the distinction between anatomy and psychology to Thomas Bartholin ('Bartholine'). It should also be remembered that the concept of 'introducing' a word to English was of far less significance in the seventeenth century than it is now, given that physicians usually read and often wrote in Latin, if not Greek as well. In any case, there is an earlier use of the word in a translation by Nicholas Culpeper, who ends Tome 1, part 3, book 1, headed "Of the Faculties and Functions of the Soul both Special and General" with "And thus much of *Psychologie*" (Culpeper 1654: 174). Culpeper also uses *psychologia* in this work. The editor of Blancard was probably referring to the translation of Bartholin by Culpeper and Cole published in 1668.

https://doi.org/10.1515/9783110639186-006

in 1702 by Boutesteyn and Jordan Luchtmans, in 1717 and 1735 (incorporating an English index as well as English glosses), and 1756 by Samuel Luchtmans. Further German editions appeared in Halle, by J. F. Zeitler in 1718, and from the Fritsch publishing house in Magdeburg in 1739. A later French edition was that by Van Overbeke, published in Lyon in 1754. Schwickert published it in 1777 in Leipzig, and it appeared as late as 1832 from the same publishing house. It had also become a polyglot dictionary through its various re-workings; the latter edition includes English, German, French, Greek, and Dutch, a development which did not take place in the English editions.

This work is basically Latin with some Greek and a little German. It seems that this lexicon quickly became acclimatised to its new country, becoming the German version, the English version, and so on. The English and German/Dutch versions were clearly distinguished from each other before the end of the seventeenth century. To illustrate this diversity, the 1718 edition produced in Halle is entitled *Lexicon medicum graeco-latino-germanicum*. This process of differentiation was briefly outlined at the end of the 1693 Leiden edition, the printer explaining the chequered history of the editions and languages involved.

While the dictionary was selling well in England, with a last edition in 1728, there were many continental editions, which included various language 'registers', including that printed in Leiden in 1690 in which the English register runs to 28 pages. This section, entitled "Englisch[sic] register, in which alle[sic] the physical terms are very accurately demonstrated" is an English finding list with single-word entries and references to page numbers. Registers for other languages also appeared, this edition having them for Dutch, French, and German. Many though by no means all entries contain glosses in the languages mentioned, so that this particular edition has taken a strikingly different direction, becoming more a polyglot lexical medical dictionary than a somewhat more encyclopaedic dictionary like its English counterpart. The market for such a book can hardly have been England, given the popularity of the local edition, so that the editors and publisher must have felt that continental readers would have found this feature useful. Was it the case that medical books in English were beginning to find their way into the continental market along with other vernacular continental publications, or was it simply that the models long since established by non-specialist dictionaries such as the polyglot Calepines and the various van Barlement dictionaries (see Stein 1989) were being used? A further question is that since the definitions have English glosses as well as there being a register, is the register simply a list of the glosses? This does seem to be the case. The index thus sends the reader to English as a target language in the text.

6.2 The English version of Blancard

Blancard's dictionary in its English garb, *A physical dictionary*, 1684, proved to be not only a good seller in England but durable as well, being reissued twice in 1684, and then republished in 1693, 1697, 1702 (twice), 1708, 1715, and 1726. It was apparently translated by 'J. G.', who signed the dedication, and who may be the John Gellibrand identified on the title-page as one of the sellers of the work. Plomer (1922: s.v. *Gellibrand, John*) indicates that Gellibrand published mainly Latin books in a career spanning 1680–1684 at the Golden Ball in Paul's Churchyard. More recent information shows that Plomer's dates are now slightly out, however, since there is a book published in Latin in 1679, and several in 1685. Gellibrand, who also published a number of sermons, was possibly the son of Samuel Gellibrand, himself a well-known bookseller. Gellibrand seems to have been learned–he issued a book catalogue in Latin in 1682. ESTC suggests that the printer, only identified as 'J. D.', was in fact the controversial non-conformist, John Darby (see also Lynch 2008; Furdell 2002: 90).

The preface first mentions Blancard's fame and the care with which he has compiled the dictionary, and attention is drawn to the list of authors consulted, a feature which was dropped in the next edition. Authorities both ancient and modern are mentioned, although the modern ones listed in the preface were all either compilers of dictionaries or pharmacopœias. This salient lexicographical fact is not specifically alluded to, however, presumably being regarded as well-known. The first is Joannes Gorræus, whose Greek-Latin medical dictionary appeared in 1564, *Definitionum medicarum Libri XXIIII literis graecis distincti*, published in Paris by Andreas Wechel. The second, Bartolomeo Castelli, was perhaps the most frequently reprinted medical lexicographer of the seventeenth century, while Anutis Foesius (Anuce Foës, 1528–1595) was best known for his research into the writings of Hippocrates, whose collected works he published in Frankfurt in 1596. Foesius also produced a pharmacopœia published in Basel in 1561. Blancard has presumably used these works as sources of his word-list and definitions, although Castelli must have been the primary text, given that Foesius's is a pharmacopœia and Gorræus's word-list is in Greek.

The head-words in Blancard are seen as Greek and Latin rendered in Latin. Definitions are in Latin, followed by glosses in Greek, etc. J. G. goes on to claim that nothing of use has been omitted from these sources. He also claims that

> things of this nature are extremely wanting, that so the terms (in which all, or the most part of Mankind has daily occasion to use) may not be talkt by rote; but may give a rational account of their discourse, than which, nothing is more rational or demonstrative than this of Physick.

The stress here is on the particular terms being in daily use, rather than the dictionaries; we need not take the claim that everyone uses such terminology too seriously. The allusion to a "rational account" appears to anticipate the idea of a systematic, inter-related lexicon, a notion which appealed greatly to the encyclopaedists of the eighteenth century. More practically, the preface ends with an appeal to cost and convenience. The book might have been bulkier and hence more expensive, but "the Buyer's Interest ought to be, and has been consulted" (The Preface). These various assertions are not entirely compatible, but the preface is also a puff aimed directly at the perceived market for the work. The dedicatee of the work is William Molins (1617–1791), a well-known surgeon and anatomist (see Morris 2008).

The structure of the entries is relatively consistent, albeit simple. Entries take the form 'X is/are is when', etc; that is, they are usually in the form of a complete or intact sentence, such as "*Pneumatosis* is the Generation of Animal Spirits, which is performed in the barky Substance of the Brain ...". The exceptions are usually entries which offer a gloss of the head-word or a synonym or variant of some kind, or a cross-reference, as in "*Consensus*, a Disease by Consent, is when ...", or "*Convulsio, Convulsion*, is a Motion whereby ..." and "*Medius Venter*; see *Thorax*." Cross-referencing is extensive, perhaps being seen as a more convenient alternative to clustering syonymns within entries.

Derivations are not generally offered, although there are a few exceptions. The dictionary is inconsistent as to glosses; they are sometimes offered, sometimes not, and sometimes more than one appears. Sometimes there is a generic (species-genus) relation like 'X is a kind of Y', which does not constitute a gloss, but a genuine definition, as in "*Viscera*, are Organs contained in the three great Cavities of the Body ...". The following entry provides a translation gloss, a synonym, and a species-genus definition: "*Medulla Spinalis*, the spinal Marrow, or the tail of the Brain, is that Part which goes down the middle of the Back by the Vertebres". At other times, there is a synonym, not necessarily in English, as with "*Miserere mei, or Chordapsis*". *Chordapsis* has itas own entry, under which we learn that *miserere mei* is a barbarous usage, and that *iliaca passio, volvulus* and *ileus* are also synonyms. Towards the end of the work, a comma after the head-word becomes normal, possibly with a change in compositor. It had occurred only sporadically before. Entries are generally short, very few entries occupying more than a page.

The job involved in translating a dictionary, especially a specialist one, is more than simple translation. The English glosses have to be inserted and managed. It also follows that the translator needed some expertise in medicine. Next, the alphabetical order has to be adjusted for any differences between Greek and Latin, such as the large block required for the third letter, C, in Latin as against Γ in Greek. Entries and blocks of entries would have to be shifted accordingly. Since English glosses are not directly available from the text, they must be supplied, presumably from a pre-existing source. Translating a bilingual dictionary is thus by no means a simply mechanical task. It seems unlikely that the Blancard translator was simply using the *Physical dictionary* of 1657, since it would have been quite inadequate for this purpose.

6.3 The first English edition and the later ones compared

There are at least two variants of the 1684 edition in ESTC: Wing B3164A (302 pages), Wing B3164C (304 pages), and Wing B3164 (304 pages). The 1693 printing is the second edition, considerably changed from the first, and the 1697 edition is the third. All these editions were printed for Samuel Crouch. The second edition incorporated a number of changes, both in the layout of the pages and in the text itself. The major changes in the appearance of the second edition are that rules now appear at the top and have been used to improve the appearance of the pages and to aid the user. The writer of the preface alludes to the provision of capital letters in the bar at the top of each page as making finding easier ("much more easie than in the former Edition"). It now has a double column instead of a single column per page, divided by a rule, this arrangement cutting the number of pages by approximately a third despite the incorporation of substantial additional material. This page layout had been used in English printed dictionaries as early as Thomas Elyot's dictionary of 1538, and on the continent by Ambrosius Calepinus (Calepine, c.1435–1509) in *Dictionum latinarum et graecarum interpresa*, a work which first appeared in Reggio Emilia in 1502. Blancard's original title-page has been supplemented by a paragraph explaining that terms relating to pharmacy have been added:

> Also the Names and Virtues of Medicinal Plants, Minerals, Stones, Gums, Salts, Earths, &c. And the Method of choosing the best Drugs: The Terms of Chymistry, and of the Apothecaries Art; and the various Forms of Medicines, and the ways of Compounding them.

It does seem that the majority of the additions are of this kind. All three major branches of the medical lexicon were thus now covered, as the preface indicated. The dedication to William Molins has been dispensed with, perhaps simply because he was dead by then, and an entirely new preface added. Not finding a new dedicatee to replace Molins was an interesting decision given that a patron was then regarded almost as a necessity for any serious work. The only other difference between the title-pages of the second and third edition is that the licensing statement has been removed. Two other items have been removed from this edition as well. The list of sources has now gone, as have the advertisements for Crouch's books. Why the list of sources should have been deleted is unclear, and somewhat puzzling. We might conjecture that either the list was felt not to be entirely accurate given the revisions with which this edition started out, a new list was to be compiled but was never completed, or that a technical complication in the printing house required its removal.

A number of changes in the preliminaries and the text itself are apparent. The writer of the new preface assumes that everyone is aware of "the Usefulness and Necessity of Dictionaries ... to every one that's in the least, conversant with Books, or studious to improve in any Art or Science" (Preface). It also now claims to cover everything in the "Commonwealth of Physic", while the appeal to the "Buyers Interest" and the low price in the first edition preface have been omitted. By far the most consistent changes in the text apply to the details of punctuation and capitalisation, which are pretty consistently applied throughout the text. There is no need to ascribe these to authorial or editorial intervention, since printing-house conventions changed with the times. Another change which involves punctuation and is consistently applied throughout is the deletion of 'is/are' at the beginning of the definition and its replacement by a comma.

A look at selected parts of the word-list shows that additions have certainly been made. These include *diagrydium* (scammony) between *diagnosis* and *dialeimma*, *dialepsis* (the middle space in wounds and ulcers) after *dialeimma* and before *diaspasma*, *diapegma* (a surgical instrument) between *diapedisis* and *diaphanum*; *melano piper* (cross-reference) between *melanagoga* and *melancholia*, three additions between *melicratum* and *membrana* are *melitema* (a honey cake with medicines added), *melosis* (searching with a probe), *melotis* (cross-reference). The multiple entry *rha, rheum, rhaponticum* (a purging root), as well as *rhabarbarum* (rhubarb), *rhabdoides sutura* (cross-reference), *rachis* (cross-reference), *rachisagra* (spinal gout), and *rachitæ* (the muscles of the spine) have all been inserted between *revulsoria* and *rachitis*. These few examples will serve to show the concentration on simples and cross-referencing as well as surgery and anatomy in the editing work.

The important changes are however in the main word-list. The claim that there have been numerous additions to it seems in general to be correct, but there are also major revisions to a number of entries in the early definitions, in which words and phrases have been changed or deleted. The changes are usually the removal of unnecessary expressions, sentences and parts of sentences which seem to take particular attitudes on controversial issues, some deletions of references to authority, and changes in word choice. To take some examples, under *acamatos* 'figuration' has been replaced by 'shape', and under *acantabolus* "Chyrurgeons Tool" has become "Chyrurgeons Instrument". The expression 'the same that', as in "*Canna minor*, the same that Fibula os", has been changed in some cases. This usage characterizes the 1684 edition, and is corrected spasmodically and inconsistently in 1693. There do not appear to be many additions to the definitions, although these can occasionally be found, as in the case of *allogotrophia*.

More detailed comparison of the entries however reveals that the second edition was an incomplete job. About nineteen to twenty-one entries in continuous blocks in the 1684 edition were compared with the corresponding blocks in the 1693 edition, these being thirty pages apart. This produced seven blocks of entries in the letters A, C, F, L, O, S, and U/V. The final total number of entries examined was determined by the number added in 1693, since only one deletion was found. A very slight exception to the thirty-pages rule was made to include *urethra* as the first entry in the last block. This investigation shows that *alcohol, alimentum, allantoides, alteratio, amphiblestroides*, and *analeptica* have been considerably reduced, *aisteterium* has been heavily edited; some references to authorities have been dropped, as under *allogotrophia*, which has been augmented as well, and a few others have undergone minor reduction or editing. Under *apoflegmasticus*, "which are excited at the Mouth" now reads "which are excreted at the Mouth", and *antidysenterica* has been deleted altogether.

Further investigation reveals that major editing work seems to have ceased early, since it largely disappears in AR-, *arthrodia* seemingly the last entry showing any major changes. No major editing has been noted in the rest of the dictionary, but of course it has only been sampled for this study, not compared to the last detail. Another way to look at this is that the major revision process stops at the end of sheet C2 rather than in the middle of a sheet, which might indicate that ending the full-scale editing was a printing-house decision, perhaps on the grounds of cost, time, or both. It would certainly have been a time-consuming process to pursue the editing to its completion. To take a single instance, *aisteterium* typically shows punctuation changes and deletions, the deletions here being quite extensive. The 1684 entry

> *Aisteterium* is the common sensory: which *Cartesius* and others his Abettors make *the glandula pinealis*; but the common sensory ought rather to be placed where the Nerves of the external senses are terminated, which is not in the *glandula pinealis*, but (as the most ingenious *Willis* has demonstrated) about the beginning of the *medulla oblongata* (or top of the spinal marrow) in the *Corpus striatum*

becomes

> *Aisteterium*, the Common Sensory: Which *Cartes* places in the *Glandula Pinealis*; but *Willis*, about the beginning of the *Medulla Oblongata* (or top of the spinal Marrow) in the *Corpus striatum*

in 1693. The first omission removes a value-judgement about the Cartesians, and the second a somewhat speculative remark, and a laudatory but probably unnecessary comment on Willis. The addition of the comma after Willis removes a possible ambiguity. Additional capitalisation of nouns as well as a capital after a colon both characterise the second edition. This was obviously a major revision process, but the attempt to re-edit that work so enthusiastically begun was thus abortive.

6.4 The repute of the dictionary

The English version of Blancard seems generally to have been well received. Allusions to his dictionary are usually positive, being cited a number of times by way of deference to an authority (the Hippocratic word is *anacyriosis*, 'authority and dignity'), although the earliest references to Blancard in English sources are to his anatomical work, not to the dictionary. Some instances include a cure for warts cited under Blancard's name on page 55 of William Salmon's contribution to the popular domestic dictionary genre, *The family dictionary: or, houshold companion*, which appeared in its fourth edition in 1710. There is a mention accompanied by a quotation in Benjamin Marten's *A new theory of consumptions* of 1720, quoting Blancard's account of the "small animals" or "worms" seen under the microscope in advancing the idea that these are the cause of fevers (62). Thomas Spooner of Lemon Street also makes mention of the 'learned' Blancard in *A compendious treatise of the diseases of the skin*, 1721, quoting his description of leprosy (11). Recent research has shown that John Harris owed a considerable debt to Blancard, making extensive use of him in his *Lexicon technicum* of 1704 (see Lonati 2007), with many references to and quotations of him, both explicit and unacknowledged.

An apparently grudging concession to Blancard's lexicographical authority occurs in the "Tabula Ætilogica" in Daniel Turner's *The art of surgery*, 1722. Under *harmonia*, he says that "with us" this word "implies a strait or equal Line, or a Conjunction of the Bones by the same; being the second Way reckon'd under Synarthrosis, as the Bones of the Nose: Blancard will have it so named, ab ἄρω, congruo, adapto." It is not easy to interpret this remark. It seems that Turner accepts either Blancard's definition or etymology or both rather unwillingly, or that he intends a distinction between Blancard and 'us', presumably the English or just possibly surgeons, on this issue.[79]

The unlicensed man-midwife John Maubray calls him "the ingenious Blancard" (110) in relation to the seat of the hypochondrium in his *The female physician* 1724, and the "famous" Dr Blancard appears in a brief reference and with a quote in Lewis Southcomb's *Peace of mind and health of body united* (1750: 68). Bielfeld, author of *The elements of universal erudition*, advises those of his readers wishing to inform themselves about medicine, among other works, "to furnish themselves with the best medical dictionaries, as those of Castell, Brunon,[80] Blancard, &c." (1771 1: 229). Again, a question of definition motivates the naval surgeon Robert Robertson to incorporate an allusion to Blancard in his account of the symptoms of a fever, since he mentions "A cardialgia. The pain and oppression about the præcordia, or in the stomach, in the Weasel's fever, did not occasion a swooning away—as Blancard defines that disease, or symptom to occasion" (15). In this case, the author begs to disagree, not taking issue with Blancard, but arguing that this was not the disease in question, since immediately after he calls Blancard "that accurate writer" (15). Robertson's declared intention is to contribute to an understanding of the various fevers and diseases which afflict British sailors in various parts of the world (The Preface). These allusions, while not very frequent, all trade on Blancard's lexicographical authority and at the same time augment it.

The use of medical dictionaries was not confined to the writings of medical specialists. References to Blancard are found in Chambers' *Cyclopædia* of 1728, for example, under *hippus*. Both Blancard and Quincy are cited in a comment on the term

---

79 Blancard 1684 reads "*Harmonia* is a joyning of Bones by a plain Line; as may be seen in the Bones of the Nose and Palate." The entry in the second edition is unchanged.
80 Jakob Bruno (Jacobo Brunone,1629–1709), who edited Castelli.

tremor cordis in a footnote on Shakespeare's *The winter's tale* in Zachary Grey's *Critical, historical, and explanatory notes on Shakespeare* of 1754 (244–245). Grey also made use of Blancard in a note on Butler's *Hudibras*, about women who have the pica ('pique') "a depraved and longing appetite of women with child" (pt. III, Canto ii, l. 80: 183). Thus Blancard could also provide a source of authoritative information in an unrelated scholarly discipline.

Laurence Sterne adroitly exploits Blancard's reputation to demolish his apothecary, Mr Bump, in *The life and opinions of Tristram Shandy, gentleman*. Mr Bump is one of Uncle Toby's assistants in the great work of fortification in his garden, and a go-between for the intrigues of the Widow Wadman. When Toby wants assurance that the repaired fortification would resist the weather, "the opinion was learnedly back'd by Mr. Bump, who practises with great success, as an apothecary, surgeon, and man-midwife". The learning of Mr Bump is not what it may seem however:

> All his medical knowledge consists in hard words from Blancard's dictionary, which he has learnt to pronounce tolerably well, by the assistance of the curate of the parish. This, and a good share of modest assurance, has enabled him to maintain a wife and five small children very decently (IX: 23)

The hard-word dictionary tradition stemming from the late sixteenth century has died hard. Mr Bump's use of Blancard as a hard-words dictionary is, however, entirely practical, self-interested, and not a little fraudulent:

> Mr. Bump is remarkable for his assiduity in feeling people's pulses, whether they will or no; and if he can by any means assure them that the vis vitæ is not in good condition, he very ingeniously will hook in two or three boluses, and an occasional julap, to the tune of two or three shoulders of mutton.—He never speaks to you without some design against your purse (24)

Never ask the barber whether you need a haircut. Sterne's pungent irony allows the reader to imagine the Mr Bumps of the real world of medical practice of his time.

The particular question of Blancard's influence on medical lexicography in the eighteenth century is more pertinent here, however. Closer study of citations of Blancard which noted him by name reveals a clear pattern in the extent to which he is exploited.[81] Obvious questions include the extent and chronology of references to him. Do they increase or decrease over the course of the century? How many appear in this period and in which dictionaries? Whether the results of this study can be extrapolated to other dictionaries and lexicographers and their compilation practices is quite another matter, and no assumptions should be made without further investigation. Another confounding factor is of course the willingness of the individual lexicographer to acknowledge sources, which must vary considerably. The deletion of

---

81 A single instance which referred to the "same author" in the previous entry was also included.

acknowledgements may itself be an editorial decision affecting a whole dictionary, as we will see.

Almost three hundred references to Blancard were spotted in James's *A medicinal dictionary*. There are undoubtedly more, but these were enough to reveal some patterns in his use of Blancard, as well as his successors. Unfortunately, James hardly ever tells us which of Blancard's works he is using as a source, but the context is helpful in most cases. Almost all of the citations, although the lexicon itself is only actually mentioned once, seem concerned with definitions and naming, and confirmation of the naming used by James. Such definitions are usually prefaced by formulae such as "A name for…" with "Blancard" at the end of the definition, "according to Blancard…" and, in a number of very short entries, "the same as…". Typical entries are "JESEMINUM. the same as Jasminum. Blancard", "LAPPAGO, according to Blancard, is the same as APARINE," and "COLLATITIUM. A sort of Food, prepared, according to Blancard, of the flesh of a Capon or Pullet bruised, and then mix'd with Mutton-broth, and exhibited with Verjuice or Lemon-juice." The lemmas concerned are almost always of a few lines only; a slightly longer one is *chema*, which runs to 16 lines and paraphrases Blancard only briefly. "Blancard's Lexicon Renovatum" is mentioned once, in the long entry for *circulatum*. The only other reference to Blancard found in a long entry was in *ganglion* (very long), but the lexicon is probably not meant. A further point is that James seems to have mined Blancard for relatively obscure terms only, and for synonyms, so that his use for this source was somewhat peripheral.

As might be expected, given that John Barrow relies heavily on James, the great majority of his entries mentioning Blancard duly appear. There are some few deletions, as in *acaron*, *acatera*, *heptapleuros*, and *pleurorthopnœa*, but these are rare. Entries in Barrow's dictionary (1749) with the reference to Blancard deleted are even more rare, *buselinum*, *kirath*, *radicule* and *vernix* among these exceptions. Given the general sloppiness of this dictionary (see Ch. 10 below), these may simply be mistakes.

George Motherby (see Chapter 11), however, despite recording much of the same vocabulary, makes relatively little reference to Blancard in his first edition compared to James. The 14 (of the total of 217 shared terms) references which do occur, with the exception of *circulatum*, are strictly to do with questions of definition, and are usually introduced by a formula such as "according to Blancard" or "Blancard says", as we have seen in James. Motherby thus seems to have consistently ignored Blancard as an authority. Only one (*pleurorthopnœa*) was found after the letter M, which might suggest that Motherby actually found Blancard increasingly irrelevant as he worked through his own compilation. However, the second edition, edited by Wallis, brought a considerable increase to thirty-three, more than double the number. Strikingly, these additions are once again all in the letters A-M, the largest concentration falling between A and C. The citation under *pleurorthopnœa* has remained. References to Blancard in Motherby's first edition appear to be in the text rather than at the end of the entry, which suggests an editorial decision to excise references generally. They also decline towards the end of the alphabet.

While the first edition of Quincy's *Lexicon physico-medicum* contains no references to Blancard, the tenth edition (1787) has 23; either single word references at end of an entry or in the "Blancard says" form. Once again, most fall into A-M, with one in N (*nisi*) and one in P (again *pleurorthopnœa*). These extras in Quincy's tenth edition largely correspond to those added to Motherby: *anamnestica signa, bipemulla, chema, cicongius, circulatum, hydropyretos, lappago, meligeion, nisi* and *pleurorthopnœa*, which suggests that Motherby may have been a source for these references. Several in the early letters appear independently of what has been added to Motherby's second edition. Meanwhile, no references to Motherby have been identified in the tenth edition of Quincy.

Allusions to Blancard which appear in all three of James, Barrow and Motherby are very infrequent. Those which do are *abiga herba, anamnestica signa, centunculus, collatitium, hydropyretos, lappago,* and *meligeion*. The indications are also that Motherby and the latter editions of Quincy were compiled with only slight reference to Blancard. A strong indication of the way the medical wind was blowing by the late eighteenth century is that, despite the increase in references to Blancard, the tenth edition of Quincy has more references to Linnaeus than Blancard by a factor of more than nine to one, and those to Cullen outnumber Blancard by about eight to one. Other indications of being up to date include the very long entry for *gas*, which incorporates a reference to Alessandro Volta.

The first edition of Chambers has only one Blancard citation (at least found so far), *palpitation*. By 1778–1788, however, this work included Blancard references under *agaric, anacatharsis* (new), *anamnestic, chema* (new), *darsis, dasymma, ecphraxis, ecrithmis, endeixis, hemlock,* and *hippus*. Thus eleven references have been added, two of which are entirely new. The use made of Blancard in medical dictionaries is thus overwhelmingly by Robert James and inevitably by John Barrow, and there is a minor revival in the 1780s but, to judge by such allusions, the influence of his medical lexicography is not great. This still leaves us with the question of why Blancard would be quoted more in such works nearly a century after his first publication, not less. Individual editorial preference and dictionary inter-dependence may be sufficient to explain this given the small numbers of entries involved.

A somewhat surprising light on citing Blancard is shed by John Harris, who feels obliged to make the apotropaic point in his Preface that

> tho' many things are well enough done in him, yet some can hardly be said to be so; so that in many Places I have been obliged to put his Name to what my Amanuensis or Assistant transcribed from him, lest the Reader shou'd mistake it for my own Words.

Not that this is unexampled, since Thomas Blount adopts a similar strategy in justifying some of the foreign terms in his dictionary: "Foraign Words ... To many of which

I have added the Authors names, that I might not be thought to be the innovator of them" (1656: To the Reader).[82] The use of Blancard in Harris's *Lexicon technicum*[83] and Robert James's *A medicinal dictionary* is diametrically opposed. There are about 500 explicit references to Blancard in Harris (by electronic search), in addition to the roughly 300 in James. Words common to both are, surprisingly, very few, however. Those with explicit reference to Blancard in James are *cuneiformia ossa, decussorium, diacoprægia, ectillotica, hidronosis, inium* (=*inion*), *phyma* (=*phymus*), and *talpa*. However, in such a large list this is a remarkably small number, amounting to well under two percent. A few more appear in James, but have no explicit reference: *bradypepsy, darsis, dassyma, ecrithmus, hemiplagia, hippus, hidroa,* and *palpitation*. If James and Harris had worked completely independently, with no preconceptions about what they were taking from Blancard, one would surely expect more overlap. The most obvious explanation is that James chose one kind of word, but that Harris chose another. There is some suggestion that the choices were more familiar terms in Harris as against the more obscure in James, which would explain the fact that James's Blancard references are largely in small entries. To take some examples, Harris cites Blancard for words such as *apoplexy, bubo, carcinoma, cathartick, cataract, cholera, crisis, cuticle, diabetes, excrements, forceps, hæmorrhoides, herpes, lumbago, mesentery, paroxysm, rachitis, sarcocele, spasmus,* and *tabes,* all basic medical terms, where James does not. Blancard was apparently and understandably far more new and relevant for Harris, while for James he seems to have become a source of material to increase copiousness irrespective of contemporaneous relevance, and perhaps even to bolster the historical aspect of the dictionary. In such a large body of entries, however, this seems to be only a partial explanation of their almost complete independence.

The translation of Blancard was the first full-scale medical dictionary in English and, in the absence of serious competition, quickly became the leading English-language medical dictionary of the early eighteenth century, at least until the appearance of Quincy's *Lexicon physico-medicum*. Although it was last re-issued in 1726, its repute and use lingered until much later. Its repute in the out-of-print period raises a few teasing questions about the way its material appeared in medical dictionaries later in the century, which apparently marks a somewhat increased conservatism in medical lexicography.

---

82 My thanks to Professor John Considine for pointing this out.
83 The precise numbers are uncertain and so are not cited since the search was of necessity mainly manual. The final figures might be a little higher. The relativities are probably acccurate, however.

7 John Quincy (1683?–1723) and the *Lexicon physico-medicum*

As Blancard's dictionary began to outlive its usefulness and fall gradually into obscurity, an apothecary who had taken out a medical degree was on hand to meet the need. The circumstances of his career and the vigour of his approach conduced to revitalise English medical lexicography. Although he only outlived the appearance of his dictionary by three years and revised it only once, his work, which advanced the role of English in medicine, soon pushed Blancard out of the bookshops, becoming the most popular lexicon of its day and the underpinning of medical dictionaries into the nineteenth century.[84]

7.1 The relative obscurity of Quincy

The Baptist apothecary and physician John Quincy has remained an obscure figure, despite his considerable though unspectacular medical contributions, and despite his rather forward-looking attitudes to the theory and practice of medicine, which proved remarkably durable.[85] The many familiar studies of eighteenth-century medical practice conspicuously fail to mention him for the most part, perhaps on the tacit assumption that dictionaries as such can have no role to play in the history or evolution of medical knowledge. His published contributions to such things as dispensatories, which were well received and widely used, to judge by the many editions, are also overlooked.

Despite the influence of his dictionary, *Lexicon physico-medicum*, spanning at least a century, he disappeared from scholarly attention surprisingly quickly. Even Benjamin Hutchinson, who published a collection of medical memoirs at the end of the eighteenth century, fails to notice Quincy, mentioning him only twice, under Hoffman and Santorius, and not according him his own entry. Even the most elementary knowledge of him remains stubbornly opaque. While his date of birth is unknown, he died in 1723, not 1722 as usually reported. The circumstances of his apprenticeship, which he completed in 1704, suggest 1683 as his year of birth. The little we know of Quincy's life and works suggests that he was professionally ambitious, producing a number of publications, despite the disadvantages imposed by his religion and his trade. As a Baptist, he presumably had a non-conformist education, and he was a competent Latinist. He began a career as an apothecary, and proceeded MD at the

---

84 Part of this chapter has recently been published in McConchie, Roderick and Tyrkkö, Jukka (2018): 149–163.
85 The ODNB account of his life is sketchy; see Moore 2010.

https://doi.org/10.1515/9783110639186-007

University of Edinburgh on November 14, 1717 (University of Edinburgh 1846). He maintained a friendship with Dr Richard Mead (see Guerrini 2008), another non-con-formist, a further connexion being that both were staunch adherents of Newtonian medicine.

Quincy's lack of a university education and his first profession as an apothecary were to be a constant source of chagrin as well as jibes from physicians. Quincy's own prickliness exacerbated the situation. His translation of *Medicina statica* by Santorio Santorio, published in 1712, may have provoked an adverse reaction from the medical establishment. Members of the College of Physicians can hardly have rejoiced to see a plain "John Quincy", who admitted to being merely an apothecary, presume in "an introduction concerning mechanical knowledge", tell them what "the grounds of cer-tainty in physic" were. Equally however, Mead, a fellow non-conformist and one of the best-known proponents of Newtonian medicine, may have found Quincy's ap-proach congenial. Quincy later weighed into the pamphlet war against the opinion-ated and quarrelsome Dr John Woodward (1665/1668–1728; see Levine 2004), on the side of Mead and John Freind (Quincy 1719a; Beattie 1935: 260).[86] Woodward had penned a controversial medical work on smallpox and the role of "bilious salts" as a cause, which created a storm (Woodward 1718). Friend and Mead attacked Wood-ward, and his supporters responded in kind. Those favouring Woodward's theory re-peatedly stressed Quincy's inferiority, even insinuating that he was merely Mead's flunkey (N. N. 1719: 6).

Quincy's affairs did not always prosper, evidence being provided by the pseudon-ymous N. N., who weighed into the flurry of pamphlets on Woodward, charging that Quincy was a "Bankrupt Apothecary", (1719: 24). The insignificance of Quincy, "an obscure Fellow" (23), is repeatedly stressed in N. N.'s diatribe. Quincy meanwhile was hard at work on his dispensatory and his dictionary, as well as his career, work which must have occupied a good deal of his spare time.[87]

Not all notice of his dictionary was positive. Edward Strother (1675–1737), F. R. C. P., who had taken an M. D. from Utrecht, poured scorn on Quincy's lack of Greek, castigating the folly of writing a medical dictionary without knowing a language which is essential to it. Strother reports that Quincy, "a certain Compiler of a Physical Lexicon" in attempting

---

86 For Woodward, see Eyles 1965; Porter 1979. For a long account of the various public quarrels Woodward became involved in, see Beattie 1935, Ch. 3. See also Langdon-Brown 1946: 62–63. Part of Beattie's opening remark is that Woodward "made himself a storm-center, and for twenty-five years was at odds with naturalists, physicians, scientific leaders, pamphleteers, and fun-makers." For the medical disputes in particular, see 242–262.

87 Anita Guerrini's claim that Quincy had studied medicine in Edinburgh with Archibald Pitcairn presumably in the years before 1717, is rather doubtful (Guerrini 1989: 237). Pitcairn, on Guerrini's own account in the ODNB, was not greatly involved in teaching during these years and was in declin-ing health, while there is no suggestion that Quincy was anywhere but in London.

> to explain the Word Euodia ... display'd his Ignorance in the very manner that could have been wish'd for ... upon Enquiry, and pressing the Question too hard upon him in a private Conversation before Witness, he was oblig'd to confess he neither understood Greek, nor had ever read the Book, and would retract his Error in the next Edition: Thus the memorable Quincy! (1729: xxvi–xxvii)

The criticism was fair in that day and age, although Strother milked it for all it was worth, and the allusion to the wished for manner displays Strother's prejudice. Strother was probably still disgruntled at having been attacked under this head-word in Quincy's 1722 edition (see below).

Quincy was on the right side of history, however, and he was still well-enough regarded by the early nineteenth century to appear in John Gorton's *A general biographical dictionary*, first published anonymously in 1826, a compliment not accorded to Robert James or George Motherby. Gorton remarks that all of his main publications have become obsolete except for the *Lexicon*, having by then become the basis of Robert Hooper's medical dictionary. There are scattered references to Quincy throughout the eighteenth century, although it is not always clear which work is meant. Noah Webster makes an acerbic comment in a letter to Dr Ramsay of Charleston in 1807 in criticising Johnson's undiscriminating and unenlightening use of quotations under the entry for *finger*: '

> Here we arrive at the end of the author's exemplification of this sense of finger—and except a little anatomical knowledge from Quincy and Ray, what have we learnt from these long quotations? Why, surely nothing—except what we all knew before (21)

Webster's accusation is that Johnson was frequently guilty of such errors of judgement. Quincy appears in entries such as *caries*, *pennated*, and *pericardium* in John Wilkes's *Encyclopaedia Londinensis* (1810). There appear to be over 80 such mentions in all, not always to the *Lexicon*. Quincy was cited with approval for his advocacy of physical medicine in the mid twentieth century in the introduction to an article by Allsopp (1957: S40), and yet again in *The Lancet* (1952: 111–112) under the title 'A Wise Apothecary'. This short piece is really no more than a very brief digest of material in the lengthy account of his writings by Howard-Jones (1951), but it does show that his progressive attitudes were still capable of striking a chord in the twentieth century.

The social status of apothecaries has been discussed at length by Burnby (1983: Ch. 6), who argues that social status for medical practitioners was more fluid than generally thought, and that to assume that an apothecary must be unlearned and of low social status was to fly in the face of reality. Burnby also outlines the reasons which might persuade an apothecary to upgrade his status to physician, as Quincy had done, such as more money and a more comfortable life-style, as well as the fluidity which existed between the two professions (1983: 22–23; see also Loudon 1986: 71–72). The imputation of apothecaries being ignorant probably stemmed in some cases from those who felt threatened and had a professional borderland to defend.

7.2 Quincy the Newtonian

The search for a convincing, rational and reasonable account of the workings of the human body as well as an account of its diseases was a quest shared by a number of physicians in the period immediately following the publication of Newton's works, which seemed to offer a way forward (see Guerrini 1985). These included, firstly, Archibald Pitcairn and, following his inspiration, Richard Mead, James Keill, George Cheyne, William Cockburn, and John Freind (see Guerrini 1987: 82), with some of whom Quincy was on good terms. Pitcairn, having been appointed professor in 1691, taught medicine in Leiden, and actively sought a mechanical and mathematical analogue in the human physiology for Newton's account of the workings of the macrocosm; a "principia medicinae" (Guerrini 1987: 80–82). Robert Boyle came to endorse this view of the role of mathematics (Debus 2001: 81).[88]

Pitcairn's views on Newtonian medicine were outlined in his inaugural address in Leiden, published in 1692.[89] Burchard de Volder, rector magnificus of the University of Leiden in the 1690s, may have found Pitcairn's views congenial; in any case, de Volder wrote that "Physicians should study the human body in the same way as Newton studied the universe", arguing in particular that "more attention should be given to fluids, which must be studied according to the laws of mechanics" (Feingold 2004: 69–70). We cannot know whether Quincy had read de Volder, but he put his exhortation into practice minutely. If the physician knew the forces driving the hydraulic machine which was the human body, as the astronomers knew the heavens, this would suffice for practical purposes, and seeking for causes would become pointless. Herman Boerhaave was to take up the Newtonian baton along with Georgio Baglivi's fibrillar theory, which makes the fibre the basic elastic constituent of the body and the means of transmitting motion, in Holland as the new century began (see Steinke 2005: 27–28: Donato and Mazzei 2014: 98). Quincy's work also shows his assimilation of fibrillar theory, promoted by William Harvey, and Francis Glisson in the seventeenth century as well (see Steinke 2005: 24–26).

The introduction to Quincy's translation of the *Medicina statica* of Santorio contains a very long and useful explanation of the principles of 'mechanical reasoning'. Very briefly, the assumption is that all bodies have solidity, extension and figure, and that these operate on comprehensible and immutable laws:

> if Matter howsoever modified cannot move it self, and there cannot be any Change brought about in it without Motion, and if that Motion is under the Influences of these Causes, and determinable only by such Rules; then it is most certain, that whensoever our Enquiries are engaged about the Powers and Vertues of the most minute and unheeded Compositions of Matter whatsoever, that, I say, we are to be guided only by those very Rules, by which we are enabled to determine the

---

88 See Brown, Theodore M. (1987) for background.
89 Published in English in 1715.

> Powers of the most bulky and conspicuous Bodies. And it is a close Application and Adherence to these Guides, in Physical Searches, that is called Mechanical Reasoning; and so far, as any of the Conditions of Motion can be discovered, sufficient to demonstrate by those Laws, those that are unknown, is justly called Mechanical Knowledge (The Introduction: xxxiv)

He argues that the human body is to be considered in precisely the same light (Preface: xlii–xliii), since it is in no sense better than the rest of creation. There is also a passage in which he indulges in ridicule, culminating in a striking image:

> It has something in it that would move ones Laughter as well as Amazement, to reflect upon the Extravagancies of some subtile crafty Heads, who, to account for the Operations of a human Body, have abstracted and spiritualized upon it (if it may be so termed) so far as to assign every particular Part some sort of Intelligence or Soul, which rules and manages it in the Performance of its Offices ... And upon this means likewise there is laid open a direct and pleasant Road to the Art of Healing ... there is no more required, than to apply such Remedies, as the indisposed Faculty delights in, and will be comforted and strengthened by. And of this kind, we never fail of being plentifully stored, by the indefatigable Searches and Discoveries of such as have been conversant with the Planets, and are versed in the occult Sciences. So that every Medicine given to rectify the Disorders of any particular Part, seems only to be a kind of Sacrifice to the presiding Deity of that Part. (Preface: xliii)

Quincy is not one to jib at a dig at such physicians, or at pet targets like the dispensatories by such as William Salmon. Persisting with the religious imagery: "the Merit of the Sacrifice", Quincy writes, "is so much enhanced by the Qualifications of the Persons who offers [sic] it" (Preface: xliii–xliv).

It is perhaps not surprising that Quincy, being a dissenter,[90] was a friend and supporter of both Freind and Mead.[91] The RCP in the early years of the eighteenth century was strenuously resisting change by restricting membership, pointedly excluding the Newtonians. That body by and large accepted the Cartesian view of physic derived from Thomas Willis, as well as the views of Thomas Sydenham, to which those trained up by Pitcairn and in the tradition of Boerhaave were opposed (see Martin 1988: 403–404). Quincy was also marginalized in several other ways, not just because of his medical views. Change was ultimately inevitable, however; the Newtonians prevailed, and eventually the irascible John Woodward was left as the sole survivor of the old order after about 1716 (see Martin 1988, esp. 408–409; Rowlinson 2007: 112).

Quincy's translation activity continued throughout his career. A translation of Archibald Pitcairn's *The philosophical and mathematical elements of physick* was issued anonymously in 1718, but the second edition of 1745 acknowledges Quincy as the translator. The application of Newtonian principles to medicine were exactly what

---

90 Quincy published a poem on the death of Joseph Stennett, a leading Seventh Day Baptist minister and a friend of Quincy's brother-in-law, Joseph Collet, who died in 1713.

91 For Mead's views on iatromathematics, see Hanson 2009: 164.

would have attracted Quincy. The two editions are essentially the same. Pitcairn, the translator claims, has introduced

> the true Method of Reasoning in the Art of Physick; which before, amongst us, was but a con-
> fused Jargon, and as equally unintelligible as absurd; insomuch that the Theory of Medicine
> might then more properly be stiled a Mystery than a Science. (Pitcairn 1718: iv)

This encapsulates Quincy's essential interests in language and in perspicuity in medicine. He also sees Pitcairn as the means of bringing Newton's solutions to "all the
Irregularities in the System of the World" (xv) into medical practice. Those who have
ignored the advances brought about by Harvey, Newton, and others, Quincy argues,
have merely confused the issue with unmeaning terminology which fails to relate to
scientific phenomena: "Charleton, Willis, Morton, and others, have only abused us
with new Words, without any Ideas, and which have no relation to the Animal Oeconomy" (Pitcairn 1718: vi). Quincy's concern is not just with the discoveries, but with a
language fitted to convey them clearly:

> When he [Pitcairn] treated of the Institutions, he exhibited an exact Idea of the Animal OEcon-
> omy, and shewed the Falshood of many Notions hitherto received as certain Truths; endeavour-
> ing at the same time to fix the Meaning of divers Terms, frequently used by the Writers of Physick,
> tho they had not as yet any determinate Signification. (Pitcairn 1718: x)

Quincy sought to clear away the unclarities and obfuscation which he saw as charac-
terising the earlier dispensatories. He saw difficult medical language as a hindrance,
and metaphorical excesses meant to bedazzle the reader as simply pointless. He
sought to avoid all metaphor, "for in Physick no Figure of Speech is allowable, which
carries off the Mind from the Images and close Representations of the thing in description" (xi). The dispensatory is the work for which Peter Shaw reserves the greatest praise in introducing his posthumous edition of Quincy's lectures (Quincy 1723:
ix).

In a dialogue between Harlequin and Scaramouche in an egregiously scabrous
pamphlet against Woodward, possibly by Mead, the author stresses two matters;
Woodward's theories concerning bilious salts, the crux of the medical dispute, and
Woodward's language which, in the spirit of Quincy's approach, he rebukes as obscure, and never simple and straightforward, whether directly, as in:

> My Clients have the whole Faculty of Physic on their side, who universally look upon Wood-
> ward's Book as stuffed with Absurdities, false Anatomy, extravagant Whims, imaginary Princi-
> ples, inconsistent Deductions, ill-adapted Allegories, and fantastical Expressions (6)

and:

> Harl: Is not Dr. Woodward's Language proper, clear and intelligible?
> Scar: No. (1719b: 14)

or by way of irony, with a swipe at Harris as well:

> HARL: ...we don't care to be defil'd with the Zibethum Occidentale,[92] or keep our Friends at a distance, by the Sulphureous Exhalations of colluctating Biliose Salts ...
> SCAR: ...I am mightily pleased with his new Terms of Art; they will make a rare Supplement to the next Edition of the Lexicon Technicum (1919b: 5)

As for Latin, Harlequin cynically asks "don't you see the Use of it, how by the Magic of a few Words, one can make a Hero of a Quack?" (1719b: 16). Quincy may have wished to be a hero, but by no means a quack; he is at pains in his dictionary to eschew such suggestions.

7.3 The *Lexicon physico-medicum* 1719

Since so little is known of Quincy and his work, his *Lexicon physico-medicum, or, a new physical dictionary* of 1719, is thus a neglected dictionary by a little-known medical lexicographer. Quincy places it within the then ubiquitous notion in English lexicography of the 'hard words' dictionary in describing it as providing an "Initiation into a Circle of hard Words" (Quincy 1719b: xii). Despite its idiosyncrasies and being rooted in a medical philosophy which had certainly run its course by mid-century, the dictionary had a long life and was very influential, not only surviving for nearly a century and eleven editions, but also forming the basis of the medical dictionary by Robert Hooper which dominated the first half of the nineteenth century. That the *Lexicon physico-medicum* has received so little attention is quite surprising. Howard-Jones of course mentions it (1951: 167–169), but does not attempt an analysis of the work. He also mentions that Hooper found it necessary to re-cast the work, containing as it did "very many of the absurdities of his [Quincy's] day" Hooper adds: "When, therefore, the present editor was solicited to undertake its revision, he thought he could not do a more acceptable office to the public, than almost wholly new model it" (Hooper 1817 Preface). As we shall see, however, the job of revision had already begun, despite Howard-Jones's assertion that it had remained largely unaltered up to Hooper's revision (1951: 167).

James Keill's *Tentamina medico-physica* appeared in 1718, and it was probably no coincidence that its title of this work is echoed by that of Quincy's dictionary, published a year later. Quincy dedicated this work to John, Duke of Montagu, a courtier who took an interest in scientific progress, was admitted as a doctor of physic at Cambridge, and had become a fellow of the RCP in 1717 (Munk 1878, vol. 2). He was also a fellow of the Royal Society. These interests may have suggested him to Quincy as a

---

92 Zibethum occidentale is a Paracelsian medicament of human dung dried and powdered as a treatment for the eyes. See Salmon 1705, 85. The term was occasionally used for the faeces itself.

patron. The *Lexicon physico-medicum* went through many editions and several revisions. The first change was a revision in 1722, a version which was issued both under the original title and the sub-title "a new physical dictionary" by Bell, Taylor, and Longman. It was then reissued under the new subtitle "a new medicinal dictionary" by Osborne and Longman in 1726.

The *Lexicon physico-medicum* is the first such work to include illustrations and diagrams, as well as a number of tables. This is no mere coincidence, but actually a function of Quincy's Newtonian agenda, as explained in the preface to Santorio. Pictures could do far more than words in the right circumstances:

> Physical knowledge is assisted by picturing and drawing to view the Figures and Dimensions of those Instruments or Agents that are under Consideration, whereby their Powers and Efficacies are the better determined and demonstrated. (Santorio 1712 Preface: xxxvi–xxxv)[93]

A basic point to make is that the *Lexicon physico-medicum* avoids remedial formulations altogether, these apparently being felt to be the proper matter of the dispensatories and pharmacopœias. An indication of the methods of cure is sometimes briefly mentioned without being very specific, as under *mania*: "The Cure of this is in refrigerating Diet, Evacuation, and especially by strong Emeticks and Catharticks." This is not necessarily so of other medical dictionaries, which may include them, as James does at great length. Furthermore, Quincy omitted a number of the generic terms found in the tables of contents of such works. They are also less frequent in the text of the *Lexicon physico-medicum*, since there is a clear qualitative difference between these genres. The ubiquitous dispensatories might have been regarded as rich sources for dictionaries, as well as their indexes, as providing ready-made word lists. In practice this seems not to have happened, however. A fundamental, practical stumbling-block is that the pharmacopœias are topically arranged, not alphabetically.

Quincy's dictionary declares its radical stand from the outset. The preface to this work begins with the claim that "the Study of Medicine has in all Ages been influenced by the Philosophy in vogue" (1719b: ix), an assertion which radically undermines the assumption that the lexicon of medicine is fixed and immutable, and that the truths of medicine are likewise fixed. Quincy might have begun more predictably and conventionally with the usefulness and honour of medicine, or the care he had for his country in undertaking such a book, but he did not, preferring to subsume the art of medicine under the uncertain and shifting aegis of the fashions in science. The stated purpose of the dictionary is to introduce the reader to "Etymologies and Derivations ... the Original Significations of each Term, and the reason of its Application to such particular Occasion" (xii); in short, Quincy sees his initial role as lexical, despite the work also being a "dictionary of things" (Tarp 2013, Tarp and Bothma 2013,

---

93 For an account of the fact that Johnson failed to use illustrations which had appeared in scientific reference works, and for their function, see McDermott 2005.

unpub. 2014; McDermott 2005: 174–175), a distinction made by John Harris in introducing his *Lexicon technicum*.[94] He continues with an appeal to a long-familiar concept of the dictionary in English, declaring that it is essential "at their Initiation into a Circle of hard Words, to understand them; because it is an inseparable Introduction to a Knowledge of the things themselves, and a convenient Testimony to others of their having such Knowledge" (xii). The 'circle of hard words' notion nicely captures the peculiarly English tradition of hard-word dictionaries, especially with their proffers of help for the not-entirely-competent, while also acknowledging the circle of knowledge which the encyclopaedia encompasses.

He further claims to introduce a body of terms not previously encountered in these dictionaries—those concerned with the Newtonian understanding of medicine—offering the reader the example of "Momentum or moment" (xii). These terms represent for Quincy "a new System of Physicks and Medicine", two disciplines which, he argues, cannot survive without each other. He assures the reader that "a great deal about Attraction, the Laws of Motion, Gravitation, Air, Winds, Tides, Light, Heat, Cold, and the like" will appear in the pages of his lexicon (xiii–xiv).

An important general point is that Quincy shows how far the particular interests and agendas of the lexicographer can influence a dictionary. Quincy makes his agenda clear on the title-page, in declaring that the work will explain the terms used in those areas of philosophy (in the eighteenth-century sense of natural science) which underpin medical theory and practice. He also declares that the terms of philosophy are drawn from "Authors … who have wrote upon Mechanical Principles" (tp.). Since early modern lexicographers have not been conspicuous for following through on their avowed purposes consistently, we should ask how this agenda informs Quincy's dictionary.

The dictionary which Quincy proposed was seen as situated in a succession of medical works, all of which respond to the most current and useful changes in and additions to the medical lexicon. These are seen as "the newest, and most fit for modern Use" (1719b Preface: x). This view is not shared by the translator of Steven Blancard's dictionary, who argues simply that the terms of medical practice are useful and necessary, but assumes that they are fixed, not that they form an evolving lexicon; in this sense, Quincy's is the new, modernising view of the medical lexicon. Quincy invokes various forms of reasoning which he sees as the basis of medical knowledge—mathematical (Preface: x), mechanical (under *baths*), geometrical (under *calidum innatum*), and physical reasoning (under *balneum*).[95] 'Mechanical reasoning' is used

---

94 "That which I have aimed at, is to make it a Dictionary not only of bare *Words* but *Things*; and that the Reader may not only find here an Explication of the *Technical* Words …but also those *Arts themselves*" (Preface: A2ʳ).

95 Interestingly, however, he does not use the term iatromathematics, which would describe not a little of what he is concerned with. This term goes back at least to the early seventeenth century, but seems never to have become widely used (see OED).

here to cover what Quincy himself describes in these various ways since that is what he uses in his preface to the dictionary, as well as alluding to 'mechanical principles' in the title. These forms of reasoning obviously overlap but are not identical in practice.

Quincy begins his dictionary with a statement of what he perceives as the terminological problem of his time in medicine and of his intentions in this work:

> since the Introduction of Mathematical Reasoning, and the Application of mechanical Laws to a Study, indeed no otherwise knowable, the Books of Physicians abound with Terms very unmanageable, and which are not explained in any one Work extant (1719b: x)

The question at issue here is how far Quincy's dictionary has been influenced by the concepts and terminology of mechanical reasoning, primarily under the influence of Newtonian principles. Quincy explains in the preface that "the Terms of Philosophical Writers have been transplanted into the Discourses of Physicians, and rendered it frequently necessary to explain such new Terms" (Quincy 1719b: x). Since the praecognita of medicine are now heavily influenced by works in mathematics and philosophy, they must be entered in a medical dictionary and defined. Quincy criticises the earlier dictionaries by Steven Blancard, Bartolomeo Castelli, and John Harris: Blancard for not incorporating these terms, and Harris for simply taking over entries from Blancard. He also finds that Blancard's definitions are outdated and need recasting, and that many of his terms are now out of use and should be deleted. As to Castelli, Quincy regards this work as more a dictionary of the terminology of the ancients than one for contemporaneous use, and it was indeed a century old when Quincy published his. This understanding was later corroborated in Thomas Amory's *The life of John Buncle: Esq*, a work which expatiates satirically upon what is required to make a physician:

> A METHOD of studying PHYSIC in a private Manner: By which means a Gentleman, with the Purchase of a Diploma, may turn out DOCTOR, as well as if he went to PADUA, to hear MORGANNI.
> THE first books I got upon my table, were the lexicons of Castellus and Quincy; one for the explication of antient terms; and the other of modern. These, as Dictionaries, lay at hand for use, when wanted. (1766: 440)

Quincy makes some further comment about the adequacy of Harris's definitions, the insufficiency of which he ascribes to the author's haste (Quincy 1719b: xi–xii). Quincy, unlike his predecessors, argues that modernity is crucial to an understanding of medicine as it is now practised and in terms of the theory on which it is based.

Quincy's interest in mechanical principles did not however arise with his lexicon, appearing, as we saw, in the translation of Santorio Santorio's *Medicina statica* (1614) of 1712. The introduction explains the principles of 'mechanical reasoning' as constituting the assumption that all bodies have solidity, extension and figure, and that these operate according to comprehensible and immutable laws.[96] Santorio was particularly concerned about "insensible perspiration" and the balance between dietary intake and weight. Measuring and calculating daily was his recommended regimen, as appears in the 'weighing man' at his meal in a weighing chair, an image widely known in Europe in the seventeenth century, which forms the frontispiece to Quincy's translation.

Quincy writes in the preface:

> Mechanical Reasoning is what is much talked of now in Physick, and by some perhaps more than it is well understood; but the greatest number of Professors in Medicine are declared Enemies to it ... It is therefore for the Information of ... these, that I have been at the Pains of shewing what Mechanical Reasoning is, and proving that all Physical Certainty depends upon the same Principles. (Santorio 1712: Preface: ix)

This shows two things—first, Quincy's placement of mechanical principles at the heart of the medical endeavour rather than natural philosophy in Latin and Greek and, second, his no-nonsense and rather gritty approach to people who have other views.

We also need to understand the significance of Quincy's title, *Lexicon physico-medicum*. The adjective *physicus* in Latin meant pertaining to natural sciences and physical nature. One of the three senses of *physical* then current for Quincy derives from this. The other two are the now current one pertaining to "The branch of science concerned with the nature and properties of non-living matter and energy" (OED *physics* n.1b; see adj. 1b), the sense which OED suggests was beginning to emerge in Quincy's day, and the sense of pertaining to medical science (OED adj, 1a).[97] Thus Quincy plays quite consciously with this term and its potential ambiguities, invoking elements of all three senses at times, especially since he distinguishes between "physicks and medicine" (1719b Preface: xiii), and "physicks and mechanicks" (1719b Preface: xiv) in his declaration of intent, as distinct from using the term in the older sense. In this respect, his differs from earlier English medical dictionaries, which had used the title 'physical dictionary' in some form, as in the dictionary of 1657 and the English translation of Steven Blancard's dictionary, the latter speaking of the discipline as "the Commonwealth of Physick" (1708: A2ᵛ). This gives added point to his English sub-title in that his work of not quite the same title as the previous two will be genuinely and uniquely new.

---

96 Santorio (1561–1636) seems to have had some currency in England, having been published in 1676 in a translation by "J. D.", and then in Latin with a Latin commentary by Martin Lister in 1701. Quincy's translation was reissued in 1716 and 1720.
97 The ambiguity in the term *physica* in Latin however goes back at least to the twelfth century; see Burnett 1988: 168; 174–176.

In this respect, it is worth considering his somewhat perfunctory definition of *physick* itself:

> Physick, from φύσιζ, Natura, is in general the Science of all material Beings, or whatsoever concerns the System of this visible World; tho in a more limited and improper Sense by many it is applied to the Science of Medicine.

Quincy may have been kicking against the pricks, however. Dr Johnson is less judgemental a little later, noting that the word, "originally signifying natural philosophy, has been transferred in many modern languages to medicine." The word *mechanical*, "a Term much of late introduced into Physicks and Medicine", is accorded a far longer exposition than *physick*. Quincy explains that the only way to understand a material body is by understanding it quite literally as a physical machine.

> For considering an animal Body as a Composition out of the same Matter from which all other material Beings are formed, and to have all those Properties which concern a Physician's Regard only ... naturally leads a Person who trusts to proper Evidences ... to consider the several Parts, according to their Figures, Contexture, and Use; either as Wheels, Pullies, Wedges, Leavers, Skrews, Chords, Canals, Cisterns, Strainers, and the like ... to keep the Mind close in view of the Figures, Magnitudes, and mechanical Powers of every Part or Movement just ... as is used to enquire into the Motions and Properties of any other Machine.

Quincy is therefore interested in explaining the newly-created configuration of physics and medicine—those new terms which for him constitute the conceptual basis of the new medicine. "I say Physicks and Medicine, because the latter cannot subsist without the former" (Quincy 1719b: xiii), Quincy claims. This differs from earlier claims such as that by John Hatchet (Securis) in 1566 that the basis of medicine was natural philosophy in general and that this should be in Latin:

> for Aristotle saith Vbi desinit Physicus, ibi incipit medicus, A man must first peruse naturall Philosophie, before he entre into physycke ... But ... we coulde neuer haue it yet in Greke and Latine perfectly ... howe thenne shoulde you haue it [in English]? (Biᵛ–Biiʳ)

Quincy's dictionary thus includes a number of terms which we would not normally associate with medicine as such, including *abstraction, barometer,*[98] *congruity, form, levity, light, musick, moment, regular body* and *tide*. His view is that unless these things, which form an essential basis for medicine, are properly understood, medicine will remain in a state of confusion. As he explains, "there is no Knowledge in Medicine but by such means" (1719b: xiv). The authors to whom he alludes in these general remarks are indicated by his references—Isaac Newton, Robert Boyle,

---

98 An entry which acknowledges Harris's *Lexicon technicum*.

Thomas Willis, James Keill,[99] John Ray, George Cheyne, John Freind, Clopton Havers, Robert Hooke, and Richard Mead—among the English authorities who are most frequently mentioned, along with a list of foreign authorities, including Ettmüller, Schröder and van Helmont.[100] Very few of them represent a countervailing point of view, the glaring exception being John Woodward, his foe in the pamphlet war, whom he mentions quite respectfully as an authority more than once. Willis, the distinguished physician and neurologist and broadly speaking an iatrochemist, could also be regarded as taking a different view.

The nature of the animal spirits was a contentious issue in the early eighteenth century, especially as medical science became increasingly sceptical about the Cartesian view of their nature and operation. They become the butt of Mead's satirical dialogue between Scaramouch and Harlequin: [101]

> Scar. ... Will you engage to prove the Existence of your beloved Mephistophili, the Animal Spirits? An apparition of any of which no one ever yet saw.
> Harl. ... dost think we mean Hob-Goblins, or Fairies, by Animal Spirits? ([Mead] 1719b: 20)

While he does seem to accept the existence of animal spirits, Quincy's own dictionary entry does not dignify this term with a full entry, preferring a roundabout route. He merely refers the reader to *nervous fluid*, which in turn refers the reader to *brain*, where the account of animal spirits appears secreted away at the end of the entry. Perhaps he was uncertain as to what view to take.

7.4 The innovatory *Lexicon physico-medicum*

We now turn to the actual entries in Quincy's dictionary to see whether and how he follows through on the promises on the title-page and in the preface. It is not practical however to attempt to categorise and classify lemmas strictly by the appearance or non-appearance of such terms and ideas, because of the many different guises in which they may appear. However, since Newtonianism and the notion of mechanical reasoning pervade the dictionary, we can pick out some of the more obvious examples. This process reveals some general points and some more particular considerations. First, the entries more likely to invoke mechanical reasoning are longer and concern the more fundamental concepts. These include *air, action, blood, centre,*

---

99 Not John Keill, the mathematician of the same period and James's older brother. James Keill wrote perhaps the most overtly Newtonian medical text of the period, *An account of animal secretion* of 1708. Keill argues that since the animal economy is driven by mechanical forces, the symptoms of diseases must be a consequence of changes in the machine (Preface: vi).

100 It is surprising that the champion and pioneer of Newtonian medicine, Archibald Pitcairn, is not mentioned at all.

101 As emanating from and being regulated by the pineal gland, the seat of the soul for Decartes.

cohesion, colour, density, digestion, elastick, energy, fibre, heat, matter, menstruum, motion, particle, phlebotomy, projectiles, respiration, vision, and *water.* Newton himself is mentioned, sometimes more than once, in at least twenty-one entries: *action, air, attraction, cohesion, collision, colour, corpuscular philosophy, density, elastick, fluidity, heart, light, muscle, nature, particle, pori, projectiles, sound, tide, vision,* and *water.* Quincy's mechanical view of the human body also explains the inclusion in the dictionary and the dispensatory of terms like *cooler, strainer,* etc. (1719b Preface: xlvi).

The *Lexicon physico-medicum* was searched for entries which appeared to be Newtonian and mechanical or mathematical. The basis for this search was less than exact, but some criteria used included mention of Newton himself, an entry which had as much if not more to do with physics and mathematics than medicine, a lot to do with motion, especially of fluids and volumes of flow, matter and gravity, applications of the laws of Newtonian mechanics, and measurement of various kinds. Secretion had after all been the "paradigm case" in Newtonian physiology (Guerrini 1989: 225). Only the clear cases are listed here, but there are others which could have been included, such as *artery, conatus, disease, gland, larynx, lemma, pain, palsy, refaction, renitency,* and *visual point,* instances in which the Newtonian and mechanical interest seemed to play only a minor role.

Promotion of the vernacular is a way in which this dictionary attempts to break new ground. Quincy creates a precedent in making considerable use of references specifically intended to direct the reader from a Latin or Greek term to an English one, as we see under *plumbum,* which directs the reader to the head-word *lead.* Others include *catamena* (menses), *acetosella* (wood-sorrel), *oculus* (the eye), perhaps less obviously in the eighteenth century *arytænoides* (of the larynx), and so on. Many more arise because a Latin or Greek term and its definition have been incorporated into a larger entry under an English head-word, as with *chylification* referencing *digestion, medulla* referencing *marrow,* and *septum auris,* which cross-references *ear.* A more conventional work would use a Latin or Greek head-word, and then employ the English word throughout the text, not only in the corresponding definition, but throughout the dictionary. This is not the only form of cross-referencing for linguistic reasons in Quincy, a complex matter which merits further research.

Polysemy is a matter which Quincy had flagged in the preface, explaining that he would cover the various uses of his terms by contemporary writers and would explain them "in their greatest Latitude" (1719b Preface: xii). An example is *explosion,* which he explicates with the sensitivity to semantics one might expect of a profession lexicographer:

> Explosion, is properly the going off of Gun-powder, and the Report made thereby;[102] but is used frequently to express such sudden Actions of Bodies[103] as have some Resemblance thereunto ... Some Writers have likewise applied it to the Excursions of animal Spirits, and instantaneous Motions of the Fibres, on the Mind's Direction; but the Term then becomes too figurative to express any determinate Signification, so as really to inform the Understanding.

Similar explorations of meaning occur in *magistery* and *fibre*, the latter being not only a very long and complex entry, but also incorporating several diagrams. On the other hand, it is a key medical term for Quincy, and thus perhaps need not be accorded too much significance in this discussion as he was bound to be thorough in dealing with it.

Under *freezing*, Quincy also evinces a characteristic interest in processes as against things:

> Although this Term is out of the Province of Medicine, yet it is concerned in such a Change of Bodies as bears a Resemblance to, and therefore may explicate the Alteration made in several Substances under the Physician's Directions; and for that reason of use to be understood.

Quincy offers a meaning for the word *intention* in three semantic domains—medicine, physics and metaphysics, while *mars* is one of four entries for iron — *chalybs*, *ferrum*, *iron*, and *mars*. The main entry is *mars*, and *ferrum* and *iron* are merely cross-references. Despite this head-word, mars is not used at all in this lengthy entry, iron being preferred, along with the adjective chalybeate. There is also a comment on the use of mathematics in medicine where Quincy discusses the effects of iron on the blood:

> This is a way of reasoning that is plain to the meanest Capacity; and altho it may be called Mathematical, a Name shocking to some in Physick; yet it has no Conjuration in it, unless to force Assent by Demonstration.

Derivations are used in the *Lexicon physico-medicum*, but are somewhat restricted to Greek rather than Latin. Greek derivations occur frequently, just a few examples being under *acromion*, *lithiasis*, *odontoides*, *oesophagus*, *oxycroceum*, *panacea*, *pancreas*, *pathology*, *polypodium*, *pylorus*, and *scelotybe*. There seem to be particularly many in the letters O and P. Derivations from Latin are also found, however, as under *adust*, *circumforaneous*, *percolation*, *petrification*, and others, but they are much less frequent, suggesting that Quincy usually assumes that the Latin, which often appears as a gloss for the Greek, is by and large known to the reader already.

Quincy makes extensive use of propositions and equations. A spectacular example is *muscle*, a ten-page entry nearly half of which is calculations and formulae. In accordance with his declared intentions, some mathematical terms such as *corollary*,

---

102 This definition also adds significantly to the record of the OED, being an antedating for OED senses 3a and 3b, 1744 and 1775.

103 An antedating for OED sense 4a, 1799.

moments, *sphere*, *spheroid*, and *tangent* are also included. There are also some conspicuous entries for concepts; e.g., *consent of parts*, *form*, *nature*, *principia*, and *quality*. He also exhibits thoughtful awareness of defining at times, as in the entry for *pain*:

> It is commonly laid down, that Pain is a Solution of Continuity, but this is not a good Definition;
> for it is the Sense of a more violent and sudden Solution of Continuity made in the Nerves, Mem-
> branes, Canals, and Muscles

where *solution of continuity* refers to a wound, fracture, or break in the body.[104]

7.5 Quincy's use of sources

There are instances of Quincy acknowledging his debts, as well as appropriating large
slabs of text with minimal change. An example occurs under his entry for *jecur* (liver).
He cites Keill (1708: 37–40) at length on the function of the vena cava, paraphrasing
both his text and figures, which are taken over wholesale but are edited here and
there and are thus discriminating adaptions to some extent. Quincy also acknowledges the debt. Keill's diagram of the artery is also used, but in a slightly more sophisticated version which incorporates shading as well as simple lines. Quincy appears to
have expanded on Keill's calculations as well, with the result that he disagrees with
Keill on at least one figure, the rate of flow in the mesenteric artery as against that in
a branch of the vena porta, while retaining Keill's text verbatim at that point (Keill
1708: 42). In this entry then, the hand of the lexicographer is relatively marked, despite the heavy inter-dependence.

By contrast, the entire entry for *muscle* is from Keill verbatim (1708: 160), but is
not acknowledged as such. The first minor change occurs at "as will appear by the
sequel of this Discourse" (Keill 1708: 158), which Quincy shortens to "as will appear
by what follows". Two more very minor changes are "distension" for "distention" and
"stopped" for "stop'd"; "and therefore since both the Blood and Fluid" replaces an
obvious error "and therefore being both the Blood and Fluid" (Keill 1708: 160), but
this is not changed later in the same sentence; further on, "and being the greatest
Contraction" becomes "and seing the greatest Contraction", suggesting that either
Quincy or his printer was unsure about what to do with a construction which is obviously consistent in Keill, but with which they felt uncomfortable. Quincy's text removes most italicisations; "what has been said in several places" replaces "what has
been said in the Theory of Secretion"; a few very minor punctuation changes have
been made; the first-person "I have sometimes observed" is replaced by the

---

104 '*Continuity* is that Texture or Cohesion of the Parts of an animal Body which they naturally enjoy,
and upon the Destruction of which by foreign Accidents, there is said to be a *Solution of Continuity*",
is an addition to the 1722 edition, not appearing in 1719.

impersonal "it may be observed"; "after this manner I conceive the Vesicles" is reduced to "after this manner the Vesicles", although elsewhere another first-person reference is left in. A minor slip, the omission of an article, is corrected when "the Velocity of Parts moved" becomes "the Velocity of the Parts moved". The treatment of first-person references is, sensibly, generally to remove them: "I shall in the next Place determine" becomes "In the next place let us determine", although there is one exception to this practice. The spelling alterations are "Threds" for "Threads" throughout; "through" becomes "thro", and apostrophised past tense forms are expanded. There is a shortening of "which is already found", which becomes "already found". Two footnote references to another of Keill's works are omitted. At "flying off of the aerial Globules through the pores of the Muscles" (Keill 1708: 166) a long deletion is made, and the text is picked up again on Keill's page 168. Keill's geometrical figures are also reproduced exactly. A table of the muscles ascribed to Keill appears at the end of the entry, but this table is in Keill's earlier *The anatomy of the humane body abridg'd* of 1703, not in the work on animal secretions. In all, the changes are minor, and most could easily be explained by the influence of compositors and perhaps readers in the printing-house, leaving aside the large deletion and the first-person adjustments, and two changes necessitated by the new context of the dictionary. While Quincy's hand is there, its imprint in this case is very light. Similar comments can be made about other anatomical entries, such as *aspera arteria* (see Keill 1703: 122–123). His close adherence to Keill's text indicates that Quincy found it concise and to the point.

7.6 Comparison with later editions of Quincy

A question to be answered is whether these terms survived in later medical dictionaries, including later versions of Quincy. It turns out that substantial changes were made in the 1722 edition, and then not until the ninth and tenth editions, issued in 1775 and 1787 respectively by Thomas Longman (1730–1797), nephew of the first Thomas Longman.[105] The ninth edition makes additions, lengthening the work considerably, but leaves most of the existing entries intact. The brief preface to this edition indicates that up-to-date terms have been added, especially those from Linnaean botany. The tenth edition makes further changes, as we shall see.

The 1719 preliminaries are the same in the 1722 edition, with the exception of a small addition at the end of the preface. This addition responds to the charge that insufficient attention has been given to a perceived imbalance in the excessive inclusiveness of entries: "It may be here necessary to excuse a Fault or two charged by

---

105 The Longmans had been involved in every edition from the third, 1726, first with Thomas Osborne, and then alone.

some upon this Work since its first Impression; viz. in not observing a due Proportion in its Parts, and including sometimes the Explanation of many terms under one" (1722a Preface: xv). The first remark seems to mean that critics have detected an over-emphasis on the realia, a point which is dismissed on the grounds that a full under-standing of the word requires a corresponding understanding of the thing signified, not just a lexical definition. That Quincy regards this is an essential element of the book and one he is not prepared to compromise on is also indicated by his remark that "this Enlargement in some Instances ... has been thought proper to take notice of even in the Title of this Book" (xvi). He further indicates that there has been extensive omission of entries for simples, which, he argues, has created space for previously overlooked head-words: "in this Edition a great deal relating to the Description of Me-dicinal Simples hath been expunged, as not proper to such a Work, and in their room such Materials supply'd, as were thro Inadvertency before omitted" (1722a Preface: xvi). Quincy's *Pharmacopœia* had been re-issued the previous year, after all, allowing him a perspective on his dictionary not shared by his predecessors.

It seems safe to assume that Quincy himself was the reviser, especially since some of the additions also show his characteristic acerbity, as well as his impatience with quackery and superstitious imposture.[106] Since the changes between 1719 and 1722 carry through to the end, Quincy was probably still editing close to his death. To il-lustrate, under *leo* we find "a Species of a Leprosy, the same as Elephantiasis; but the Chymists have most grievously tortured it by its Application to several of their Whim-sies, now too much in contempt, to deserve any notice here." Likewise, Paracelsus, Quincy's favourite whipping-boy, is castigated under the new entry *magia* for the use of magic to invoke supernatural powers:

> chiefly Paracelsus, Crollius, and Helmont, have treated it in this manner, alledging much to be done in Medicine by Magick, or Inchantment: and hence arise likewise our modern Legends of Witchcrafts, and Exorcisms, which it is to be feared have not a little been encouraged by Priest-craft.

Among previous entries which have been augmented, the entry for *adept*, defining the term as those who "pretend to some uncommon Mysteries in Chymistry", is ex-panded in the 1722 edition with the reflection that "these prove either Enthusiasts or Imposters: and such were Paracelsus, Helmont, and their Followers." *Abracadabra*, a formulaic incantation dating from Roman times, has also been inserted, with the explanatory comment that it is "a magical Term with which some pretended to cure Diseases ... such Tricks are now in just contempt."[107]

---

106 For more on quacks, see Loudon 1987.

107 This word has an equally contemptuous but, surprisingly, considerably expanded entry in Quincy's ninth edition, concluding with "But such Tricks are now justly detested as unlawful, by all Physicians who call themselves Christians, and laughed at by the more rational Part of the rest."

Some adjustment was made to the alphabetisation, although the improvement was only partial. The head-words *adeps*, *adeposum membranum*, *adeposa vena*, *adeposi ductus*, incorrectly ordered in 1719, are correctly alphabetised in 1722, *but conjunctiva tunica* and *conniventes valvula* (cross-references only) now fall out of order. Some further changes found include the correction of the alphabetisation of *abcess* [sic], which has been restored to its rightful place before *abdomen* where it had previously been placed after *abductor*, etc. This was perhaps the result of a typographical error in the first place, but the spelling has not been corrected.[108]

A closer look reveals that Quincy keeps his promise of omitting the names of plants and simples: some deletions include *abrotonum*, *absinthium*, *adianthum*, *dens leonis*, *marjoram*, *malabathrum*, *matricaria*, *pæonia*, and *violet*. *Deciduous*, purely botanical in 1719, has the bodily sense of relaxation added, and the long entry for *manna* has gone. There are a few other deletions as well, the reasons for which are unclear; these include *acetosa*, *acetosella*, *acetum*, *conjunctiva tunica*, *lemnian earth*, and *maturantia*; rather against his stated principles about simples, entries for *malicorium* (pomegranate peel) and *veratrum* (hellebore) have been added. Some of the additions seem typically Quincian, such as *continuity*, *consequentia*, *conservatina medicina*, *contingent*, *deambulation*, *palato-staphilinus*, and *ventriloqui*. *Matter subtle* is now described as a "figment" of the Cartesians designed to avoid postulating a vacuum, which was thought abhorrent to nature. Some entries have had references added, some to the ancients, as under *adiapneustia* and *deleterious*, and others to the moderns, as in the case of *absorbents*, where a reference to Waldschmidt's *Institutions* has been added. Finally, there are some editorial improvements to a few entries.

Much later, significant changes appear in the ninth and tenth editions. Major deletions are effected and additions made, but these are not as thoroughgoing or detailed as in 1722. A heavy hand has simply deleted large chunks of entries to make way for the new material. Minor changes are made to the text now and then. The overall impression is that the Longmans decided to resuscitate and modernise this perennial favourite by the most brutally efficient methods available. The entry for *elastick* will illustrate some basic procedures. Comparing the 1719 entry for this word with that in the tenth edition of 1787, we find that the first page is verbatim, but that lengthy calculations and theorems constituting most of the next four pages are entirely omitted. There is a summarising conclusion to the entry in 1719, which is also omitted in 1787; in other words, the entry has been cut completely at the point where Quincy begins his demonstrations and equations, without any corresponding adjustments.

Exactly the same has happened to the entry for *fibre*, effectively reducing four pages to half a column, although the section omitted does not contain calculations

---

108 OED does not record *abcess* as a variant spelling. Quincy does use the correct form elsewhere, as in *adenosus abscessus*.

and formulae.[109] Nevertheless, the discussion does contain a great deal about the effect forces exert on fibres, their elasticity, and so on. These omissions were primarily made to allow for a larger number of head-words, rather than to update entries in detail. In these circumstances, as the anonymous editor comments rhetorically in his own preface "though a familiarity with the whole circle of Science, may be ornamental … the omission of several processes merely Algebraic, will not be censured", and mathematical knowledge is declared to constitute only a minor part of what the practitioner needs to know (Advertisement to the tenth edition). An exception is *particle*, which remains a very long entry, is retained verbatim in its entirety, as well as retaining a diagram, apparently one of only two kept by the tenth edition, the other being under *spiral line*.[110] We see a similar pattern in the entry for *motion*, where the calculations and diagrams are removed, and the theorems retained. This entry also shows some minor editorial changes—occasionally in punctuation and italicisation, past tense '-'d' by '-ed', and spellings such as replacing 'thro' by 'through', and 'strait' by 'straight', changes only partially present in the ninth edition. *Projectiles*, another very mathematics-based entry, is reproduced verbatim in edition nine, but is cut about halfway in the tenth edition and loses its diagram. Thus some of this pruning was conducted for the ninth edition and the process was continued in the tenth. The reduction of what Quincy argued was indispensable to the status of an ornamental accompaniment was a telling part of the renewal of the dictionary.

The advertisement to the ninth edition (1775) suggests that significant changes had been made. It declares that recent discoveries have been taken account of; in particular, the terms of chemistry, and that the Linnaean botanical system, "the most universally received", will be properly represented, and plant names have indeed been restored. A number of the mathematical parts of entries, which are "repugnant to Anatomical Truth" such as under *muscular motion*, have been shortened or omitted altogether and more up-to-date entries inserted.

One further conclusion is that even after the lapse of over half a century, the editor did not see fit to change Quincy's language in any substantive way. There seem to be no serious attempts to add, simplify, reduce verbosity or repetition, and so on, as was frequently the case in other such works, an instance being the changes between the first and subsequent editions of Blancard, so that Quincy's prose had proved clear, flexible, and durable, and his definitions and information had continued to be regarded as sound.

Chemical theories and practices in medicine had already come under attack in England, particularly by physicians Quincy admired such as Freind, Keill, and Cheyne.[111] Throughout his writing career, Quincy demonstrated a sceptical disdain for

---

109 No editor is acknowledged on the title-page.
110 Some of the tables are retained however.
111 See Rowlinson 2007: 110.

claims that could not be based on some form of evidence or depended simply on unsubstantiated traditional notions. This cannot have pleased his opponents, let alone those who thought that an apothecary publishing on medicine was getting above himself. In the main, however, it is Paracelsus and the iatrochemists who suffer the lash of his tongue. *Archidoxis* (not in the first edition) he defines as "a whimsical Title given to a book wrote by Paracelsus of Chymistry, and which Libavius ... says looks more like Magick than Knowledge."[112] Sometimes the use of the term is under attack, as in *conjugation*, added in 1722: "being by some used in the same sense as Conjugium, and Copulation, Paracelsus and some other Chymists whimsically enough apply it to particular Mixtures of several things together", and sometimes the practitioners themselves, like the "jugglers" mentioned under *carminative*. Although Paracelsus is his customary whipping-boy, Quincy is not above putting some of his compatriots such as Robert Boyle to the sword, despite their reputations. To cite an example, he adds to his definition of *amulet* that "These were in esteem antiently amongst some Enthusiastick Philosophers, and have been last supported by the Credulity of Mr. Boyle; but now have none to appear in their behalf but Empiricks and Mountebanks."

Iatrochemists are given short shrift under *luna*, which, "in the Jargon of the Chymists, signifies Silver, from the supposed Influence of that Planet (the Moon) thereupon. The medicinal Virtues of this metal are none at all, until it has undergone very elaborate Preparation." This doctrine of resemblances is also treated sceptically under *sputum*. Likewise, iatrochemists are under attack in the entries for *aquila alba*, *balsum*, and *balneum*. Under the latter, Quincy adverts to the well-known tradition of hard words, which he pointedly rejects, complaining that "a Sand-Heat is also sometimes called Balneum siccum, or cinereum, so much do they delight in hard Words." Under *clavis*, we hear of the auger, a device sometimes used to relieve headaches, so that "Some Chymists also from the use of this Instrument very whimsically apply it to many things, to which they ascribe strange Virtues in opening or unlocking other Substances."[113] And under *spuma*, an entry added to the second edition: "The Chymists likewise according to Custom do use it in a very whimsical manner for many things, as the Spuma Duorum Draconum".

The whimsy of Paracelsus is also mentioned under *confluxion*. 'Whimsy' and 'whimsical' seem to be Quincy's favourite expressions of disdain. "Noli-me-tangere ... is ... thus called from its Soreness, or Difficulty of cure; but either seems upon so whimsical a Foundation, that it is not much matter which." Another target appears under the head-word *climacterick years*, which he calls "this whimsy". Empirics are accorded similar treatment for fatuous language as well, although less frequently:

---

112 The word 'whimsical' appears only in the second edition.
113 This remark added to the second edition.

"Magisterial remedy, is yet sometimes retained in the Cant of Empiricks, more for its great Sound than any Significancy."

A somewhat obscure category is those whom Quincy calls "institution writers". He is not at all clear about who they are, but we may perhaps assume that he means those who set out the basic principles of a subject (its 'institutions'), although I have not found an instance in Quincy which makes this perfectly clear.[114] We find them under *acme*, where their account of the four stages of a disease are quite neutrally mentioned; under *acute disease*, however, they come under attack: "Institution Writers define this very confusedly", for example, and in general this appears to be his own mildly negative expression. In any case, its use is of a piece with his usual perception of himself as a professional outsider. Further criticism appears under *chirurgery* (1719, 1722): "Some Institution-Writers divide this Art into several distinct Branches, but such are not worth notice." The entry for *critical days* (1719, 1722) seems to offer some help: "The Writers of Institutions have strangely perplexed this Part of a Physician's Province" helps a little since institutions often took the form of classification. The OED lists at least two instances of this term applying to medicine in the eighteenth century under sense 5.

Sometimes he is less specific about the kind of writer he means. *Occult quality* he describes as "a Term that has been much used by Writers that had not clear Ideas of what they undertook to explain, and which served therefore only for a Cover to their Ignorance," an accusation repeated almost verbatim under *quality*. *Daemon*, only in the 1722 edition, is a word which "hath not likewise escaped Torture from the Application of some Writers in Medicine, most of which are too ridiculous to take Notice of". Quincy's later editors must have taken him at his word on the value of this entry.

Great stress is put on the misuse of words, especially that which makes exaggerated claims. Quincy also uses the London dispensatory as an implied authority in this example, another addition in the second edition: "Divinum, is used variously by the Physical Writers ... but the Chymists and Medicine-Makers have most deviated from the proper Meaning of the Word, by applying it very conceitedly to several things, of whose Virtues they had extravagant Opinions." Neither is Quincy above sometimes approving of an author on whom he normally turns his scorn, such as Van Helmont under *cement*. Under *arbor Diana* (added to the second edition) he writes that "Helmont very conceitedly gives the Name of Arbor Vitæ to a Medicine, by the Help of which he pretended Life would again shoot out like a Tree." In this case, the objection is to an inflated and inappropriate, not to say misleading metaphor. Terms like this are, in Quincy's opinion, simply used to puff the nostrum in question. An addition in

---

114 This conjecture is corroborated by Dr Thomas Knight in his *A vindication of a late essay on the transmutation of blood*, 1731, 116, who mentions a "famous Institution Writer" offering a footnote reference to the *Anatomicæ institutiones corporis humani* (1611) by Caspar Bartholin the Elder (1585–1629).

1722 was the entry "Sanctus, holy. This hath been applied to many things both simple and compound, as whimsical Persons have conceited of their Virtues; as the Guaiacum is called Lignum Sanctum". The word alone creates the supposed medical efficacy, not the characteristics of the simple.

Archeus falls into the same category of hyperbole, and is thus fraudulent in Quincy's view.

> Archæus, a Term much used by Helmont to express an internal efficient Cause of all things; which seems no other than the Anima Mundi of his Predecessors ... But these are such abstracted Terms, and convey such confused Notions, that they rather serve the Purpose of Ignorance and Imposture, than any useful and generous Knowledge (1722a)

This rather neutral entry in the 1719 edition, where it was described merely as an "enthusiastick" term used by chemists, has been expanded, and criticism added to give it new edge in the second edition. We have seen sufficient such additions to the second edition to suggest that Quincy had embarked on a campaign to explode such nonsense entirely given that there is no practical medical reason for entries like this. Not even more familiar terms are exempt: *Caro* (flesh) is a term for which "some Anatomists make very perplexed and useless Distinctions". Quincy is quick to debunk almost any concept, no matter how familiar. He mentions the creation by the poets of an eponymous goddess under the head-word *hygieia*, but then brusquely claims that this notion is no more or less than an appropriate rate of blood-flow in the living body.

Quincy often rejects out of hand notions that in his view lack rational justification. Magnetism and its supposed benefits comes in for its share of opprobrium.

> Magnetical Virtues, are much used by some who find their Account more in Amusement than useful Knowledge; and some affect to explain or recommend by such Terms, those Remedies, for the Application and Operation of which, they have no better Reasons at hand.

Other forms of verbal manipulation which he finds objectionable include inflating the price of a remedy by exploiting the connotations of a particular word, as under *bezoardick* "a Term given to many Medicines, only the better to palliate the Price they go under, than to express any extraordinary Virtue", a case in which Quincy is quite prepared to sacrifice the actual definition in order to fire his shot. Another term widely used to describe an undiscriminated range of supposed panaceas is *catholick*, "but such are now laughed at for Impositions." Perhaps it is no surprise that no nostrum bearing Quincy's name has been identified so far.

7.7 Quincy and Blancard

Since a comparison between the entries marked in the *Lexicon physico-medicum* as Newtonian and the corresponding entries, or lack of them, in other dictionaries of the period could be revealing, a comparison between Quincy and Blancard for Newtonian entries was conducted. It is perhaps as well to recall Quincy's assessment of Blancard's dictionary in the preface to the first edition of his own.

> BLANCHARD's Lexicon Medicum has been ... much in request among ordinary Readers, and is yet much the best of its kind for such; but it is grown now extremely defective ... because there is so much of a new Turn of Reasoning and Speaking among modern Physicians, that it is of no manner of Assistance in reading them with understanding. He also abounds with Terms long since intirely out of use, and now of no other possible Service, but to puzzle good Sense (1719b Preface: ix–x)

A comparison was made to see whether entries corresponding to a list of Newtonian entries appeared in the fifth edition of Blancard's *The physical dictionary* of 1708 and the edition of 1726. Thus 69 entries in Quincy were sought in Blancard's work. Blancard's dictionary had already reached its fifth edition by 1708, and so had pretty much ruled the roost in England in medical lexicography for a generation before Quincy published. In this study, words were sought in Blancard, much more a Latin–English dictionary than Quincy's, under several possible corresponding head-words where it seemed necessary. Some were obvious and straightforward, but some needed to be sought under a range of possible Latin equivalents. Other discrepancies were that Blancard has *motus conuulsivus*, but not *motus* alone for Quincy's motion, as happens with several other terms as well, none of which are therefore recorded as matches. Some entries were problematic—I have left *cylinder/cylindrus* on the list, but the meanings given were rather different, Quincy defining it as the geometrical figure, and Blancard as a cylinder-shaped plaster.

Only five additions were made from this modest list in Blancard 1726, but all of them could be seen as under the influence of Quincy in some respect. The first, *barometer/barometrum*,[115] is described rather more fully in Blancard 1726 than in Quincy 1719:

> Barometrum, or Baroscopium, A Barometer, which is a certain Instrument so call'd by the curious Enquirers into Nature, in which by the Assistance of Mercury put therein, the Weight and Pressure of the Air, according to the minutest Variations, may be observ'd and seen.

This is a definition which clearly relies on Harris without copying verbatim but independently of Quincy. Meanwhile, Quincy 1722 has

> Barometer, and Baroscope, from βάροσ, Onus, a Weight, and μέτροσ, Mensura, a Measure; is an instrument to measure the Weight of the incumbent Atmosphere

---

115 Called a baroscope in the proposal issued by Harris in November 1702. The *Lexicon technicum* was published by subscription, and was announced in this proposal as already being in the press at several printing houses.

which also seems to rely on Harris.[116]

An especially intriguing entry is that for *demonstratio* in Blancard 1726.

> Demonstratio, hath been reckon'd rather a Philosophical than a Medicinal Term; but since it
> signifies a Proof taken from certain and undoubted Evidence, as well from Sense as the Intellect,
> those Physicians undervalue the Art and themselves who do not think it a proper Term.

While this is in no sense derived from Quincy's entry verbatim, the fact that it has
been added so recently, and so pointedly picks up the question of the properness of
such a term makes the Blancard entry read like a comment on Quincy, and a concession to his innovations. Quincy waspishly adds at the end of his own entry: "But when
this is apply'd to Purposes not attended with equal certainty, it is with great impro-
priety; tho too often done by Persons too opinionated of their own Abilities and Speculations." This is somewhat reminiscent of the entry in Quincy for *hypothesis*, a notion he rejects as a method in medicine, which he claims must rely on "demonstrable
Principles, which our Senses are Witness to, and will not allow any thing suppositious". In this regard, he remains the faithful follower of Newton, whose disdain for
hypothesis and speculation was well-known and constituted almost a moral impera-
tive for his acolytes. James Keill had already written in 1708 that "the raising of Theories and Hypotheses is but the building of Castles in the Air" (Preface: xi).

Another addition to Blancard 1726 is *fluidity*, a head-word which has not been
Latinized, which again hints at Quincy's influence even though the definitions are
quite dissimilar.[117] The inclusion of *elastick* (*elestica*), an important notion for the then
current theory of muscular contraction (Steinke 2005: 33), also suggests Quincy's influence in general terms, since it is rather a term in physics and mathematics than
medicine. *Menstruum* ('solvent'), the last of these additions, is a term directly associated with the apothecary and his manufacturing processes.

The differences between the ninth and tenth editions of Quincy require some
comment. If, as claimed, Blancard is falling inexorably out of date, and possibly out
of favour, why increase the number of references to him, two generations after the
first appearance of Quincy? Quincy's ninth edition has two citations of Blancard in
the entries (*anacatharsis* and *soporales*), as do most of the previous editions. Quincy's
tenth edition adds twenty-nine new ones. Some instances are *meligeion*, of which no
usage could be found in any other eighteenth-century text, or indeed any earlier text,
not even in Blancard; *lappago* was found fourteen times in a handful of botanical
texts in lists and usually not in English; *cicongius* was only found in Blancard; *bothor*
was located three times in the translation of Luisini's *Aphrodisiacus* but hardly

---

116 The opening of Harris's five-page entry is "BAROMETER is an instrument for estimating the Minute Variations of the *Weight* or *Pressure* of the Incumbent Air".
117 A definition of *fluid* has also been incorporated into the Blancard *fluidity* definition, a head-word
which Quincy does not have.

anywhere else; *amblotica* in Lewis's materia medica, Blancard, and various editions of Nathan Bailey's *An universal etymological English dictionary* under the head-word *ambloticks*, but hardly at all elsewhere, and so on. The only one with any currency was *impetigo*, and even there it was limited to medical discourse, dictionaries and grammars, usually of Greek and Latin. It is hard to know why the editor of Quincy's tenth edition would introduce so many terms from a dictionary considered out of date in 1719; terms which for the most part were never in general medical use and some of which can hardly be evidenced at all, especially with the claim in the original preface still in place in 1787, virtually unaltered except for a change in capitalisation practice. This claim was of course a means of paving the way for Quincy's own Newtonian agenda, but why it should be retained through nine further editions and half a century after the compiler's death is unclear.

7.8 Quincy and language

The significance of the title of the *Lexicon physico-medicum*, alluding as it does to Quincy's Newtonian view of medical theory, has already been commented on by Wimsatt (1948: 77), but not so much should be read into this given the existence of the pre-Newtonian *A physical dictionary* of 1657 and the fact that the translator of Blancard had used the same title in 1684. By implication, the particular collocation Quincy uses may suggest that he does indeed have a theory of the præcognita of medical practice, as opposed to the laxity of the empirics (Wimsatt 1948: 77), and as opposed to the rather incoherent and increasingly discredited assumptions of medical works in general and the dispensatories in particular. Quincy alludes to the familiar and long-exploited concern about revealing the secrets of the profession in the preface to his *Pharmacopœia*, arguing that "If any should charge us with laying open hereby the Mysteries of their Profession too much; they may reflect, that nothing of this nature has yet been suffer'd to remain in a Language unknown to the common People" (1718: vii–viii). This argument was however a straw man for Quincy, who was entirely convinced of the appropriateness not only of using English, but of using the simplest and most straightforward English in his works. This concern about maintaining the mysteries of the profession by linguistic means goes back at least to the sixteenth century, and was almost a required disclaimer in prefaces to medical works in English. The point was more germane in the sixteenth century than it was for Quincy, however, who can be seen as merely exploiting the recollection of a well-worn cliché.

Quincy also pointedly eschews the use of metaphor:

> And in this has been study'd the utmost Plainness and Perspicuity, avoiding all those Figures, and metaphorical Ways of Expression, which the best Writers have too much abounded with. For in Physick no Figure of Speech is allowable, which carries off the Mind from the Images and close Representations of the thing in description; because tho they may amuse, and give a confus'd Notion, yet they add not at all to true Knowledge (xi)

In this he followed commentators such as George Castle, a physician who embraced the recent discoveries in science, and who attacked the "thousand such conjuring unintelligible words of the Chymists" (Castle 1667: 6). Quincy also shared Castle's view that "a man is as Mechanically made as a Watch, or any other Automaton" (Castle 1667: 5; see also Debus 2001: 96–98). Wimsatt quotes Quincy's entry for *heterogeneous*: "This is a Term of a very lax Signification, and by the Chymists is come to serve almost for any thing they do not understand" (1948: 6). Quincy's tolerance of pseudo-learned pomposity and its use to conceal ignorance was slight.

Quincy's attitude to language, particularly the use of florid rhetoric, also stands in contrast to the kinds of expressions often used by the quacks of the period to sell their nostrums (Barry 1987: 32). Regular physicians parodied the use of such language by quacks (Barry 1987: 30–31), although it is also clear that many were not above using such devices themselves. Indeed this is precisely what Quincy accuses the iatrochemists of. This was not new, however; no less a figure than John Wilkins had already attacked the language of the chemists in his *Mathematicall magick* as being "so full of allegories and affected obscurities" (1648: 227–228).

A number of rhetorical strategies designed to denigrate theories and persons with whom he disagrees are also used. If such beliefs are not supported by some underlying form of reasoning, Quincy is quick to dismiss them. He describes things as 'whimsical' when he finds them fanciful, incredible, or credulously accepted; hence, under *euodia* (1722; not in 1719) we find "But we have not heard of this Term latterly, unless prefixed to a Book, the Contents of which are as whimsical and unintelligible as the Title". Quincy clearly alludes here to the work on fevers by Edward Strother (1716), which, having a Catholic dedicatee and including an attack on mechanical medicine, cannot have recommended itself to Quincy.[118] He is not shy about the kind of language used in previous publications, for which he expresses disdain. He also clearly despises superstition, regarding such practices as suppositious: "Amulet, any thing ... supposed to be a Charm against Witchcraft, or Diseases." "Our common Term of Conjuror, who is a Person supposed to deal in diabolical Inchantments"; this under *conjuration*, yet another medically dubious addition to the first edition. In yet another addition to the second edition: "Saxonicus, is an Epithet ...[for] a compound Pouder, yet retained in some Dispensatories, for its supposed Efficacy in breaking the Stone". An even harsher dismissal is reserved for *alchemy*: "Alchymy, is reckoned to be a sublimer sort of Chymistry ... but is found to be mere Jargon and Imposture."

Quincy has no patience with the use of imagination, which always seems to be a negative process for him: "*Animation*, a Term used by the hermetick Philosophers, to express an imaginary Perfection of something new brought into their Processes; but such Jargon is now quite in neglect" (the second edition). He also describes both language and beliefs as 'cant' and 'jargon', as we saw under *magisterial remedy* and

---

118 Dedicated to Don Isisdro Casadro.

mercury "They also talk much of the Mercuries of Metals; but they conceal their Notions in such a peculiar Cant and Jargon, as to run no hazard of being contradicted by being understood." Such usage is merely a stratagem intended to forestall more reasoned and reasonable objections. Similar scepticism is suggested in "*Lunatick*, [which] signifies being mad, from Luna, the Moon; because it has antiently been an established Opinion, that such Persons were much influenced by that Planet", although here it is not spelt out so explicitly. Under *fuga vacui*, Quincy writes that it is "an imaginary Abhorrence in Nature of a Vacuity: but a more reasonable Philosophy has expunged such Phantasms," alluding to the Cartesian notions of the universe as a series of interlocking vortices, which was a theory designed to support the notion that nature abhors a vacuum—a belief decisively exploded by Newton.

There is also a long semantic comment under *carminative*, which he claims has been taken to derive from carmen (song), "a very good Covert for their Ignorance as well as their Knavery", and thus to have been medicines which operated by a sung incantation: "more particularly termed carminative, as if they cured by Inchantment." Quincy finds this inappropriate, explaining the functions of such medicines in terms of the mechanical characteristics which allow them to expel flatulent material from the body.

Other strategies for structuring lemmas include incorporating some terms into the sentence as new lemmas, as under the entries *præcipitantia–precipitation* joined by "these are what cause", as also happens between *rare–rarefaction, stamen–staminous flower*, etc. These are also links between Latin or Greek terms and their English glosses in many cases, where the sentence and the lemma divisions overlap. The sequence *ptylaism–ptyalon–ptysma–ptysmagogue* represents simply a list linked by 'and' within a single sentence, the last two items being linked to the underlying derivation: "are all from".

An important point about Quincy's criticisms is that they are generally confined to language. Even where discussing processes and ingredients based on alchemy, he does not necessarily debunk the processes themselves, merely the use of obscurantist language. Robert Boyle made similar criticisms, although making an exception of the language used to describe the most arcane processes (Debus 2001: 83). While indulging in what looks like blanket denunciation of alchemy (as above), his own profession and his recipes accept alchemical notions like reiterated procedures to obtain increasing degrees of refinement in the end product.

Quincy is clear in other works as well on the need for an uncomplicated approach and simplicity in language, objectives which characterise all his publications:

> when an unprejudiced Person is resolved to venture of himself, upon the strength only of those Capacities his Maker has thought fit to bestow upon him, and pursues his Enquiries with that Simplicity, and upon such Evidences as the Nature of his Subject will admit of, so far as he[sic] advances will be attended with Plainness and Conviction, and be as easily made appear to any other Person of tolerable Sense, as to the common Stagers of that Subject. (Santorio 1712: iv)

He is also aware of the shortcomings of previous translations, picking up especially on the retention of Latin terms:

> These Aphorisms have formerly appeared in English under the Title of Rules of Health; but the Translator has retained so many Terms and Latin Phrases, that the Original I should think as easy to an Englishman as the other (Santorio 1712: 4)

Quincy also finds Santorio's explanations of medical phenomena ("Systematical Helps", (4)) obscure. He explains his own methods thus:

> I have translated them [the Aphorisms] as close as I am able, I mean as to the Author's Sense, and taken as much care as possible therein not to transplant any hard physical Terms; and where that could not be avoided, I have been particularly careful to make them intelligible in the Explanations. (Santorio 1712 Preface: 5)

There is a consistent stress throughout this preface on what a reasonable intelligence will be able to comprehend, and a particular insistence on the claim that the human body and the ways of coping with various ailments is within the grasp of the common man. Just as Santorio has in his view cleared away much of the medical obfuscation, so Quincy hopes to breach the language barriers (Santorio 1712 Preface: vi).

7.9 Quincy's legacy

It may be of interest to consider the way in which later works have made use of Quincy, since doing so should reveal something about both him and the later work at the same time. I do not intend to embark on an exercise in dictionary archaeology here. Tracing the descent of Quincy's entries through the multifarious dictionaries, pharmacopœias, dispensatories, materia medica and other medical works through the eighteenth century would be very time-consuming, and may not in any case reveal all that much. One might expect, in the course of nearly a century, that quite a lot would change. Language conventions, spelling, and punctuation will have changed in some respects, while grammatical structures, always in some degree of flux, might also change. The content might also alter to reflect more recent findings, especially given the large increase in the number of specialist medical treatises and the increasingly sophisticated research they report as the eighteenth century proceeds. We must also assume that the objectives of an encyclopaedia, however overarching, cannot be the same as those for a medical dictionary, so that one might expect highly specific medical information to be omitted. Note that equivalence between dictionaries in these comparisons may be elusive, since practices vary as to spelling, endings, relevance or not of doubled letters; likewise i/y, i/j and u/v, and through alphabetisation of binomials or not. All this makes perfectly reliable comparison more difficult. Hence one encounters such variations as *malva viscum/malva viscus/malvaviscum* (marshmallows), etc. Not to mention incomplete and inconsistent accounting for polysemy and homonymy.

The sincerest form of recognition in the eighteenth century was use of an author's material, whether acknowledged or not. A complete account of this for John Quincy is beyond the scope of this volume, but some idea of how he was used may be gained from a brief selection of those indebted to him. Ephraim Chambers (1728) acknowledges Quincy in a number of entries, including *ague, alkermes, antimonials, bile, caustics, dispensary, elixir, erysipelas, hellebore, hiera picra, hydragogues, hypocistis, hystericks, lotion, malt, palsy, pharmacopoeia, purgative, rhaponticum, rheumatism, ructation, salivation, saxifrage, sperma-ceti, teeth, temperament,* and *testaceous.* Under *temperament* he is called a "Mechanical writer" who rejects most of Galen; a good deal of Chambers' entry for *fibre,* including the figures, is *verbatim* from Quincy but with no acknowledgement. The 1778–1788 edition of Chambers also mentions Quincy under *amber, aqua aluminosa bateana, camphor, emetic tartar, fever, fibres, lentigo, mechanical, methodists,* and *nervous,* most of the original acknowledgements having been retained. Chambers does not indicate whether his references are to the lexicon or other works, except under *dispensary* [sic], where he explicitly mentions Quincy's *Dispensatory.*

Adverting now to the early nineteenth century, comparing early editions of Quincy with the entries which appear in the *Encyclopædia Londinensis* (1810–1829) edited by John Wilkes (hereafter EL) reveals a number of pertinent considerations, both in terms of language and content. The EL set grandiose objectives for itself, not the least of which was to be a kind of universal lexicon, incorporating all words from all dictionaries into its pages: "all the words and substance of every kind of dictionary extant in the English language" (tp.). This ambition also represented "the most powerful encyclopaedic vision: a work containing the collective knowledge of a community which might be put together again if all other books were lost," as Yeo puts it (2001: 3) in relation to Diderot's aims half a century earlier.

I have chosen several entries for examination among the 73 identified which are derived from and actually mention Quincy. Several general points are immediately obvious. Spelling conventions have changed in that the capitalisation of nouns has disappeared from the EL, and the use of the apostrophised past participle ending '-'d' has also disappeared. Some adjectival endings in '-ick' are now '-ic'. Some miscellaneous changes include Quincy's "Wall-Nut Tree" becoming "walnut-tree" in EL. These are changes which may with equal confidence be ascribed either to the author/compiler or the printing house. The first of the entries for consideration is *cooler.*

First of all, the head-word is in the plural in *Lexicon physico-medicum,* but the singular in EL, in accordance with the tendency of the earlier medical dictionaries to use the plurals of count nouns for the head-word. The opening of the *cooler* entry is more dictionary-like in EL ("That which has the power of cooling the body"), and more encyclopaedia-like in the *Lexicon physico-medicum* ("These may be consider'd under these two Divisions"), which perhaps suggests that Wilkes or his editor/co-writer saw the entry as another of the comprehensive word-list promised on the title-page. However, the two entries fall together shortly after, and are verbatim, excepting the orthographical changes already mentioned and minor changes to the numbering conventions, until "all substances producing Viscidity", at which point the EL cites Quincy, but not the work from which this comes, the *Lexicon physico-medicum*.[119] That work goes on at this point to offer some practical advice to practitioners that both kinds of coolers "may be used by a knowing Physician to answer many good Inventions in Medicine; and both do a great deal of Mischief in the hands of the ignorant." This comment is hardly the kind of thing which is needed in an encyclopaedia aiming at even a comprehensive generality in scope, although it would be instructive to know whether the encyclopaedist omitted it simply for this reason, or more specifically knowing that it had become outdated or irrelevant advice. The EL at this bifurcation takes another direction, offering a dictionary-like second sense of the word "A vessel in which any thing is made cool".

Under *corymbiferous*, we encounter another strategy of change. The entry is basically the same as in *Lexicon physico-medicum*, but the lists of flowers in Quincy are all in Latin, and these are all translated into English in EL. A few have also been removed. Thus the shared part

> Corymbiferous Plants, which are distinguish'd into such as have a radiate Flower, as the Flos Solis, Calendula, &c. and such as have a naked Flower, as the Abrotonum fæmini, Eupatorium, Artemisia; to which are added the Corymbiferis Affines, or those a-kin hereunto, such as Scabious, Dipsacus, Carduus, and the like (*Lexicon physico-medicum*)

appears as

> Corymbiferous plants are distinguished into such as have a radiate flower, as the sun-flower; and such as have a naked flower, as the hemp-agrimony, and mug-wort: to which are added those a-kin hereunto, such as scabious, teasel, thistle, and the like. Quincy. (EL)

As in other entries, a lexical definition has also been added at the beginning.

In assessing these two entries, the conventional modern scholarly ploy would simply be to accuse the EL of plagiarism, but we see that there has also been a strategic omission, as well as a re-constructed opening involving the addition of a lexical definition, and a second lexical definition added at the close of the entry. The 'plagiarism', while absolutely blatant in itself, is only a part of a more complex entry. Added to the orthographical changes, this makes the process which has produced the EL entry, whether directly from *Lexicon physico-medicum* or indirectly mediated through other works, a multi-layered conceptual restructuring. Similar considerations apply

---

119 I have cited the second edition here.

in turn to Quincy's entry, which is clearly a paraphrase of that in Harris's *Lexicon technicum* of 1704

7.10 Quincy and Johnson's dictionary

The largest body of head-word citations of Quincy is in Johnson's dictionary (1755), however, there being 292 in all. All but fourteen of these appear in the first edition.[120] Although Johnson was prepared to work with James on his *Medicinal dictionary*, Quincy's is the one he leans heavily on for medical terms and their definitions (see Wiltshire 1991: 106–107). Some of the many definitions used are acknowledged, but others, such as *adenograph*, which is cited verbatim, are not. Sometimes the head-word is used, but the definition has been rewritten; Johnson obviously had little use (or space) for lengthy encyclopaedic entries, although there are some exceptions, especially among the plant names from Philip Miller. Others, like *plethora*, are quoted verbatim, and still others, including *acousticks*, are almost so. In *alcahest*, Johnson deletes Quincy's editorial comment that it is "a ridiculous notion long since exploded". Johnson quotes Quincy partially in some cases, such as *alteratives*, and in some cases changes the head-word, usually replacing Latin or Greek by English, as with *cuticula* (recorded as *cuticle*), *extensores* (recorded as *extensors*) or *hemicrania* (recorded as *hemicrany*), or by changing the morphology, as in *efflorescence* (recorded as *efflorescency*). Another striking feature is that Johnson is often led to insert an adjective but not the corresponding noun, possibly for reasons of perceived non-Englishness, as with *cichoraceous*, but not *cicoreum*, *crural* but not *crura*, *diaphoretick* but not *diaphoresis*, *papaverous* but not *papaver*, *pappous* but not *pappus* (Quincy 1719b), *umbilical* but not *umbilicus*, and so on. Finally, there are virtually no plant names from Quincy which, along with the fourteen terms not found in Quincy's first edition, suggests that Johnson used a later edition, since the second edition of Quincy in 1722 expunged almost all plant names, for which Johnson overwhelmingly uses Miller.

7.11 Conclusion

It does appear that in many respects Quincy and his work remained on the margins, being a dissenter with a somewhat unconventional approach to his subject and his profession and not really prepared to compromise on what he saw either as common sense or principle; noted in passing by some, with admiration and respect by a few, and occasionally reviled. In the end, however, he was a man amply justified by the

---

120 Johnson was manually checked for acknowledgements of Quincy.

course of subsequent history, whose major works influenced medical lexicography as well as practice for over a century. We will see that, despite the sheer gravitas of Robert James's dictionary, it had far less influence.

It is hard to avoid the conclusion that Quincy is very consciously taking a bold step forward with this dictionary. He has a modernising agenda which is adumbrated in the preface and implemented throughout the text; indeed it was pursued with increased vigour in the second edition. He silently accepts the need to use the vernacular where possible, despite this not being consistently followed through; in this respect he is the inheritor of Andrew Boorde and Nicholas Culpeper. He is also critical of those who retain outdated and obsolete terminology. The diagrams included in the dictionary are intended to enhance comprehension of the principles being explained. Quincy also shows the interest in language and the niceties of meaning and semantics that one would expect of a genuine lexicographer. Quincy saw mechanical principles as potentially explaining the structure, power, and articulation of bones, ligaments, muscles, and arteries, and the flow and regulation of bodily fluids. Unlike many dictionaries, this one makes a genuine attempt to put its declared principles into practice, instantiating Quincy's claim that *mechanical* is 'a Term much of late introduced into Physicks and Medicine, to express a way of Reasoning conformable to that which is used in the Contrivance, and accounting for the Properties and Operation, of any Machine' (1719b: s.v. *mechanical*).

8 Aids to memory: Surgical dictionaries

The eighteenth century saw the publication of many surgical works, but only two dictionaries dedicated to surgery, as well as a significant glossary. Despite the fact that surgical works came off the presses by 1700 at a rate of at least one a year, no English surgical dictionary designated as such had been published in the seventeenth century. A work by the German surgeon Johannes Scultetus (1595-1645) was translated into English as *The chyrurgeons store-house* and appeared in 1674. The multiple glossary by Randle Holme had also contained surgical terms. Both these works were rich with surgical terminology, and were profusely illustrated as well.

8.1 *Prosodia chirurgica* (1729)

The first dictionary proper, by an anonymous author, was *Prosodia chirurgica* (1729), which contains 1230 head-words, and is perhaps the most purely lexical of the dictionaries surveyed in this book. The sub-title of the work indicates the extent to which this is a linguistic exercise, rather than simply a list of the realia of surgery, since it announces that a definition of each term will be given, as well as a guide to their pronunciation and quantity. Marks over each relevant syllable are provided. The title particularly suggests that a large part of this work concerns the syllabification/accent (prosodia) of the surgical lexicon. This also suggests that the compiler has given close consideration to the needs of students, his target audience. In this respect, the work is pointedly envisaged as not intended for trained professionals; indeed they might have little to learn as the dictionary contains no encyclopaedic content. It is essentially an aid to memory for the terms alone. The notion that the work is an artificial aid to memory relates it to the later surgical dictionary by Benjamin Lara, who explains that this was the origin of his own work.

The unsigned dedication to the *Prosodia*, which begins by acknowledging help received, is to the well-regarded surgeon John Shipton (1680–1748; see Power 2004) who, the author claims, had a hand in correcting the text. The preface is a document of special interest. Allusion is first made to the multitude of already-existing dictionaries, but this is not strictly accurate—medical dictionaries, perhaps, but certainly not surgical dictionaries. The author goes on to explain his intentions surprisingly clearly for the age and in some detail. The work is to be circumscribed by these criteria: all words used only by one author will be omitted, as will those words only used by a few authors. All obsolete words will likewise be rejected. The compiler undertakes both to avoid "pompous Definitions" and to eschew conjectural definitions, of which there are too many already. No 'physical' (that is, medical) terms with no relation to surgery are to be allowed. Furthermore, descriptions of body parts, medicines, qualities of medicines, or instruments not relevant to the etymology of a lemma being defined

https://doi.org/10.1515/9783110639186-008

will be omitted. This is a remarkably succinct account of the kind of lemma to be excluded from this work. Finally, it is intended to be a volume designed for the convenience and pocket (in both senses) of the student, an "assistant" as the title page declares. The author then claims with some justice that "in every one of these Articles, it differs from most of the Dictionaries in use among us" (vi), at which point he proceeds to explain this in terms of both the characteristics and defects of earlier works. While we expect authors to compare their predecessors unfavourably with their own publication, this one amounts to a brief survey of the dictionaries previously published, which is unusual:

> For instance, Gorræus's Definition. Medic. is a large Book, expensive to the Buyer, and though a Book in Esteem, of no Use to an English Reader; Castellus is subject to some of the foregoing Objections, besides, that you are forc'd to take up frequently with the Physical Sense of a Word, when you are hunting for an Etymology. Blancard I must own I have a stronger Objection to; who so often takes an Etymology upon trust, that it almost looks like a thorough Inacquaintance with the Language he deals in: the Version of him is every way more Defective. Dr. Quincy, I own, has bid fair for an useful Book; but one may trace Blancard throughout him, so much as to shew his Complaisance has made him copy even his grossest Absurdities. Another, in which it differs from all, is, in settling the Pronunciation of every Word, in regard to Quantity, by proper Marks over every Syllable that is subject to any alteration, and this is the chief Consideration that induced me to take this Trouble upon me (vi–vii)

The absence of any firm evidence renders it difficult resolve the question of the authorship of the *Prosodia*. The work has been ascribed to Benedict Duddell (c.1695–1759x67), the surgeon and pioneering oculist.[121] Wyman discusses the attribution to Duddell in his 1992 article, which apparently arose with Albrecht von Haller's *Bibliotheca chirurgica*, published in 1775 but, without offering any further explanation, Wyman suggests that the style is not Duddell's. Albrecht von Haller's attribution to Duddell has the dual advantages of being nearly contemporary and the fact that Duddell's continental reputation was greater than that in England. Wyman's claim that the style of the *Prosodia* is not that same as Duddell's other texts may merely confirm that style in a dictionary, especially one with many very short entries, is likely to be very different from fully articulated running text (Wyman 1992: 414), as in encyclopaedic entries.

Another possible means of investigating this question is to see what and how many entries there are to do with the eyes and their diseases, especially in relation to comparable dictionaries. In doing this, we are forced to look at Lara's later surgical dictionary, despite their obvious differences. The *Prosodia* has eighty-three entries for the eyes, whereas Lara has only twenty-three, seven of which are not in the *Prosodia*. One might thus think that there is a preponderance of eye entries in the *Prosodia*,

---

121 See Wyman (1992: 414, 2004), who does not make this attribution, however, for Duddell's life. ESTC does not make this attribution either.

but it is not quite that simple, as this has to be taken in the context of the *Prosodia* having far more entries, despite being a lot shorter than Lara's text. The *Prosodia* contains 1228 main entries, while Lara has only 151, that is, a mere 12.2 percent of the figure for the *Prosodia*. The figures for the percentage of eye entries for each dictionary are thus *Prosodia* 6.8 percent and Lara 15.2 percent, but Lara's absolute figures for entries are so low that this may well be misleading. A further consideration is that Lara's long entries contain many other terms which are not given lemma status, and the *Prosodia* has less in its much shorter entries. On the whole, the large number of eye entries in the *Prosodia* suggests but certainly does not prove Duddell's authorship.

A second edition was issued in 1732, selling for the modest sum of two shillings. The declared target market for this work changed somewhat between the two editions. The title-page now suggests that it is intended not only for students, but as "a memoria technica, calculated for the use of old practitioners", and those already established as well, but the question remains whether this is simply a publisher's puff rather than a genuine description of the contents. Although the title-page has been altered and augmented, the dedication has not; in fact, the whole of the second edition contains the same sheets as the first, suggesting that copies remained unsold and that the publishers were anxious to move them. The allusion to the book's use for young students (Preface: vi) has not been altered to accommodate experienced practitioners and match the claim on the title-page, confirming that these are the original sheets re-packaged. Finally, there are none of the minor compositorial changes throughout the text, intended or unintended, which one would expect in a reset text.

8.2 The surgical glossary by J[ohn] S[parrow] (1739)

A translation of the surgical work of Henri-François Le Dran (1685–1770), *Observations in surgery*, appeared in 1739, thought to have been translated by John Sparrow, also contains what is called a dictionary, but is in fact a glossary running from to pages 402–443, entitled "A general chirurgical dictionary."[122] This extensive surgical dictionary might have been dealt with in the chapter on glossaries but, given its scope, seems better placed here, and examined in relation to other immediately preceding dictionaries. It is glossary-like in being lexicographically simple, merely headword and either gloss or definition, entirely without linguistic data. On the whole, there are more definitions than glosses. Occasionally there is both gloss and definition, albeit elementary, as in "*Chorea Sancti Viti*, A Species of Madness call'd St.

---

122 Sparrow does not appear in ODNB. He published a dissertation on lues venerea in 1731. His full name and profession are noted in various booksellers' catalogues and other near-contemporary bibliographical notices and advertisements.

Vitus's Dance," The major source of this work is apparently the *Prosodia chirurgica*, although with a considerable number of omissions. Not all entries are verbatim, there being a number which are paraphrased. Where definitions in the *Prosodia* are longer, only the first part is used.

Between these two dictionaries, there are 1679 head-words, 911 being shared. This sharing suggests a dependent relation between them, especially given that the sharing relation between other such dictionaries and glossaries is so much lower, as we will see. The relation between Sparrow's work and Duddell's entries is that Sparrow's are usually cut-down versions which take only the definitional part, remove etymologies and trim away any extra explanatory text from Duddell, as in *cornua uteri*, *modiolus*, and *nephritis*. This material is most often verbatim, as with *acceleratores*, defined in both as "Muscles so call'd from their Use", but Sparrow deletes the remaining "which is from accelerare, to hasten the Urine."[123] A lengthy example is *pampiniforme corpus*. Duddell's entries with no derivation are often rendered complete and verbatim, as with *mons veneris*, *respiratio* and *salivales ductus* or simply with the deletion of an example, as in *organica pars*.

A few other illustrations of the relationship will have to suffice. At other times the entry is not quite verbatim, as in *nodosus* and *nyctalopia*. Sometimes Sparrow deviates entirely, as under *acores* (achores) which he defines simply by way of the gloss "A Scald-Head", while Duddell has "Ulcers of the Head, running from a small Orifice ..." after which a longish explanation follows. Under *coxendix*, Sparrow cross-refers to the alternative head-word *coxæ os*, a term not in Duddell. Under *cuticula*, defined by Duddell as

> The Scarf-Skin; a Diminutive of
> Cutis, the Skin

his text runs on to create a separate head-word for *cutis*. Sparrow makes this a single entry.

Further editing is applied to Duddell's *gastrocemion* "the Calf of the Leg", which Sparrow alters somewhat in meaning, rendering it as the plural *gastrocnemii* "The Muscles of the Calf of the Leg." Sparrow and Duddell offer completely different meanings for *meconium* ("Juice of Poppeys" in Duddell as against "The Excrements of the Fœtus after the Delivery" in Sparrow), and the connexion between their definitions of *meliceris* is present, but loose. Sparrow is medically correct about *meconium*, and Duddell linguistically so. There is disagreement as to the meaning of *sarcoepiploocele*, Duddell describing it as a 'tumour' and Sparrow as a 'rupture'. Sparrow will sometimes add an extra gloss, as in *necrosis*, glossed by Duddell as 'mortification', to which Sparrow adds "Deadness of Parts'"; under *omocotyle*, he adds that it is the

---

123 'Verbatim' in this section ignores minor punctuation changes.

socket of the scapula. *Scaleni* is augmented in Sparrow, who has "A Pair of Muscles which extend the Neck' where Duddell has only 'A Pair of Muscles of the Neck" followed by an allusion to their shape. Summing up, the great majority of Sparrow's shared entries are verbatim or near verbatim excerpts of Duddell, but he also exhibits a willingness to deviate, delete or add to what he finds, deletion being the most usual. Some deletions however remove potentially useful information. The deletion of derivations is consistent throughout.

The source of the remainder of Sparrow's entries is another matter. One would expect to find many of them in Blancard, Quincy, or perhaps Harris. Establishing relations between dictionaries is not always easy, especially when multiple potential sources are available. One or two-word glosses appearing in each are certainly not indicative, since they usually represent what is obvious and likely to be repeated in any such dictionary. There is little to suggest that Sparrow used Quincy, although an indication of the fact that he was copying from some source and less concerned with completeness is that he cross-references *suprascapularis*, which head-word he omits to include. Quincy makes the same cross-reference and has the corresponding head-word. Among those terms in Sparrow but not in Duddell, only about twenty appear to have any relation to what appears in Quincy, and only one (*pectinis os*) is verbatim; there is little here that cannot be explained by what is common to familiar glosses or simply by an antecedent lexicon at one or two removes.

The relation between the remaining Sparrow entries and Blancard is certainly closer than that with Quincy, although only eleven were verbatim, leaving aside a number which were simply verbatim cross-references.[124] This entry seems typical of the putative Sparrow-Blancard relation:

Coctio, Concoction or Digestion, is the Fermentation of the smallest Particles which our Nourishment consists of ... (Blancard)
Coctio. A Fermentation in the smallest Particles of the Aliments (Sparrow)

The same consideration applies to *critica signa* and many others. Many definitions in Sparrow not found in Duddell, such as *corone*, are short verbatim excerpts from Blancard. While there are agreements between Blancard and Sparrow, there are also glaring disagreements in some definitions. Sparrow defines *lipodermus* as "One that has lost his Fore Skin", but Blancard declares that it means "A Disease of the Skin, covering the Glans of the Yard, so that it cannot be drawn back", which we would now call phimosis.[125] *Soleus musculus* is another conflict, on which Sparrow is incorrect,

---

124 A separate study of cross-references both within and between these dictionaries seems justified, although it lies beyond the level of detail possible in a survey work like the present one. This study has not been extended to cover Harris either.
125 Blancard defines *phimosis* as being the same as *paraphimosis*, the condition of the foreskin being too short to cover the glans.

calling it a muscle of the sole of the foot, not the calf. An obvious error in Sparrow is that *phlegmagoga* is described as a medicine purging choler, not phlegm, as in Blancard. Sparrow has "any preternatural Humour" for *phyma*, where 'tumour' was obviously intended, as in Blancard; perhaps this is a compositorial error. In short, it seems that Sparrow has used Blancard only sparingly, and it may still be that most of the correspondences could be explained by the use of an intermediary text such as Harris's *Lexicon technicum*.

8.3 Benjamin Lara's *A dictionary of surgery* (1796)

Benjamin Lara (1769–1848), who compiled *A dictionary of surgery* (1796), the second stand-alone surgical dictionary, is unrecorded in the ODNB, but a little about his activities can be recovered from the record. Lara seems to have taken an early interest in paediatrics and midwifery. *The Laws of the society for the relief of widows and orphans of medical men, in London, and its vicinity*, probably published in 1788, lists Benjamin Lara in Leadenhall St as one of its members (23), Lara's first published work, entitled An essay on the injurious custom of mothers not suckling their own children, 1791, was a little tract on breast-feeding, the title-page of which describes him as a surgeon, and as a "Member of the Corporation of Surgeons in London", as well as a "Practitioner in Midwifery". "This Essay is written in a familiar style, and totally free from technical phrases, and is well worthy the attention of the Ladies" is how Lara's publisher, James Ridgway, advertised this work at the end of Daniel Dancer's *Biographical curiosities* of 1797. Reuss mentions that this work had been translated into German and published in Leipzig in 1799 (1804 II: 6). The work was written in a plain style, the same claim being made by Lara in his introduction with the proviso that if technical terms must be used, they will be explained.

Ridgway was also the publisher of Lara's surgical dictionary, which followed in 1796 and was advertised repeatedly by the publisher. In a catalogue of his books, he added the following endorsement in about 1800: "Mr Pearson, of Golden-square, Head Surgeon of the Lock Hospital, has, in his public lectures, recommended to the attention of his numerous Pupils Mr. Lara's Dictionary" (4). Recognition for these two works came quite quickly, since David Rivers, the author of *Literary memoirs of living authors of Great Britain*, mentions Lara's two "useful performances" (1798 1: 355–356).

Lara's *A dictionary of surgery* is directed at students, and is described by its author as a pocket dictionary and a vademecum; hence the work is not explicitly located by its author within the circle of learning, nor as a substitute for or compendium of a competent professional library, but merely as a handy companion. Lara's stated readership is students, especially students and young surgeons working for the army or navy. Ridgway made less modest claims for it. The title-page mentions more of Lara's appointments : "Surgeon to the Royal Cumberland Freemason School, and Late Surgeon to the Portugueze Hospital", Stepney Green. The work is targeted at younger and less experienced surgeons, and was, Lara tells us, prepared in the first place simply as a compilation for his private use. Colleagues who saw the manuscript urged him to publish (v–vi), but, as we shall see in looking briefly at his sources, this may be somewhat ingenuous given the overwhelming reliance on Motherby. This process of writing word-lists and indexes to assist learning is also mentioned by the physician John Coakley Lettsom in a letter of 1791: "I never possessed genius; my memory was bad; I made dictionaries and tables of my own invention; to assist memory, I formed indexes of what I read, and by industry acquired something" (Thomson 1929: 3).[126] Lara probably found himself without an up-to-date and viable surgical dictionary since the only other stand-alone one produced in the eighteenth century was modest, and by this time was certainly inadequate, given the advances in the science. Dictionaries jog the memory of the practitioner, and writing them assists the memory of the learner.

Lara acknowledges his most obvious debt in his preface. "To Dr. Wallis's improved edition of Dr. Motherby's very excellent Medical Dictionary, I am indebted, for the arrangement I have adopted; as also, for many valuable facts; these are detailed nearly verbatim" (vi). This declaration probably understates the case. A later puff from Ridgway appended to Samuel Child's *Every man his own brewer* (1798) declares enthusiastically that the work "is compiled from the original Papers of some of the most eminent Surgeons of London and Paris, the best Authors extant, and the result of the Compiler's researches during a long and extensive line of practice" (30). We have to take Ridgway's word for this, as there is no corroboration from Lara himself. A reviewer in *The English review* of 1796 saw Lara's work as admirably compendious, praising the author for "collect[ing] particulars in as narrow a compass as possible" (27: 546–547), reducing them to a convenient and practicable form.

Lara's dictionary, with its lengthy entries and many sub-lemmas, reads rather like a medical common-place book, whereas the *Prosodia chirurgica* is essentially a word-list. Entries like *fractura hæmorrhoides* and *lithotomia* in Lara run for many pages, while the *Prosodia* does not contain an entry which extends to one column of the page. Lara's work is rich in text and poor in lemmas, so much so that the letter M has only a single entry, *mortificatio*, while the letter R has only two, *ranula* and *rectum intestinum*. In this elementary respect, the *Prosodia* and Lara's dictionary could not be less alike. *Prosodia chirurgica* has very short entries confined to definitions and derivations, hardly ever touching on medical concepts, procedures, cures, remedies, and so on, while Lara, following an even more restricted lexicon, is expansively

---

126 Another dictionary which began life as a similar set of notes is James Keir's *The first part of a dictionary of chemistry* (1789). As he writes in the preface: "I was much pleased with ... Mr. *Macquer's* Dictionary of Chemistry above all the books then existing in the science. I began to make extracts ... but I found they soon became so numerous, that, I thought, I could not take a better method of fixing in my mind a knowledge of chemistry than ... making a complete translation, and giving it to the public."

encyclopaedic, sometimes ignores derivations and definitions, and has far fewer head-words than the *Prosodia*. Lara's does indeed look like a fair copy of orderly working notes, while the *Prosodia* is an attempt to educate in the linguistic basics of the profession. The brevity of Lara's word-list is a striking indication of the incompleteness of the work, and the probability that he did not work consistently from a pre-existing word-list other than Motherby, identifying all the surgical terms. His prefatory comment that his readers may be those "who, perhaps, neither have the means not the opportunity of access to more elaborate and systematic works" (1796: vi), might well be the voice of experience given that he served on various ships himself.

Lara made extensive use of Wallis's editions of Motherby (1785, 1791), but there is little indication that he used the *Prosodia chirurgica*.[127] Despite the brevity of Lara's word-list, he has words not contained in the *Prosodia*, including *anaphrodisia*, *blepharoptosis*, *bursæ mucosæ*, *castratio*, and *cerebri compressio*, so the word-lists are apparently not interdependent. Lara also includes many relatively up-to-date notes on the entries, including comment on treatment, nomenclature, and so on, as in *bronchocele*, *hernia ventralis*, or *paronchyia*, additions which are quite frequent. Some errors appear in Lara, such as *achyls* for *achlys*, *carcuncula* for *caruncula*, and attention is not accorded to less official usages, as in *cataracta* "used only by the barbarous Writers" (*Prosodia chirurgica*); there is no mention of this in Lara, who quotes Cullen instead. Lara does not appear to mention barbarous usage at all.

While Lara relies heavily on Motherby, he does make judgements about what to include and what not, especially at the beginning of entries, so that one may legitimately discuss his own lexicographical practices as distinct from Motherby's. Lara frequently gives a number of synonyms, while sometimes omitting derivations, both these forms of information derived from Motherby. Examples of the derivations in Lara include *amblyopia*, where the discussion is largely taken up with synonyms such as *dysopia*, and the way in which nosologists and others have understood the term, as well as its various sub-species. Some of these are given Latin or Greek terms with their corresponding English terms, such as *myopia* "shortsightedness", and *nyctalopia*, "seeing only in the night". This entry is thus primarily concerned with classification and thus, indirectly, terminology. Lara offers no opinion as to which of these may be correct. The opinions of various authorities are usually at the centre of such discussions, a typical example being *psoas*, but not all of those in Motherby are reproduced, especially where the discussion concerns description of the disease.

Lara's entries characteristically define minimally, and sometimes, as in *pneumatocele*, have an extended discussion of the anatomical and surgical phenomena, which may generate quite a lot of additional terminology. Language questions,

---

127 For a discussion of Motherby in relation to James's *A medicinal dictionary*, including some detailed examples, see Lonati 2017: 78–88.

however, are very much secondary. Some other entries, such as *labia leporina*, spend very little time on the definition, and a great deal on the surgical procedures. One minor formatting change is that Lara uses small capitals for the head-words, whereas Motherby uses full capitals. The presentation of Lara's entries is inconsistent, those like *abscess* and *ulcer* each having a number of sub-entries, while *inflammation* treats its divisions as main entries. Consistency in this respect would reduce the number of entries under the letter I from nine to three.

The fact is, however, that comparison between Lara and the 1791 edition of Motherby by George Wallis reveals that Lara's compilation consists largely of the surgical entries from Motherby, lightly edited, if at all. There is occasional editing, such as a change of wording, the addition of authorities or of a recipe/treatment, cross-referencing, as under *ambusta*, where there is a reference to *sclopetoplaga*, or the deletion of Motherby's inter-textual references where they have become irrelevant. *Ambusto* has a considerable addition about treatments at the end, while *amputation* shows substantial additions and a few deletions. There is an occasional reference to Lara's own cases, as occurs under *anaphrodisia*, an entry which also adds a possible treatment. Other entries, such as *calculus*, are largely verbatim, but show that Lara can be picky about what he deletes. On the whole, he prefers to take over procedures and remedies verbatim, but will add to them here and there, and delete more general descriptive comment as he does under *carbunculus* and *cancer*; a large section on the types of cancer in Motherby is also omitted. Excisions are usually of paragraph size, which perhaps indicates the subject coherence of the Motherby entries, although there are instances where the excisions are only a sentence or so, an obvious example of this being *genu*. Initial sections are rather more likely to be omitted than others, a process which can leave entries with no definition at all and, in the case of *trepanatio*, repositions a warning about the limitations on the use of this procedure to cases of depressed fractures of the skull in a re-organised first paragraph. The first part of this entry is more heavily rewritten than most, describing the same procedures but not relying greatly on Motherby. There is also an added section on the use of the trepan and trephine at the end. By contrast, *pernio* begins with a newly-added definition where Motherby does not have one at all, returning to Motherby only in paragraph four. *Caries* also starts with a different source, not identified so far, and returns to Motherby after a few short paragraphs; the section deleted is descriptive and in this case partly concerned with definitions by various authorities. *Furunculus* and *gonorrhoea* are entries in which there are short deletions on treatment. *Trachoma* involves a different kind of change in adding a recipe for an ointment mentioned but not described in Motherby, and changing another medication in Motherby from the *London pharmacopœia* for a different one; presumably this is a conscious professional choice since this entry is otherwise verbatim. We turn now to a comparison of a few selected words between Lara and Motherby.

A comparison may be made between the entries in Lara and Motherby for *paracentesis*, consisting of slightly over two pages in Lara. The first change is that Lara omits a synonym from the lexical part "called also compunction", leaving only the Greek etymon and the gloss "to make a perforation." Lara appears to replace "integuments" by "teguments" in "This operation is commonly called TAPPING, and is used for discharging water through the teguments of the belly". This is unlikely to be merely a typographical error, since tegument (Latin *tegumentum*) is certainly attested in this period, including both a medical and botanical sense. The latter is not all that frequent, but neither was integument in the same sense. This may in fact be a shortening to save space. The OED entries for these words obscure the fact that integument is appreciably more frequent in medical and botanical use than tegument, but the frequency of both in all senses is about the same in the eighteenth century. Lara next makes a small editorial improvement in that "from the cavity thereof" becomes "from its cavity", which both saves a little space and makes the tone somewhat more familiar. After four lines, he suddenly leaves his source, at the point where Motherby introduces precise instructions for what is needed in this operation–Lara ignores most of this, switching now to the method of testing for the presence of fluid in the abdominal cavity by percussion and the use of one's fingers in Bell's *System of surgery* (II, 1783: 338).

Editorial change does not always serve increased clarity and brevity, however, as the symptom "by a difficult or laborious breathing" becomes "by the breathing being difficult and laborious"; similarly, "especially in a horizontal posture" is somewhat expanded to "especially when in an horizontal posture", which suggests that minor changes in space are immaterial, the savings in general probably being made through excising whole chunks. There is a change in preposition as the placement of the fingers is described as "in one side of the abdomen" becoming "on one side of the abdomen", and "a concurrence of these circumstances will always point out the real nature of the disorder" is somewhat shortened, becoming "a concurrence of these circumstances point out the real nature of the disorder". At this point in the entry, Bell is dropped, and is succeeded by "As soon as a fluctuation is distinctly felt, the operation may be performed. Perhaps if it was always recurred to at an early period, an effectual cure might frequently be obtained" is added, a remark which appears to be Lara's own. The following section of ten lines dealing with the dangers of the sudden release of fluid from the abdomen is a loose paraphrase of Bell. He next mentions a bandage invented by Dr Monro, information which is in Bell (1783: 383) and Milman (1786: 56), but is not quoted verbatim. This contains the same information but is not close enough textually even to be called a paraphrase. Lara gives a reference for the text and illustration provided by Bell, and most of the rest of the text closely paraphrases him. Lara has references to Bell's *Surgery*, White, and Sharp; Motherby to Le Dran and Heister as well.

The entry for *anaphrodisia* is verbatim down to the end of Motherby's first paragraph, except for minor changes in punctuation and italicisation which seem so trivial as possibly to be mistakes in copying. One, however may slightly change the meaning. Motherby has "where impediments occur to prevent the act, from piles, or some fault in the urethra", while Lara has "where the impediments occur to prevent the act from piles, or some fault in the urethra" the adverbial "from piles" now being restrictive.

The first significant change from Motherby occurs in

> when it arises from paralysis, such medicines as are necessary for the conquering that complaint must be had recourse to, particularly to eat stimulants. Sauvages gives us an account of a man being cured by immersing the penis often in the day in a strong decoction of mustard seed

Lara renders this as "when it arises from paralysis, such medicines as are necessary to subdue that complaint must be employed. Sauvages gives an account of a man being cured, by immersing the penis often in the day in a strong decoction of mustard seed." Three changes in all are involved here: "us" is deleted, "had recourse to" shortened to "employed" and the remark about stimulants is omitted. While the latter may represent a medical judgement, it also leaves the main clause bordering on tautology. At this point Lara abruptly breaks off from Motherby, mentions that he once had such a case, and gives a recipe for the liniment he used. Lara returns to Motherby immediately with "If it is occasioned by a simple gonorrhea" adding the "a" to Motherby, thus employing "gonorrhea" as a count noun, and changing its spelling. In the very last line, Motherby writes "such means must be used as the nature and particular circumstances of the case demand." Lara simplifies this somewhat to "such means must be used, as the nature and particular circumstances may demand."

8.4 Comparisons

In making meaningful comparisons, it is best to consider the surgical glossaries, including Traheron and Turner, as well as the stand-alone dictionaries. Comparing the word-lists of Traheron's translation of Vigo, the *Prosodia*, and J. S.'s Le Dran immediately reveals two important points: first, there is only very slight overlap between Traheron and the others, and lemmas shared between all three are rare, let alone definitions. Only nine terms are shared between Traheron and the *Prosodia* but not with J. S.–*clyster*, *diacodon*, *diagredium*, *diapomfilicos*, *euphorbium*, *focilia*, *infusion*, and *oximell*, and *vesicatorie*, while as few as six are shared between Traheron and J. S., but not Duddell–*diuretike*, *inflatio*, *inspiration*, *pessarie*, *pustles*, and *varices* (Traheron's forms used). Second, Traheron has an obvious tendency to prefer English forms as head-words. To take an example or two, *flebotomye* and *excrescences* in Traheron appear as *phlebotomia* and *excrescentia* in the *Prosodia*.

A comparison between the head-words of Traheron, Duddell, Turner, and Sparrow shows a very restricted range of words in common. Daniel Turner's surgical glossary was discussed in Ch. three. Those appearing in all four are, using Turner's spelling, *albuginea*, *apostema*, *cancer*, *cataplasma*, *cicatrix*, *collyrium*, *diaphoretica*, embrocation,[128] emunctorium (in English form only in Traheron), epilepsia, erysipelas, excrescence, fistula, fomentatio, fracture, gargarisma, mesenterium, phlebotomy, and phlegmon, This amounts to a mere 0.81 percent of the total, which does not suggest that there was a widely agreed surgical lexicon through this period. The comparable figure for the three eighteenth-century lists is much greater at 119, that is, 5.08 per cent.

Comparing the definitions shows that there is no obvious relation between them– diuretike, inflation, and oximell show the kind of similarity that would be expected in very brief entries while the rest show no relation at all. To illustrate, while Traheron predictably has "Inflation Puffed vp, swellyng", J. S has "A puffing-up". A further interesting point is that Traheron and the Prosodia disagree as to whether oximell is made of roses or poppies. Under infusion, Traheron mentions that the Latin form is an apothecaries' word, but J. S. makes no such distinction, merely offering infusion as a gloss for infusio.

Further work on the items shared between all four reveals some further distinctions which are worth noting. Cataplasm is glossed by Traheron as emplastrum, but by the later compilers as poultice. All four agree that a cicatrix is a scar and that epilepsy is the falling-sickness. Diaphoretica for Traheron has to do with the discussion (breaking up) of humours generally, while for the latter three it concerns sweating only, and gargarism means for him the act of gargling, while for the later three it is the liquid used for this purpose. Traheron does not gloss erysipelas as St. Anthony's fire as the others do, offering ony the Latin ignis persicus. Under collyrium there is disagreement between the basic gloss, being variously medicines, wash, remedy, and medicine. Traheron alone distinguishes between a wet collyrium (hydrocollurion) and a dry one (perocollurion).[129]

There is little or no connexion between Traheron and the eighteenth-century compilers leaving aside the obvious glosses. Between Sparrow and Duddell, however, there is considerable overlap and interdependence, which suggests that Duddell was a major source for Sparrow. Fistula will illustrate the point:

> Duddell: Fistŭla. Is any Pipe or oblong Cavity; but with us, signifies a hollow Ulcer in any Part, whose Sides are callous and hard.
> Sparrow: Fistŭla, Any Pipe or oblong Cavity.

This nicely illustrates Sparrow's usual editorial method, Sparrow supplying just enough for a working definition and retaining Duddell's diacritic in the head-word. Sparrow and Duddell fail to agree however under erysipelas and excresence, although

---

128 There is an argument for accepting embroche, the form found in Duddell, Sparrow and Traheron, as an independent lemma, but they share the same derivation and meaning, and so are accepted as the same here.
129 Neither of these terms occur in the OED.

excrescence lacks a definition in Duddell, leaving only the derivation.[130] They agree only loosely about *emunctorium* and *mesenterium*.

The significance of this rate of sharing is hard to assess. It is tempting to extract a surgical list from, say, Blancard or James for comparison and to establish the potential size of a surgical lexicon for this period, but not all will agree on which terms are properly surgical, and the surgical lists do not claim to be exhaustive and clearly contain some non-surgical terms. The increased percentage may at least indicate a more stable surgical lexicon by the first half of the eighteenth century. Lara's list, as we have seen, is so small that adding it to this comparison may not be revealing.

---

130 Duddell notes elsewhere (preface viii) that: "The Absence and Indisposition of the Author may possibly have occasion'd some few Mistakes; which the Reader is desired to excuse."

9 Robert James (1703–1776) and *A medicinal dictionary* (1742–1745)

In assessing the dictionary of Robert James, we need to ask how a physician in the eighteenth century might establish a professional position and a reputation. There were several means available—a professional qualification, patronage, publications, experience, a prestigious appointment, and a nostrum or two; requirements which were not necessarily sought in that order, and might prove of varying importance (see Cook 1986: 49–69). An Oxbridge degree was not essential and might be gained long after practice began; likewise a licence to practice. A Scottish or a foreign degree was not hard to obtain. An English degree could be gained by royal mandate, but only if one attracted the appropriate patronage,
[131] which might arise from the successful cure of an important patient, as in the case of Baldwin Hamey (Cook 1986: 53). Publication would bring the aspirant's name before the public, whether the work in question was strictly medical or not (Cook 1986: 53–54), and Robert James and John Quincy both followed this route—one already well worn by the likes of William Salmon, George Cheyne, and Richard Mead. As Mead put it:

> Should you have an itching to make your name known by writing a book on physic, yet so cus-
> tomary, I will advise you to choose the subject by which you think you will get most money; or
> that will bring you the most general business, as fevers, smallpox, etc. (cited in Cook 1986: 54)

One such publication might be a medical dictionary. Robert James certainly employed publications, including a massive medical dictionary, may have had patronage, and he found handy experience from an early date.

Experience could be gained from working with another physician, surgeon or apothecary, and further repute might accrue from the sale of one or more nostrums under the physician's name. James's best-known nostrum, Dr James's Fever Powder, became one of the most successful of the eighteenth century and well beyond. A considerable number of medical publications, including some by James, were little more than extended recommendations for the nostrums of their authors. Some digging into the circumstances under which James came by this money-spinner reveals something of the character of the man, as well as raising the further question of the extent to which the person of the medical lexicographer might be reflected in the dictionary itself. We have already seen that John Quincy's dictionary was driven by his own personal agenda both as an ambitious non-conformist Newtonian and as a practitioner.

---

131 On mandated and foreign degrees, see Cook 1986: 213.

https://doi.org/10.1515/9783110639186-009

9.1 Life and works: The dictionary context

Not a great deal is known about James's personal life, and some of this comes through his long friendship with Dr Samuel Johnson, who contributed to the proposals for the *Medicinal dictionary*, and provided a dedication for the dictionary itself. There is at least an image, since an eighteenth-century engraving reproduced in Warbasse 1907, shows the laureated image of James surmounting the three volumes of his *Medicinal dictionary*, and the caduceus, the symbol of his profession.[132] There is more to know about James, but that will have to wait for a separate monograph. He published a number of other works, several of which were apparently intended for the dictionary, and he collaborated with the canny publisher John Newbery in marketing his famous nostrum.[133]

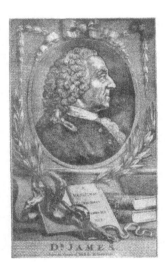

Fig. 5: Dr Robert James

Wiltshire also claims that Johnson began to collaborate with James on the dictionary in 1743, the articles with the publisher having been contracted several years before.[134] Perhaps all that Johnson contributed was the dedication and the life of Boerhaave.

---

132 Available at the Wellcome Library, London: Robert James. Line engraving by W. Walker, 1778, after Peter Scheemakers (1691–1781), the Flemish sculptor who moved to London in 1716. Collection: Iconographic Collections Library reference no.: ICV No 3239. Scheemaker's bust of Richard Mead, among other works by him, is in Westminster Abbey.
133 See Corley 2004, Timbs 1876: 114–115; for Newbery, see Maxted 2004, Welsh 1885.
134 But note that the fascicles of the dictionary had begun to appear in February 1742, as Wiltshire correctly points out (1991: 74).

James paid Johnson for the dedication, a model of brevity which stands in stark contrast to the prolixity of the dictionary itself, and his other contributions seem to have been minimal at best. James also had other paid assistants, as we shall see.[135]

Wiltshire's assertion that the dictionary proposal's intention of "cutting a swathe through the jungle of early eighteenth-century medical folklore and the various received knowledges of classical and medieval medicine" (Wiltshire 1991: 5–6) is overstated, and ignores earlier trends. Since Quincy had already undertaken this in his various works, James is merely recycling a familiar aim; at the same time, the dictionary itself achieved no such thing, simply imparking the jungle rather than re-designing it. Finally, the assertion that James was one of the leading physicians of this time (Wiltshire 1991: 65) may be true, but his reputation is compromised somewhat by what we know of his life from sources beyond the Johnson circle. It would be hardly less justified to claim that Johnson was taken in, as were many others, by one of the leading medical fraudsters of his day, who bought Johnson's skills to serve his own ambitions. As Johnson, reflecting on the public under- and over-appreciation of physicians, quipped in the life of Mark Akenside "a very curious book might be written on the Fortune of Physicians" (2006: IV: 173 and note on 472).

Samuel Johnson's early relations with James were obviously very good; he recalls, through Boswell, the many pleasant hours spent at the home of Gilbert Walmsley, convivial events remembered warmly by Johnson in later years: "At this man's table I enjoyed many chearful and instructive hours, with companions such as are not often found" such as "one who has gladdened life", David Garrick, and the company of "one who has lengthened … life … Dr. James, whose skill in physick will be long remembered" (Johnson 2006 II: 179).[136] If later scholars overlook or scant one of this threesome, it is inevitably James. Turberville, for instance, devotes only a paragraph of his two-volume work on Johnson's England to James (1933 II: 27). Johnson expressed his respect for James's abilities more than once, as Boswell reports: "Johnson now had an opportunity of obliging his schoolfellow Dr. James, of whom he once observed, 'no man brings more mind to his profession' " (Boswell 1791/1953: 1743; 116).[137] Johnson also pays James the considerable compliment of claiming that he taught him about medicine. "My knowledge of physick, (he added,) I learnt from Dr. James, whom I helped in writing the proposals for his Dictionary, and also a little in the Dictionary itself" (Boswell, James (1791/1953: 733; Friday April 5, 1776). That they were close to begin with is also clear from Johnson's later remark to Hester Thrale that James knew his earlier life very well. The summation offered by Boswell concerning

---

135 Benjamin Martin also mentions having an amanuensis in compiling his *Lingua Britannica reformata* (1749), but whether this assistant was paid or not is unknown (Preface: viii).
136 Walmsley, who lived in the Bishop's Palace, was Registrar of the Ecclesiastical Court of Lichfield Cathedral.
137 See also Waingrow's edition of Boswell, 1994, vol. I, 116, fn. 6.

the publication of James's dictionary and Johnson's involvement with it is broadly verifiable, apart from the claim about the 'several' articles, which has been called into question more recently:

> James published this year his Medicinal Dictionary, in three volumes folio. Johnson, as I understood from him, had written, or assisted in writing, the proposals for this work; and being very fond of the study of physick, in which James was his master, he furnished some of the articles. He, however, certainly wrote for it the Dedication to Dr. Mead, which is conceived with great address, to conciliate the patronage of that very eminent man. (Boswell 1791/1953: 116; 1743)

James moved to London in September 1740 (Anon. 1754?: 8), and was receiving Johnson's assistance with the proposals and perhaps other parts of the dictionary about 1740–1741, suggesting that they were still close.

James published quite a lot apart from the dictionary, a flurry of works coming off the presses in the 1740s, the period at which he is claimed to have worked as a publisher's hack. Much of this seems, however, to have been originally intended for the dictionary or to have arisen as a result of his work on it. His method is characteristically to stitch together the work of others, sometimes in translation, and sometimes epitomised or reworked, and to provide a new or revamped contextual framework for the whole rather than to rewrite texts extensively. He reuses his own material on occasions; sometimes that of others. In short, his method is that of a typical eighteenth-century encyclopaedist or even a lexicographer. In *The modern practice of physic*, he is largely a translator, and to some extent a re-arranger, but in general the extent to which he is an original translator remains rather obscure. We do at least know that he was trained in the classics, and had learnt French and Italian as well. Before we rush to judge James as a plagiarist, or at least as excessively derivative, however, we ought to recall that he was rather conservative in outlook, his profession was by nature conservative, and a proper respect for the authority of previous writers was accepted practice in medical writings, as indeed in dictionaries. The re-use of material in other publications should be seen in a different light, as it was in early modern dictionaries, and the methods exhibited here are probably a fair indication of what he did in the *Medicinal dictionary*.

Further works by James included an introduction to Thomas Moffett's *Health's improvement* (James 1746b), much of which was transferred from the dictionary, sometimes with minor deletions and simplifications. These changes include some mentions of authorities, Latin and Hebrew names, and cross-references to other dictionary entries. The entry for *alcali* provides a considerable chunk, from pages 28–62, pretty much verbatim. James or Osborne, his publisher, or both seem to have been anxious to re-use whatever they could of the dictionary entries.

A rather different publishing venture was the *Pharmacopoeia universalis* of 1747. Two passages are of particular interest:

> In the whole Course of the Work, I have industriously suffer'd the Names of Bate, Fuller, Quincy, and even Salmon, with the rest of the Dispensatory Writers of our Country, to rest in Peace; neither disturbing them by Censure, nor perfuming them with Incense; because I apprehend that meer Books of Prescriptions are of too little Importance to be taken Notice of, much less to be transcrib'd (Preface: vii)

In claiming that he will not acknowledge such compilers because he will not apportion praise or blame, James takes a somewhat novel approach. At the same time, the claim that such books are of little inherent value confirms the attitude that Quincy had complained about, and that Peter Shaw had expressly criticised in his introduction to Quincy's *Praelectiones pharmaceuticæ* of 1723, arguing that a physician without any knowledge of pharmacy was no physician at all (Quincy 1723: xiv). James's view also patently runs against the fact that he himself had compiled one and knew quite a lot about pharmacy himself, and that such works had been endlessly revised and reprinted since the mid-seventeenth century, obviously in response to a genuine need. His dictionary proposal had also made a point of including cures and remedies.

Employing the word "transcribe" in relation to these "meer Books of Prescriptions" also raises some questions. Did James actually transcribe parts of such works himself? Does he mean by this what we might now mean by plagiarise? These matters are discussed in more detail below.

The second excerpt concerns his index:

> In a Book not intended so much to be regularly perus'd, as occasionally consulted, an Index should seem to be absolutely necessary; I have, therefore, procur'd one, which appears to be more extensive and useful, than any that have occur'd to me in Books of this Kind. As it consists of near ten thousand plain References, the Reader will without Difficulty turn to whatever Subject he pleases. (vii)

Aside from their obvious benefit as a ready reference, alphabetical indexes are potential sources of dictionary word-lists, and James could have worked on both this index and his dictionary simultaneously. The meaning of "procur'd" suggests that it was a printing-house job by another indexer, or perhaps that James employed someone privately to do it. The dictionary and the pharmacopœia are four years apart, however. The familiar modern sense seems most likely here, but the sense of bring about or arrange, especially doing so with care, is also a possible reading. Too little has been done thus far on the possible relation between indexes and dictionary word-lists.

The index, which is quite as extensive as the preface claims, gives the Latin words in italics and the English in Roman. Latin head-words in the text are glossed, but not in the index, with a few rare exceptions. Where a succeeding head-word in the text is a binomial, such as "Bolus ... Bolus armena", or "Tamariscus ... Tamariscus germanica", only the first of these is listed in the index, the species being omitted.

A lexicographical point which is particularly germane to the present study is that the head-words in the various sections are in Latin, followed in book three on simples by the synonymy and the English gloss. As James declares (preface: vi), the corresponding English is also to be found in the index. *Bolus* appears in the index as *bole*, but *tamariscus* remains the same. We find "Sloe, or Black-thorn" in the index, which refers to *prunus sylvestris* in the text, for which the corresponding index entry is *prunus*. For the text entry "Motacilla, Offic. The Water-wagtail" we find index entries for both terms, and so on. Thus the index has been offered as not merely a rough subject guide in the usual sense, but as a cross-referenced 'double dictionary' on the model of the *Bibliotheca scholastica* by John Rider (1562–1632), published in 1589, which is actually an English-Latin dictionary followed by a Latin index. James has a Latin word-list with a Latin and English index. His index also incorporates other textual references than head-words.

Another publication combines a translation of a work by Bernardo Ramazzini (1633–1714) on the diseases of tradesmen with a second treatise by Friedrich Hoffmann (1660–1742) on endemial diseases (James 1745a). James indicates in his preface that the work was originally intended for his dictionary, but that pressure to complete it both from readers and from the publisher meant that it was excluded:

> The following Sheets were intended for the Medicinal dictionary; but the Desires of the Publick to see that Work compleated, and the Impatience of the Booksellers to have it finish'd, oblig'd me to omit it, tho' of Importance sufficient to deserve the Notice of the Publick. (Dr. James's preface: ix)

The text is the same as *Health preserved* 1750, which looks very much like an attempt to package up unsold copies under a new title page. Nothing else has been altered; indeed, the sheets are identical to those of the Hoffman dissertation.

Only two mentions of Ramazzini have been located in the *Medicinal dictionary*, once under *cassia*, and a second under *icterus* (jaundice), neither of which have any obvious relation to the matter of endemial diseases, suggesting that as much of the Ramazzini translation as was intended for the dictionary was indeed excluded by the publisher in its entirety despite James's protestations about the public good, although how much of the *Health preserved* James wanted to include remains unknown. There is only an extremely brief entry (s.v. *endemius*) in the dictionary, consisting of a one-sentence explanation. The claim that this material was indeed intended for the dictionary is suggested by that fact that James has added an etymology of the term *endemial* to the beginning of Hoffmann's treatise which is not in the original.

James certainly appears to have been active as a translator throughout the 1740s, although how much is genuinely his own and how much was the work of his amanuenses is impossible to know. The flurry of translations immediately following the appearance of the dictionary in its three-volume form continued with the *Modern practice of physic* (James 1746c) which consists of translations of Boerhaave, with Van Sweiten's commentaries on him, along with Friedrich Hoffman, as well as "such Parts of Dr. Hoffman's Works as supply the Deficiencies of Boerhaave" (tp.), and then with Prosper Alpini's *The presages of life and death in diseases* (James 1746d), a version of *De praesagienda vita et morte argrotantium libri septem* (Venice 1601). Since Alpini

(1553–1617), a physician and botanist, was best known for botanical works, why James translates him is an obvious question. Alpini recorded many plants from Egypt and the Greek islands not previously known, and also described the sexual reproduction of the date palm, thus anticipating Linné. There is little to help us with our enquiries in the preliminaries of this translation. There is no preface by James, the text moving straight to Boerhaave's own preface, which explains the circumstances of the source text, a corrected version of his Frankfurt edition. Since history has regarded Alpini's botanical works as his most valuable and enduring, James may have been moved to render it into English by Boerhaave's recommendation of this work: "the World was never yet favoured with one of greater Worth" (vi). James's respect for Boerhaave is apparent throughout his publications.

9.2 "Inopem me copia fecit" (Ovid): *A medicinal dictionary* (1742–1745)

James's *A medicinal dictionary* is very large, comprising 3327 pages in three hefty folio volumes.[138] Despite its impressive bulk,[139] this dictionary is largely forgotten apart from the very occasional article, which usually relates primarily to Johnson and his contributions, modest though they were.[140] Fortunately, this work has attracted some recent scholarly attention, including a published analysis of its entries (Lonati 2017: 59–63, 68–79). An exhaustive analysis is currently being conducted by Dr Alexander Wright of the University of Birmingham. This medical dictionary is by far the largest published in English in the eighteenth century, dwarfing all others. Its scope was not challenged again until the appearance of the New Sydenham Society's *Lexicon of medicine and the allied sciences* (NSSL) at the end of the nineteenth century, edited by Henry Power and Leonard W. Sedgwick (1879–1892). If James intended it to become a standard work of reference, however, it failed to achieve this. It needs to be seen in two contexts; first, the encyclopaedic tradition exemplified by John Harris, Ephraim Chambers, the French encyclopaedic tradition, and the dictionaries of the arts and sciences and, second, in terms of James's personal ambitions and methods. This section will concentrate more on the latter.

The dictionary was originally issued in parts, as we have seen, by the successful and wealthy bookseller Thomas Osborne (1704(?)–1767). Osborne was primarily a

---

138 "Inopem me copia fecit": Ovid, Narcissus in Met. 3.466: 'plenty made me poor' (cited in Parr 1809: 6), or perhaps in this case 'copiousness made me helpless.'
139 A copy weighs about 17 kilos.
140 For more on the dedications and prefaces Johnson wrote for James, see Hazen 1973: 68–73.

bookseller,[141] but many books were published for him.[142] A contract for the *Medicinal dictionary* was signed, presumably with Osborne, on the tenth of June 1741 (Anon. 1754: 8).[143]

9.3 James's assistants

It is apparent that James employed assistants in the process of compiling his dictionary. Johnson did claim to have been paid for the dedication, but his assistance may have otherwise been gratis and based on friendship. Since James was reputed to have a considerable income, even before the fever powder patent, this presumably was no great difficulty for him. His investments with Lewis Paul in the late 1730s, unproductive as they ultimately were, suggest that he had means at his disposal. The few surviving records do not indicate how many assistants there might actually have been, but we hear about two in the pamphlets concerning the fever powder patent.

The first is John Maitland, who worked as a translator for James (Baker 1754: 32–33), but we do not learn which language he was employed on to put into English. Maitland is discredited as a next-to-useless drunk in an anonymous pamphlet of 1754 on James's disputed patent for his fever powder, but this claim must be taken with a grain of salt, since breaking down the credit of the deponents for the plaintiff, Walter Baker, is a major purpose of that publication. Another assistant was William Schwanberg, supposedly the inventor of the fever powder which caused such legal conflict. James's affidavit declares that

> William Schwanberg ... appearing to be in very indigent circumstances, and this deponent being then engaged in writing the medicinal dictionary... in which work this deponent employed several hands, and the said William Schwanberg understanding the High Dutch, this deponent employed him for some time, in translating several passages out of the German writers, to insert in the said dictionary, and by which the said Schwanberg got his bread at that time. (Baker 1754: 93)

---

141 A word applied to both booksellers and publishers in the eighteenth century; OED leaves this rather unclear, but evidence abounds; e.g., "The good Reception which the former Part of these Collections has met with, as it has encourag'd the Bookseller to venture on a Third Edition; so it has laid upon the Author a Generous Obligation of endeavouring to be further serviceable to the World" (Kettilby 1724 Pt. II: preface).
142 Osborne also sold a number of libraries, including the famous Harleian library, for which Johnson wrote the *Bibliotheca Harleiana* proposal (1745) (Kaminski 1987: 174–184; see also McKitterick 1992). Johnson also did the Latin entries of the finished catalogue. Some indication of Osborne's wealth and success appears in Reid (1880: 424–425), which describes an extravagant entertainment at his new house in Hampstead. See also Brack 2008; Plomer, et al. 1968b: 185–186.
143 For bibliographical details of the dictionary, see Hazen, 1973: 71–73.

This has not prevented James claiming credit for these translations by inserting the first-person comment under *aves* in the iatrochemical sense that "the High Dutch Interpretation of the same Author is rather greater Nonsense than the Latin; for which Reason the Reader need not regret, that I have not translated it." James also claims that Schwanberg learnt how to make the powder from a German chemist, but had not invented it himself (Baker 1754: 93). "Several hands" does indicate that more than Maitland and Schwanberg were on James's payroll.

9.4 The *Proposals for printing a medicinal dictionary* (1741)

It is clearly worth considering the proposals issued in 1741 for the dictionary in detail, as well as the relation between them and Johnson's for his dictionary, especially where they bear on James's own. The James proposals are in two sections; first, the conditions laid down by the publisher for the subscribers and, second, the "General Account of the Work". The subscription list had long been established as a way of funding a publication. Subscriptions would be sought in advance, and, once enough money was either collected, or in the case of the *Medicinal dictionary*, promised, printing would commence. A list of subscribers would allow those contributing to have their names in print, along with those of the learned, the good, and the great (see Yeo 2001: 51–52), although this list seems never to have been added to the *Medicinal dictionary* in its final three-volume form. It was also a more democratic form of the use of a patron—"a form of patronage in which the 'middling sort' of people might participate" (Yeo 49).

   The publishers' conditions for the *Medicinal dictionary* were, first, that the work should come to about 400 folio sheets, and were to be printed "on the same letter", that is, in the same type-face as the account of the work, as well as on the same paper. Second, five sheets per fortnight, stitched together in a cover, and each priced at a shilling, were to be delivered to the subscribers; hence 20 pages per cover, amounting to 1600 pages and hence 80 numbers in all, and making the whole cost five pounds. An argument is added here about the reasonableness of this arrangement—although some publications delivered a sheet more at the same price, the publishers argue that since in those cases the "copy-money", the price paid to the author for the manuscript, has already been recouped along with other expenses, and a profit has already been made, the subscribers will find the present arrangement good value. It was also pointed out that James's pages contain a great deal of substance.

   The publishers go on to say that "every Folio Cut shall be reckoned as one Sheet of Print, without additional expense to the Subscribers" (James 1741b), so that the plates, which were much more expensive to produce, would be charged to the subscribers at a reasonable rate. A further assumption is seemingly that in general binders would bind this dictionary in fives, rather than the frequently-used sixes, simply because to do it in sixes would require unnecessary and tiresome sorting of sheets.

Next, the first number is to be issued on the first of January next (1742), and then fortnightly "without any Intermission" (James 1741b) until completed. In order to meet this condition, the publishers agree to keep ahead of this schedule, so that the next number is always in hand. The promise to the subscribers was thus that the publication would be completed in the second fortnight of 1745. James and his publishers could not stick to this, however, since to issue the final, greatly increased count of 168.5 numbers in the same time required producing a number every week, a change which was rapidly made.

The final condition was that gentlemen who wished to encourage this publication were invited to send their names to Mr James Crokatt or Mr T. Osborne (addresses given), so that the publishers would have an idea of how many to print. Payment was due on delivery of the individual number, not before. The whole was to be a production of the Society of Booksellers for Promoting Learning (see below), a rather short-lived society which had already produced James's work on mad dogs (1741a), and would go on to publish a further eight works.[144] In the event, the name of this society did not appear on the title-page, however.

The proposals for the dictionary also include a statement of James's intentions. He stakes a claim for disseminating knowledge, declaring that "whatever is generally useful should be generally known; and he therefore that diffuses Science, may with Justice claim, among the Benefactors to the Public, the next Rank to him that improves it" (James 1741b). Since a medical dictionary cannot be expected literally to improve science, James thus arrogates the next rank of importance for himself in his dictionary. Instructions about how to cure are also an explicit part of the purposes of his dictionary, a feature not necessarily shared by other such works. Certainly he saw this work as more than a mere list, following Chambers in attempting the diffusion of better knowledge "to establish juster Notions in the Bulk of Mankind"; on the other hand, his attempt "to supply all the Defects of those [medical dictionaries] that have gone before us, and at once to familiarize the Knowledge, and reform the Practice, of Physic" (James 1741b) misses the point of the encyclopaedic endeavour to compress and encapsulate the best of scientific knowledge, as Harris and Chambers had done.

The argument that previous dictionaries have been insufficiently extensive is reminiscent of the puff employed on so many title-pages and in so many prefaces to lexical dictionaries that the predecessors have been insufficiently copious and comprehensive and that the current publication is the best yet, a statement often made

---

144 Advertisements for this curious 'society', perhaps best understood as an attempt by Osborne and others to salvage their reputations from accusations of profiteering at the expense of authors, appeared in *The country journal; or, The craftsman*, Saturday, July 18, 1741 [Issue 785] (see Spedding 2009). Its last two publications, a work by Benjamin Parker on divine scriptural authority, appeared in 1742, before the *Medicinal dictionary* was complete. The title-page of this work adds after the name of the society "by purchasing *Manuscripts, Copies*, &c. design'd for the Press", as also appeared on the title-page of its other religious offering, *The christian philosopher* (1741).

whether the current performance was a material improvement or not.[145] Like most lexicographers addressing their public, James naturally wishes to distinguish his work from that of his predecessors, and is not above some degree of hyperbole:

> the best, equally with the worst, have proceeded upon a Scheme which our Design resembles in nothing but persuing, like them, the Order of the Alphabet. They endeavour to explain the Terms only; we, together with the Terms, the Science of Physic. They enable their Readers to name Distempers, which we instruct them to cure. (James 1741b)

In doing so, James offers the user a therapeutic compilation as well as a lexical one. He may wish to balance it against the notion of the art of physic. His claim that his work only shares alphabetical order with his predecessors is of course grossly overstated. What exactly he means by the "science" of physic is less than clear. He does not seem concerned to distinguish nicely between the art (practice, experience, intuition) and science (knowledge, theory, rules) of physic, a distinction maintained by many in the early modern period.[146]

Many terms, James points out, have been added, such that "what is not to be found in this Dictionary, it will be generally in vain to seek in any other; but what is wanting in others, may be more successfully inquired for in this" (James 1741b), although it is worth keeping in mind that the relative number of head-words in James is small in relation to its bulk. He is nevertheless prepared to give some credit to his predecessors, pointing out in a rather circuitous way that not to accept good lexicography for what it is is contemptible:

> Their Attempts were indeed useful, and are therefore to be mentioned with Gratitude: The Knowledge of Words must necessarily precede the Study of Science ... often nothing can be added to the Accuracy of their Explications; and such Passages we have carefully translated without the weak Ambition of concealing the Benefit by unnecessary Variations (James 1741b).

His further claim that he has endeavoured to reform the practice of physic by publishing this work now stands, however, as a testament to his failure to do so (James 1741b).

James stresses the presence of a large section on anatomy which forms an anatomical treatise in itself, as well as comprehensive coverage of anatomical terms. He claims, in the interests of inclusiveness, that "nothing shall be willingly omitted, that

---

145 The title-page of *Cocker's English dictionary* (1715) enthusiastically declared "The like never yet extant", but this was certainly one of the worst publications of its time and kind. This work is generally agreed not to have been by Cocker, a well-known and widely published arithmetician, but probably by hacks employed by a publishing conger.

146 The usage of the early eighteenth century in medical and scientific texts heavily favours the disjunct 'art or science' over the co-ordinating 'art and science'. This mainly seems to be an attempt to be inclusive, especially since the whole is quite often in the singular, as in 'an art or science'. 'Any' occurs very frequently as well, leaving it ambiguous as to whether the whole is a singular or not.

has been transmitted by the Antients, or discovered by the Moderns" including "all the minute Inquiries of the Microscope" (James 1741b). Surgery will be treated in similar fullness. Veterinary medicine is also accorded a place, an area James claims has been badly neglected. This he describes as "a System of Comparative Physic", since it will conduce to the advancement of other kinds of medicine as well as having its own use. He is unable at this point to resist a mention of his mercury cure for rabies.

James also points out the pervasive confusion in the terms in the materia medica, especially plants, claiming to have gathered together the various names of the same plant. This does actually seem to have been done, at least for entries like *ambrosia*, *ammi*, *carduus*, *cepibira*, *cedrus*, *costus*, *herniaria*, *ipecacuanha*, and *rhagadiolus*, or for those in which authorities are cited sometimes, but not always, at the start of the entry; less so for plants like *cardinalis flos*, which simply cites two other names for the plant and Blancard at the end of the entry. Other authorities may not have been available.

At every turn, the stress is on inclusiveness at the expense of judicious selection— a full account of anatomy, all the variant names of plants, "every Article of the Materia Medica now in Use", "all the British Plants", and so on, and all this, James declares, is merely preparatory to "the great Hippocratic Art of Curing Diseases". This part, James avers, will be organised according to five categories: select cases, accurate description, prognostics, method of cure, and "Select Cases in Confirmation of the Doctrine laid down". His dictionary will also cover "every Medicine, of the Efficacy of which we are convinced by Evidence or Experience", "all the Empirical Remedies"; only cases are to be selected from what is available. Hence such things as the long "treatise on aliments" (*alimenta*), which occupies about eighteen pages of the *Medicinal dictionary*.

Other claims are predictable and familiar, such as the one that a person remote from medical help can make use of the dictionary, and that fraudulent practices can be avoided by referring to it. James then moves on to the inclusion of "A body of surgery" but placed in alphabetical order and with the entry for the corresponding anatomical part; this problem is to be overcome by the use of a catalogue of surgical items under the head-word *chirurgia*. Lives of physicians are to be included, and a history of medicine. Previous compilers have overlooked their sources, James asserts, not unjustifiably: "we shall secure our Performance by an accurate and regular Quotation of the Authors whose Doctrine we shall adopt" and he offers to supply a general index as well. How far he remedied this deficiency remains open to question, however. Once again, he is moved to mention new cures for hydrophobia, albeit modestly not naming himself, and by way of making a general point about recent advances in medicine.

9.5 James's proposals and Johnson

The problem of Johnson's authorship of the James proposal has been widely discussed, and the matter is not yet closed. John Wiltshire ascribes the whole of the proposals to Johnson, arguing that because their aims are not even remotely achieved in the pages of the dictionary, that the specific proposals may be Johnson's. An examination shows, however, that James's aims are indeed fulfilled in a number of ways, such as giving directions for cures, the historical preface, alternative names for plants, and so on and so forth, and there is little reason to suppose that Johnson would have thought his ability to construct a medical classification for the dictionary was better than James's, let alone that James would have agreed that this was so. In the end, Wiltshire is only confident in ascribing two of the lives to Johnson (Boerhaave and Trallian), and admitting another as possible. The reliance of the life of Aegineta on Freind's *History of physick* (1725–1726: I) is also discussed (Wiltshire 1991: 104–106).

A general observation is that this proposal shares very little with Johnson's, except that both are plans of dictionaries; in fact, James's demonstrates the clearer idea of how the work and the entries should be structured, a matter hardly mentioned by Johnson at all, who concentrates largely on the idiosyncrasies of the English lexicon and morphology, and the problems to be thus encountered. If Johnson had been so clear for the structure of James's dictionary, why would he not do it for his own? However, perhaps this should not come as a surprise for proposals six years apart and for dictionaries of very different kinds. What has apparently riveted the attention of scholars is simply the possibility that some part of James's text may have come from the pen of Johnson. A fairly typical comment is that the proposals "bear many signs of Johnson's style, especially in their first eight paragraphs" (Kaminski 1987: 173). The ninth paragraph is, after all, the point at which the text shifts from introductory remarks to a description of how the dictionary is to be structured, so that a change in tone and approach is only to be expected. Hazen merely draws the reader's attention to particular paragraphs, commenting that "A study of the text makes it quite clear that Johnson was largely if not wholly the author", but without supporting this claim (1973: 69). To argue that it has characteristics of Johnson's style is not proof that Johnson did in fact write it, and any assumption that James was incapable of writing anything other than the turgid prose he is generally assumed to have written simply begs the question.

Brack summarizes this in a recent essay, in which L. F. Clifford, Hazen, and Arthur Sherbo are all mentioned as contributing to the discussion; all seem to have found writing which they thought was unmistakably Johnsonian, although Brack suggests that there are parallels in style to the *Proposals* here and there in the preface to the dictionary, which "is almost certainly by James" (Brack 2009: 252–253). Perhaps some have assumed that Boswell's report of Johnson having helped James a little was Johnsonian modesty, and that in reality he wrote all of what has been ascribed to him, but there seems no strong reason not to take Johnson at his reported word, such as it is. Perhaps it is best cautiously to suggest that what was received was by and large help rather than finished text.

The work was, as we saw, produced under the aegis of the Society of Booksellers for Promoting Learning, on whose publications the names of Thomas Osborne, Smith,[147] and J. Crokatt appear,[148] the latter of whom seems to have acted as its secretary.[149] They claimed to have an office near St Bride's in Fleet St. Osborne in particular had been attacked for exploiting authors to their detriment and his own profit, not that this was by any means a new complaint. The notion of promoting learning seems to allude to the wording of the copyright act of 1710 in which the provision of copyright was proscribed by this worthy aim.[150]

9.6 The preface to the dictionary

The preface is immensely long, and was published after the main dictionary had begun to appear; exactly when is not clear, but there is evidence that it was towards the end of the letter A. The intention of the preface is to outline the history of medicine and to indicate the major shifts in theory, knowledge, and practice. It is a rather rambling account of the history of medicine, beginning with what James understands to be the earliest mentions of instances of healing. Thus the initial impetus to healing provided by God moves to the Egyptians and then by a series of loosely connected episodes to the Greeks, and so forth. In a way, this excursus is classical legend and history mined for whatever medical stories and allusions they can provide, stripped of their original narrative coherence, and coloured and re-interpreted by James's own predilections. To take just two examples:

---

147 Not identified. See Plomer et al. 1968b, s.v. *Smith*.

148 Plomer at al. 1968b, s.v. *Crokat*.

149 Precisely why such a grandly-named society should also publish a work like *The levee: A farce*, by John Kelly (1680?-1751) is not clear if it wished to live up to its name, and was more than simply an exercise in public relations. Avoiding some provisions of the copyright act seems possible. This society is seemingly alluded to in Henry Fielding's *Joseph Andrews*: "Adams informed *Joseph* [that] ... he was making to *London* ... to publish three volumes of Sermons; being encouraged, he said, by an Advertisement lately set forth by a Society of Booksellers, who proposed to purchase any Copies offered to them at a Price to be settled by two Persons." (Fielding 1742: Bk. I, 94). Crokatt also published another medical work, J. Taylor's *The case of Sir Jeremy Sambrooke* 1743, giving his publishing address as "near *Garraway's* Coffee-House in *Exchange-Alley*".'

150 Full title: "A Bill for Encouragement of Learning, and for Securing the Property of Copies of Books to the Rightful Owners thereof."

> we are told by antient Historians, that Egypt was full of Physicians ... But 'tis scarce probable that the Medicine of the Vulgar extended further than Prevention by Vomits, Purges, and Clysters ... but we are told by Diodorus Siculus, that none durst profess Physic, without being admitted as a Member of the College of Priests (iv)

That physicians in Britain were in fact organised into colleges whereas surgeons and apothecaries were formed into companies lends extra significance to the "college" James mentions (see Jacyna 1983: 96–97). The notion of an exclusive college of priests in Egypt is uncannily reminiscent of the status accorded the Royal College of Physicians, and the somewhat archaic "durst" here is also loaded with implications of upstart pretension. Despite James's collegiate assumptions, he is also at pains to declare that his dictionary is intended for the edification of mankind at large and the assistance of families, as Lonati correctly points out (2017: 60). He also covers medicine in "remote Nations" (ix), including China, Japan, Malabar, and Mexico, among others. In the next quotation, part of the story of Troy is related simply for the reference to the knowledge of physic of Achilles and Patroclus, the latter not very convincingly distinguished from what anyone might be expected to know about wounds:

> About seventy Years after the Argonautic Expedition, the confederated Armies of Greece invaded the Trojan Territories ... Achilles ... was, in consequence of his Education under Chiron, acquainted with Physic, and is mentioned as the Inventor of some Remedies, which are specify'd under the Article of his Name. Nor was his Companion Patroclus ignorant of this Art, as we may infer from his dressing the Wound of Eurypylus, at the Request of the last-mentioned Hero. (v)

James finally declares that "my Design in this Preface is to specify the principal Revolutions Physic has been subjected to by the Introduction of new Theories, and the Influences these have had upon Practice" (xli), a remark which might usefully have appeared at the outset.

The preface also contains some quite long quotations marked as such, as on xliii–xliv. There are some longish passages on antimony (lxxix–lxxx, lxxxvi), a subject James had obviously spent some time on, confirming at least some of the claims made in the anonymous pamphlet of 1754 against the accusation that the patent for the fever powder was simply theft.[151] James must have seen an opportunity, based on his previous reading and work.

An extremely long quote from Boerhaave starts on page lxxxix and runs to xciv, outlining Boerhaave's defence of mechanical reasoning in medicine. The stress on the mechanical approach suggests that James had some sympathy for it, as does his

---

[151] The discovery of metallic antimony was often ascribed to Basil Valentine (Basileus Valentinus), whose identity is disputed. The name may have been a pseudonym for a group of alchemists. James accepts the traditional view, adding that "this Author ... first used Antimony internally, and enrich'd Medicine with many Preparations of this Mineral" (lxxx). James uses the anglicised form of the name throughout.

remark that this is more likely to benefit progress in medicine than anything arising from mere speculation, although in general he is a medical conservative. He cites Boerhaave on the fundamental principle of mechanical medicine: "the human Body is of a true mechanical Structure, and, therefore, possessed of all the Properties which belong to a Subject the best qualify'd for mechanical Speculation" (lxxxix). A concern which he repeats more than once is the danger of abuse of these principles: "The Abuse ... of mechanical Learning in Physic is highly to be condemn'd, as the Tinsel of the Art, which makes a Noise and a Shew, without communicating any real Value" (xciv).

Mentions of the moderns are relatively rare, except in the last few pages as he surveys recent developments, by far the most often quoted being Boerhaave. There are two or three references to John Freind, one to Thomas Willis, and a couple to Peter Shaw, mentioned in relation to his translation of Boerhaave's *Chemistry* (1741) on page lxxxii. The discoveries of William Harvey are put into the context of mechanical medicine, since James sees Harvey as providing the impetus for this approach. "In the Beginning of the seventeenth Century, the ever memorable Dr. William Harvey discover'd the Circulation of the Blood. And this gave Occasion to the Introduction of Mechanics into Medicine, upon the Ruins of the chymical Theory" (lxxxviii).

James incorporates a very lengthy quotation from "the Substance of an Oration wrote by the celebrated Boerhaave" (lxxxviii) on mechanical medicine, adumbrating the advantages of such an approach at length. It also becomes apparent that James is concerned with simplicity in medicine, a matter we have already encountered in relation to Quincy and his attitude to obscure language as a factor obstructing progress. James applies the same concern to medical truth, which, he claims, always represents "intelligible Simplicity" (xcvi). An instance he cites in support of this is the circulation of the blood:

> Scarce had the famous Harvey led the Way in which he was so well seconded by the industrious Malpighi, to the Discovery of the human Machine, when those imaginary Beings, and Creatures of the Brain, vanished like Mists before the Sun; and so clear was the Evidence, so great the Simplicity, that the Discoverers themselves could hardly believe their own Eyes (xcvii)

Thus James argues for reduction to essential truths and for the stripping away of misguided and superfluous theories, in this respect taking up the banner from Quincy.

Despite his own experience of chemical experimentation and contact with people such as Schwanberg and the Wallingford apothecary Cudworth Bruch, with whom he lodged in about 1726 (Anon 1754: 6), not to mention the fortune he later made from his medications,[152] his own massive dictionary accords the entry for *apothecarius* the

---

152 Others were added, as we see from the 1778 edition of the dissertation, but this may have happened posthumously. Dr James's powder for cattle is advertised at the end of this edition as well as his analeptic pills.

curt four-word definition "A Preparer of Medicines." This is stripping away bordering on disdain, especially compared with his own characteristic battology.

He comes a little nearer to the fundamental problem of the medical lexicon when he considers diseases.

> But is not Medicine oppressed and overloaded with the Copiousness of its Subject Account? The Number of Diseases is not yet settled: Of these there is such a Mul￼ ety, and they impose upon us in so many Shapes, that a whole Age woul￼ enumerate them; consequently these alone must create an infinite deal ￼ (xcvii)

The use of the word copiousness here is striking, having long been a key term in lexicography and a concept which greatly inflated the number of entries in such dictionaries as those of John Florio (1598 and 1611), Thomas Blount (1656), and Edward Phillips (1658). This may go some way to understanding the evident instability in the medical lexicon that is suggested by the low rate of agreement between the word-lists of medical dictionaries in the late seventeenth and early eighteenth centuries. The uncertainty in the terminology must have bedevilled more than simply the names of diseases. James does in fact extend this to the humours in the body, but his essential insight is that "the more we know of the human Machine, the more simple it appears" (xcvii). At the very least, this implies the rejection of terms which serve to maintain and exacerbate the confusion, but his own lexicographical copiousness does little to alleviate the problem.

9.7 The problem of length

From the beginning, there seem to have been difficulties with *A medicinal dictionary*, as with all such large dictionaries. There was clearly some concern among the subscribers once the first few numbers had appeared that the letter A was excessively long and the whole dictionary would run far beyond what had originally been proposed. James offered a justification for its length at the end of his preface. A separate single-leaf explanation dated October 4, 1742, that is, between numbers XXXII and XXXIII, was however issued by the "booksellers concerned in this work". The first person is not used at all in this explanation, while it occurs frequently in James's own account explaining this problem and attempting to allay the fears of the subscribers.[153] The publisher's sheet begins by declaring that:

---

153 This notice has been tipped in between the dedication and the beginning of the preface in a copy in private hands to which I have had access. The Cambridge University Library copies were checked (Path.bb.16; 7300. bb 1-), but neither included this page.

Whereas a number of Complaints have been made, that the first Letter of the Medicinal Dictionary runs out to so great a length, that the subscribers are apprehensive the whole Work may be
much more voluminous than originally proposed, the Booksellers concerned in this Work, have
thought it necessary to apprise the Publick of the following Particulars

The details explained to the public are that James had incorporated cross-referenced
entries in the earliest letter available, pushing material forward; the letter A contains
some lengthy lives of anatomists such as Aegineta and Aretæus; the entries for *alkali*
and *acid* contain a great deal of material which is merely cross-referenced later, such
as fermentation, and so on. Nevertheless, we know from elsewhere that material prepared by James had been omitted to expedite the work. In general, the letter A is relatively long in medical dictionaries in any case given the weight of A- borrowings
from Latin and Greek. The figure below shows this preponderance:

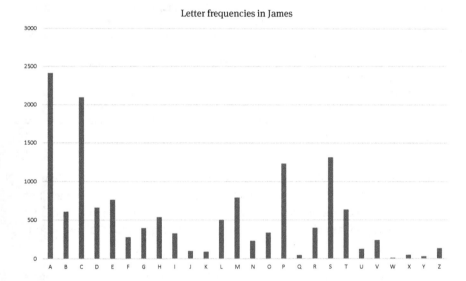

Fig. 6: Letter frequencies in James

The letter A finally ended in the 39th number, counting from the beginning of A. The
preface occupied a further five and a half numbers. The end of this announcement
assures the subscribers that the dictionary will not exceed 500 sheets, an increase of
100 over the original promise, as well as declaring that the letter A will be completed
in three numbers. The booksellers also promise to include a copperplate engraving
with every weekly number (originally fortnightly) until the plates are complete. The
rate of issuance had been increased to weekly after number IV, and that this accounted exactly for thirty-two issues by the first week of October 1742 when the notice

was printed. The promised fortnightly rate of issuance was impractical and was obviously never kept to.

James's own discussion of the question of length at the end of the preface therefore probably postdates that issued separately by the publishers, and offers much the same reasons as appear in the sheet mentioned above, albeit in a rather more condescending context and with a good deal of personal reference:

> I must not finish this Preface, without taking Notice of some Complaints which the Booksellers concern'd in this Work have sufficiently teiz'd me with, relative to its Length. As it is not possible to alter the Plan of the Work at first laid down, and since pursu'd, without utterly embroiling the Whole, and rendering it much less valuable and useful, I should have very little Regard to their Remonstrances. But for the Satisfaction of the Purchasers, whose Interests, in the present Case, I apprehend to be inseparable from my own, I shall submit the following Reasons for my Conduct to their Consideration:
>
> First, As it was absolutely necessary for every one who reads this Work for Information, to have a perfect Idea of what Authors mean by Acids and Alcalis ... I judg'd it proper to give full Information upon these Subjects in the Beginning of the Work; and this Consideration oblig'd me to anticipate several things, which would otherwise have come under other Articles in every Letter ...
>
> Secondly, As all the Parts of the Materia Medica are call'd by different Names, for the sake of Method I have made it a Rule ... to treat of every Animal, Vegetable, and Mineral, under the first of their Names which occurs in the Alphabet.
>
> Thirdly, Under every separate Article of any considerable Importance, I have endeavour'd to include every thing relating to it, tho' properly belonging to some future Article, in order to save the Trouble of turning to a Multitude of Articles, and to give the Reader a full Idea of the Subject at one View

He gives the examples of *alcohol* and *acetum*, both of which contain and anticipate the entry for *fermentation*. This is pretty much Chambers' idea of the 'systems'; but whether James actually carried it through consistently is less clear, as his intentions seem more purely alphabetical and comprehensive than systematic. James continues:

> Fourthly, The Lives of the antient Physicians have swell'd the Letter A considerably ... Instances of this are Actuarius, Ægineta, Æsculapius, Aetius, Aretæus, Albucasis, Avicenna, Averroes, Avenzoar, Archagathus, Asclepiades, and some others.
>
> That the Work is a single Sheet longer than at first proposed, is owing to an unforeseen Accident, which, though it has given me an infinite deal of Trouble, will ... be advantageous to the Purchasers ...After a few Numbers of the Medicinal Dictionary were publish'd, I observed in the foreign Papers the following Title of a Book ...
>
> Introductio in Notitiam Rerum Naturalium & Arte factarum, quarum in communi Vita, sed præcipue in Medicina Usus est. Per Alphabeti Ordinem digessit Joannes Christophorus Rieger. Hagæ Comitum 1742.
>
> I found Means to get this Book ... and as it is a most excellent Performance, I thought myself oblig'd to insert in the Medicinal Dictionary whatever I had omitted in my Collections; and to cancel what I had wrote upon several Articles, in order to make Room for better Materials (xcix)

Being struck with the value of Rieger's work, James felt that he should incorporate some of it into the dictionary, late in the process though this was, and that some entries should be rewritten. Rieger's influence was nevertheless restricted, the eighteen references to it (not counting the index reference) occurring between *camphora* and *cotyledon*; that is, volume two of Rieger's tome.[154] James goes on to explain that he believes that Rieger had been employed in Russia by Peter the Great, and later lived with a bookseller in Holland, where he had access to "the best Collection of Medicinal Authors that was ever exposed to Sale in Europe" (xcix). His exculpation is that the reader will excuse an author who has had to sacrifice large chunks of his own work, and has attempted to "divest myself of Prejudices in favour of any Theory, System, or Mode of Practice whatever". While the addition of this material from Rieger has expanded the work by one sheet, that is, four pages, this is far less than the final increase in the number (to 168.5 in all). James's final excuse for the long preface is that the reader must understand the essential history and practice of those quoted in the dictionary to make proper use of it (xcix).[155]

The two versions of James's disclaimer raise some questions. The one in the preface, assuming for the moment that the preface was issued first, must have been by many weeks the later, delivered as the last part of number five of the preface. The separate sheet appeared between the 32nd and 33rd number, as we have seen. The preface was not in fact issued as the first five numbers, but appeared much later, as is corroborated by the mention of the work by Rieger which James had already incorporated into the dictionary by the time he penned the end of the preface. Further evidence that the preface was not written before the letter A of the dictionary itself comes on page lxxix, on which he mentions an error under the entry for *antimonium*. It is immediately striking that the separate sheet does not employ the first person at all, while James's own uses it copiously. The tone of James's exculpation is also rather patronising, suggesting throughout that he knows best what the reader ought to be provided with better than the reader does.

9.8 The micro-structure of *A medicinal dictionary*

James's lemmas, despite their length and complexity, are relatively easy to access since the publishers have taken considerable trouble over the typography, which is relatively sophisticated. Head-words are indented and in large capitals, and are usually followed by either a definition or a derivation or both. Descriptions of diseases and major body parts are often extensive, and suggested treatments and procedures

---

154 Volume one was published in 1742, as was the second part of volume two; possibly too late for James to incorporate new material. Rieger's work seems never to have proceeded beyond the letter C. Needless to say, there may also be unacknowledged debts in James as well.

155 The readers' complaints were also noted in the *Daily post* as early as 20 Apr. 1742.

generously supplied, making their sheer size daunting. Botanical entries, which are numerous, often incorporate a lengthy synonymy and references, followed by the common name in large capitals. The description and use then follows. Longer entries may have one or more centred sub-headings, as under *coelia* and *pulmo*. Sub-lemmas such as *nepa*, a case of polysemy, are given small capitals, and within-text synonyms meant for cross-reference are treated the same way.

Head-words are largely Greek or Latin. James glosses some words in English immediately after the head-word, but not others. Likewise, some Latin words have Greek glosses as well, the most usual arrangement being to proceed to the Greek equivalent immediately after the head-word. Many, particularly the larger ones, include etymological comment, which is sometimes extensive, as in the entries for *laudanum* and *milium*, while others, like *os*, are completely lacking such information, moving straight to diseases following the one-word gloss.[156] Some entries contain little else than remarks on language, an example being *cardiogmus*, which might well have been dealt with as a by-form of *cardialgia*. The entries for *prostheta* and *protasis* are also almost entirely taken up by linguistic comments. This appears to be a strong tendency towards the end of the letter P, as in *psapheros*, *pyrrhos*, etc. Such remarks do also occur under other letters, however, *thaleros* and *thorexis* being instances. Recipes are indented and given a hanging indent to make them easy to find.

In the case of botanical entries, this is done in full capitals after the synonymy. Note that the practice in some entries is to include the English equivalent of the head-word, if there is one, at the end of the synonymy in full capitals., as in "ARISARUM ... friers-cowl" or "CACUBALUM ... berry-bearing chickweed" and "MATRICARIA ... feverfew". These are distinct from cross-references. Note however that this arrangement also appears in some other entries, apparently for minerals, earths, etc., such as "BISMUTHUM ... marcasite of silver, or tin-glass"; likewise *bezoar minerale*, *auripigmentum*, and so on.

A typical structure for botanical entries appears to be character, synonymy, description, use, and species, as we see illustrated under *lingua cervina* and *orchis*, but this is by no means consistent. Under *cardiobotanon* (possibly the motherwort), the confusion is outlined without being resolved. Species are often listed and numbered under the main entry, rather than given separate head-words, as in the case of the thirty-three numbered divisions under *carduus*. Not all species of thistles are listed this way, however, as a further nine appear under their own head-word (*carduus altilis*, *carduus benedictus*, etc.). Among many others, *ptarmica* lists nine species, and so on. Where there are separate head-words, as after *carduus*, they are often cross-references. However, an independent name may be used as a head-word; hence the carline thistle appears under *carlina*, not as a sub-lemma of *carduus*. *Apium* has generated a corresponding but much shorter entry under *celery*. *Ionthlaspi* has only very

---

156 This has recently been underscored as an "etymological principle" by Lonati (2017: 62, 66).

brief mentions of Tournefort as the source text with no reference, and Miller, with a reference. Miller is often mentioned, but these are to Joseph Miller's *Botanicum offic-inale; or a compendious herbal* of 1722, not to the better-known dictionary by Philip Miller, first published in 1724.[157] James's extracts from Miller expunge the quotation marks from what appear to be Miller's unreferenced quotes, but may simply be his way of indicating the section on the uses of the herb concerned, so consistently are they used. How precisely James's referencing of plants reflects the scholarship available at the time and how closely he has followed it cannot be canvassed here and is a matter for further research.[158]

Recipes are often included at length, as well as indications for cure, and not all entries are strictly relevant. James thinks nothing of incorporating scores of 'observations' from the work of others, as under *abortio*, in which cases reported by Mariceau, La Motte, and others take up about nineteen pages, while those of Wiseman fill the pages of the entry for *abscessio*. James also includes a great many entries for plants for which he admits knowing no medicinal value, such as *anblatum* (greater toothwort), *barleria*, *crotalaria* (rattlepods), *garidella*, *limonium* (sea lavender), *opulus* (guelder-rose), and *rapunculus* (possibly the rampion bellflower). In some entries, no medicinal quality is mentioned, as under *kempfera*. Other apparently medically pointless entries include "Bronte ... Thunder ... I don't know, that this relates to Medicine, further than as it purges some People by the Fright." The longish entry for gunpowder, *pyrius pulvis*, has no obvious medical relevance. The *Medicinal dictionary* is also sufficiently expansive as to incorporate glossaries and bibliographies such as that under the entry for *botany*, which contains just under 300 words, as well as a list of botanical references cited in the dictionary. This also applies to various other things such as animals (*hippopotamus*) and birds (*halieætos*, the osprey). There are limits, even for James, however. At the end of the lengthy entry for *dyspnoea*, he mentions Sir John Floyer, whom he knew, and who suffered from asthma most of his life.

---

157 Joseph Miller (?–1748?) does not have an entry in ODNB, although he is mentioned under Isaac Rand as becoming demonstrator at the Chelsea Physic Garden about 1738 or 1740. The Chelsea Garden website (http://chelseaphysicgarden.co.uk/the-garden/history-of-garden-staff/) gives 1740–1748 for this appointment, as well as Praefectus Horti 1743–1747. Miller, who was living in Bishopsgate in 1738–1742 and in Hoxton by 1746, was Warden of the Society of Apothecaries in 1737 (Society of Apothecaries 1737, 1738, 1742, 1746). His name appears as an occasional contributor to the *Philosophical transactions* up to 1750 and as a subscriber to various publications into the 1750s, but identification of the latter as the apothecary and gardener is doubtful in several cases. Miller was one of the original lessees of the Chelsea Physic Garden in 1707, along with Isaac Rand (see http://en.wikipedia.org/wiki/Isaac_Rand). The National Archives item PROB 11/761/385 may be his will.

158 The 'characters' for *linum* are loosely similar to those in Miller 1731 and somewhat reduced. The rest of the entry is not so; after all, it is about cultivation in Miller. Similarly under *lithospermum*, and the same with *melilotus* but there is a small verbatim quote: "pregnant with one or two roundish Seeds". *Mitella*, *orchis*, *sclarea*, etc., are seemingly not dependent on Miller at all. There are some botanical entries not in Miller, such as *myrobalani* and *rhagadiolus*.

James recommends the reader to consult Floyer's work on this disease "which is too long to be inserted in this Place."

The discussion of the notion of the animal spirits offers some examples of the editing process involved in the handling of dictionary sources. Under *spiritus* James quotes George Cheyne's *The English malady*, chapter IX "Of the Existence of animal Spirits" (77–89).[159] The first thing to note about how Cheyne is handled is that James acknowledges him, although not the particular work, a common referencing practice at that time. Next, James removes all of Cheyne's section numbers. There are then a number of minor editorial changes, such as

> they appear ... even when dry like crack'd Glass-wire, Horn, or any other solid Substance (Cheyne 1735: 79)

becomes

> they appear ... even when dry, like crack'd Glass, Wire, Horn, or any other solid Substance (James III s.v. *spiritus*)

possibly correcting an error in Cheyne. Another editorial alteration is

> But how ... seems very hard to explain, from the Nature of Fluids known here below. (Cheyne 1735: 83)
> But how ... seems very hard to explain from the known Nature of Fluids. (James III s.v. *spiritus*)

This next may represent a grammatical change, by which

> their containing Tubes and Canals the Nerves (Cheyne 1735: 82)

becomes

> their containing Tubes, and Canals of the Nerves (James III s.v. *spiritus*),

changing Cheyne's meaning somewhat. Others, more likely compositorial, include an omitted prop do, *tonick/tonic*, (Cheyne 1735: 79) (James III s.v. *spiritus*), *specifick* replaced by *specific* (Cheyne 1735: 87); *as* replacing *viz.* (Cheyne 1735: 83) (James III s.v. *spiritus*), 86 "&c" omitted at the end of a list, and Cheyne 89 "fœtids" replaced by "fetids". The sentence on page 84 of Cheyne "Of this last the Reader will be a better Judge, when he has consider'd the whole of this Treatise" has been completely omitted, presumably as being internally referential and not germane to James's entry.

James is normally willing to allow borrowed first-person references to stand unaltered. He certainly allows himself by this default to share Cheyne's conclusion that

---

[159] For this comparison, I have used the sixth edition, 1735, being nearest in date to *A medicinal dictionary*.

"we may, I think, pretty firmly conclude, that the Notion of the *animal Spirits* is of the same Leaven with the *substantial Forms* of *Aristotle*, and the *cælestial System of Ptolemy*" (85). The whole entry concludes with a brief dismissive comment, presumably James's own, however:

> Upon the whole, it should seem, that whoever lays any Stress upon the precarious Doctrine of Animal Spirits, in accounting for Distempers, or investigating Remedies, is either weak enough to be imposed upon himself, or malicious enough to amuse others.

A second example is from Richard Hale's "The humane allantois fully discovered", published in the *Philosophical transactions* of 1700 (see Andrews 1990: 172; 2008).[160] A closer look at James's procedure will shed some further light on his practice as a compiler, as well as the way such compilations were assembled more generally. James's quotation of Hale's tract is, as one might expect, not entirely verbatim, making the predictable punctuation and orthographical changes: "Hence Hippocrates says, that Twins lie in Sinus's, and that the *Uterus* has *Cornua*" (Hale 1700: 835) becomes "*Hippocrates* says, That Twins lie in Sinusses, and that the *Uterus* has *Cornua*." There are also minor changes in sentence structure, and even re-ordering sentences and paragraph structure. He also replaces Hale's opening sentence with a paragraph of his own about the controversy over the existence of the human allantois. Again, "For the accounts the Ancients have left of many Parts" (Hale 1700: 836) is simplified and shortened to "For the Ancients Accounts of many Parts", but the succeeding pages are close to verbatim. Other minor alterations include "Figure" for Hales's "Fig.", "Secondly" for "2dly", and "no-where" and "any-where" for "no where" and "any where" (Hale 1700: 837). Altering Hale's references to the figures in the original publication, James reproduces them as Fig, 2, Plate III in volume 1 of the *Medicinal dictionary*.

The treatment of anatomy (s.v. *anatome*) had been anticipated in the proposals, in which James has promised a full treatise on the subject and well as separate headwords. The entry itself runs to about forty-three pages, incorporating, inter alia, both an explanation of the concept, a history of anatomy, and a list of the major writers on the subject, including some quite recent ones.

James's index lists those words whose Latin form is different from the English; no doubt a matter of personal judgement in many cases, but the list is still revealing as to what was regarded as naturalized at the time and what was not. This list may be unique in medical dictionaries of the period in being set out in this way. Its purpose was obviously practical, providing a finding list for the unlearned. Some are pretty familiar, such as *bran* for *furfur*, or *coleworts* for *brassica*, but some are less so, including *coddy moddy* for *larus*, the black-headed gull, particularly in East Anglia,

---

160 For more on Hale, see Andrews 2008.

saintfoin for *onobrychis* (holy clover), or *sensific* for *sensificus*.[161] James also distinguishes carefully between words of English and Latin form but of the same etymon.

A further point us that James apparently did not attend very carefully to ways to rationalise and streamline his entries. The discussion in the next chapter on *mania*, *melancholy*, *erratic melancholy*, and *lycanthropy* will illustrate the point. These entries should overlap and complement each other, but do not, suggesting that material went into the *Medicinal dictionary* as it came to hand and undigested. Although *lycanthropy* is called a species of *melancholy*, and of *mania*, *melancholy* is dealt with under *mania*, but the other two have separate head-words, while that for *melancholy* deals mainly with *erratic melancholy*, i.e., *lycanthropy*. James makes no connexion between the latter two under *melancholy*, only under *lycanthropy*. By contrast, *ozæna*, which would now more normally be called chronic atrophic rhinitis, is described by James in detail under *nares* (nostrils), but is simply listed as a separate head-word, defined as a "disorder" and cross-referenced. Barrow on the other hand, gives *ozæna* a derivation and a brief, but more succinct, albeit unsourced definition.

9.9 The success of *A medicinal dictionary*

James's dictionary has been described as successful (Martin 2008: 184), but it is hard to agree that this was the case. Sales were rather sluggish, Newbery advertising bound copies for £6 nearly twenty years later in 1764 (James 1764, advertisement). Hazen mentions that in June 1765, Osborne advertised the remaining sheets for sale, and even later Newbery and Carnan were still selling bound copies (1973: 73). More than twenty years to fail to sell out the first printing does not sound like success. *A medicinal dictionary* was not reprinted in England, but it did have its successors in the translation into French by Diderot, Marc-Antoine Eidous and François-Vincent Toussaint published in six volumes in 1746–1748, and then into Italian,[162] published in eleven volumes in Venice in 1753. James does seem to have been anxious to publish everything he prepared, however, since, as we have seen, later publications made use some of the translations, both incorporated in the dictionary and rejected. James ascribes this rejection to the desire of both the readers and publishers to see the work finished (Dr. James's preface: ix), although of course the motives in each case might have been rather different.[163] In a review of the second edition of George Motherby's dictionary, the reviewer alludes to the sheer bulk of James's work and to his objectives, as well as the connexion with France:

---

161 *Sensific* is an OED antedating from 1822. *Stone-gluer* for *lithocolla* is unrecorded, and *lithocolla* is an OED postdating.
162 The Italian translation is from the French, not the original English.
163 There has also been a modern edition.

In a neighbouring kingdom ... a dictionary has been thought most convenient to treat of sciences, in their fullest extent; and this seems to have been the intention of Dr. James, in his very voluminous, and now very expensive work (Robinson 1785: 476)

The reception of the dictionary seems to have been muted. One striking later assessment was by Bartholomew Parr, in the introduction to his own *London medical dictionary*. While praising James's assiduity, Parr also comments perspicaciously on James's rather indiscriminate methods of collecting material and the sheer bulk of "contending opinions", which lead to difficulty in establishing "a decisive and discriminated practice", as well as "the diffuseness of his language" (Preface: vii). These are clearly matters which a medical dictionary ought to resolve rather than exacerbate. In more recent times, Hazen remarks that *A medicinal dictionary* has been called "a mass of ignorance and conservatism" (1973: 71; no source given). More recently, however, the historian Paul Kopperman (2012) has made extensive use of James's dictionary in providing an apparatus for his edition of the manuscript *Regimental practice* (1746) by John Buchanan.

The references to *A medicinal dictionary* in eighteenth-century printed works are relatively few and, from about 1760, appear mainly in booksellers' sale catalogues; unsurprisingly, given its lack-lustre sales. Among the scattered mentions are those in the surgical work by Dale Ingram (1710–1793), published in 1751, in which he refers to it as "elaborate", quoting it at some length on the relief of a discharge of matter in the chest and another, oddly enough, in a discussion of longevity and the Jewish diet in volume 5 of Benjamin Martin's magazine (Martin 1755: 112). There is a passing reference in an article on amber in the works of John Fothergill (1712–1780), published in 1783, and he is quoted in relation to the history of apothecaries as cited in Celsus (see Good 1796). This seems a poor return for such a massive tome, especially since Quincy was far more widely noticed and used. James is mentioned occasionally in *A new and complete dictionary of arts and sciences* of 1754, under *hydrophobia, impotence,* and *opiates,* for instance, although it is unclear in most cases whether the reference is to the dictionary or another of James's publications. One reference clearly designates the dictionary, that under *surgery.* More recent use has been made of James; for example, in a study of his entries dealing with nephrology. As is normal, this is research is based primarily on the medical phenomenon and how it is portrayed in the dictionary rather than James's work itself (Bisaccia et al. 2011).

Likewise, references to James in the *Encyclopaedia Londinensis* of 1810–1829 are few, once again especially by comparison with Quincy. One immediately obvious reason for this may simply be that there were no up-to-date editions of James, as there certainly were of Quincy, the most recent being the eleventh in 1794. The first American edition of Quincy under the editorship of Robert Hooper appeared in 1811. One of the rare quotes from James comes from the entry for *allantois.* The *Encyclopaedia Londinensis* ascribes the quotation to James, although at this point he is citing Richard

Hale's "The humane allantois fully discover'd", submitted to the Royal Society in 1701 (see Andrews 1990: 172; 2008).

Mark Twain's piece in *Harper's Magazine* (1890) provides a more jocular view, describing it as an outdated, forgotten monstrosity. A more modern account, in essence much the same although in an entirely serious vein, is that by Charles W. Burr (1929). Burr instances a number of the entries which demonstrate how outmoded the work is, standing as it does at the very beginning of what might be called modern medicine. Burr does not however provide any substantial analysis of the work, on the whole embracing the anachronistic view of it rather than trying to avoid the consequence of making the dictionary appear quaint.

A very positive recent view of the *Medicinal dictionary* however is that that the high quality of the work was what recommended it to Diderot and his fellow translators. "Die hohe Qualität des Werks war sicherlich der Grund dafür, daß nahezu unmittelbar nach dem Erscheinen des Werks eine französische Ausgabe in Angriff genommen wurde" (Stolberg s.a.). It may also have received a boost from the then current fashion for all things English in France (see Feingold 2004: 111), a fashion driven partly by the achievements of Newton, Locke and others, as well as by Voltaire's advocacy.

9.10 Derivative or not? James's sources

The general view is that expressed by Kaminski (1987): "'Compile' rather than 'compose,' is certainly the proper term, for the *Medicinal Dictionary* consists largely of translations, abridgements, and extracts from the best-known medical texts of the day" (173). He goes on to point out that the sources of James's work include "Boerhaave and Friedrich Hoffmann ... Daniel Le Clerc's *Histoire de la Médicine*, James Douglas's *Bibliographiae Anatomicae Specimen*, and John Freind's *History of Physick*" (Kaminski 1987: 173). Kaminski also points out that there are occasional hints of Johnson's style, listing as Johnsonian the life of Boerhaave (which Johnson published independently anyway), Alexander Trallianus (from Freind), the lives of Actuarius and Aegineta, in which the openings seem Johnsonian, and the dedication to Richard Mead.[164] Apparently Johnson was paid for this last. The stress on what is Johnsonian is typical of scholarship up to this point. There seems to be an assumption that Johnson alone is worth consideration; the consensus that James is merely derivative simply confirms this view as well as rendering the argument circular. Kaminski's remark on compilation also conveys the impression that James might have been the only one to be so derivative, but in fact what Kaminski describes is the norm for the period, as we have seen. The same might be said for Harris and Chambers as well as

---

164 Kaminski 1987: 173; see also fn 4, 246.

for the various lexical dictionaries. This being so, we need to rethink what James was doing to reflect the contemporaneous practices more accurately.

Derivative, let alone plagiarised, is not necessarily the most apt description of either this work or indeed any other such reference work in the eighteenth century. James himself makes little or no attempt to conceal the nature of what he calls "my Collections" (1743 I: xcix). Yeo has pointed out the connection between encyclopaedias and commonplace books (2001: Ch. 4), a centuries-old tradition in which the point was both to collect and to impose order on snippets of useful material (Yeo 2001: 101). This emerges in the encyclopaedic tradition as the use of 'systems', especially as they appear in the works by Harris and Chambers (Yeo 2001: 122–130). The collection of already existing material was approved by precedent and not in itself a bad thing; the crucial question about James is how astute a collector and organiser of his material he was. Was he a sufficiently discriminating and judicious compiler to assure his success? We need a more detailed look.

Switches of source within an entry are frequent. The entry for *oscitatio* (yawning) begins with an acknowledged passage from Boerhaave, but after the first paragraph, James abruptly switches to Quincy's translation of Santorio, at aphorism 74 (41). He also ignores the shift from Santorio's aphorism to Quincy's explanation of it, simply merging the two into continuous text. The only change in the aphorism itself is that James removes some but not all of the medial capitals. The beginning of the explanation, which deals with yawning and stretching and the loss of humours, excises some superfluous words, changing

> These a Person is most inclined to just after Sleep, and the Reason is, because during Sleep, a greater Quantity going off by the Pores of the Skin

to become

> To these a Person is most inclined just after Sleep, because, a greater Quantity going off by the Pores of the Skin

sensibly removing some repetition and restructuring this part of the sentence, but degrading the sense by deleting "during Sleep". Only two changes are made in the remainder of the paragraph: "such little Irritations as incite Yawning and Stretching" loses "little" but this section retains even the capitalisation. The other is to create a new paragraph where Quincy had none.

This section is now followed by a long paragraph with very little change apart from punctuation and a very few omissions and changes of word, and the familiar recasting of the opening phrases. James has no qualms about appropriating Quincy's (and hence Santorio's) first-person address: "I cannot easily pass by here, the vast Advantages of some little Exercises just after waking in the Morning." However, he is also happy to alter Quincy's wording to "I cannot here omit". At the end of this entry, after several more verbatim paragraphs, the source is finally simply identified as

"Sanctorius." The major editorial decision here is thus to take the aphorism and the explanation and decide to place them under the *oscitatio* head-word.

A reference to a source need not mean it has been quoted, since there are many entries in which it simply means that there is a parallel entry in the other source, particularly with the numerous botanical head-words. Botanical sources are particularly likely to be quite perfunctory entries and contain long lists of such cross-references, as in *rhodia radix*. *Rosa damascena* has ten such references, including both Ray and Tournefort. These references also tend to predominate numerically. Although there are many references to Boerhaave in the *Medicinal dictionary*, there are in fact almost twice as many to the botanist John Ray. References to another botanist, Tournefort, are slightly fewer but still outnumber Boerhaave, a ratio which seems to be consistent between the volumes.[165] The ratio for Philip Miller's influential *Gardener's dictionary* (1731), first published as *The gardeners and florists dictionary* (1724), then relatively recently republished, however increases by a factor of about ten between volumes 1 and 3.[166]

The translation of Simon Paulli's *A treatise on tobacco, tea, coffee, and chocolate* (James 1746e) shows familiar characteristics in that the section dealing with tobacco largely reproduces the material in the dictionary which James got from Nicholas Monardes, partly verbatim and partly in paraphrase, although not all of it is used. We can perhaps guess that the translation either preceded the dictionary or was done in the course of its compilation. After using some of the quote from Monardes in Paulli, the dictionary (s.v. *nicotiana*) entry breaks off into other matters.

We saw above that James claimed to regard dispensatories as not worthy of notice, let alone worth transcribing. A closer examination of his practice in the *Medicinal dictionary* shows that he did in fact refer to some of those he specifically mentioned as wishing to eschew (Bate, Fuller, Quincy, and Salmon), although not very frequently. References to Fuller in the *Medicinal dictionary* seem to be relatively few (*abortus*, *cantharides*, *cibus albus*, *diabetes*, and *pertussis* are examples), as are those to Bate(s) (*canis*, *creta*, *gutta rosacea*, *labrisulcium*, *mixtura simplex*, and *opium*, among others).[167] Salmon appears under *sperma ceti*. One of Bate's recipes is cited under *canis*, one of Fuller's is given under *cantharides*, and a second under *pertussis*. He is also mentioned under *abortus*. Quincy is in fact mentioned frequently—by and large these are allusions to the various pharmaceutical works, particularly the dispensatory, for entries such as *syrupus è meconio sive diacodion* and *laudanum*. On

---

165 While electronic word-searches are not very accurate, I assume that ratios are more reliable since counts for different names share the same inaccuracies, bar those for individual letters such as 'f' and long 's'.

166 Miller (1691–1771) had already produced *The gardeners and florists dictionary* in 1724.

167 The extent of the ECCO OS inaccuracy is indicated by the misreading of *suffer* for Fuller (twice), and *base* for Bate frequently. These numbers must be taken as merely indicative, since there are clearly tokens of such names that the search function does not find.

several occasions, James comments on Quincy's excellent judgement in pharmaceutical matters (see *diascordium*, for instance). *Carminantia* contains a longish quote from the entry for *carminative* from Quincy's *Lexicon physico-medicum*, which breaks off about half-way. I have not been able to identify a source for the last half of this entry, but since it contains a number of references (Etmüller, Forestus, Boerhaave, etc.), it may be a collage of those sources. The *Lexicon physico-medicum* passage is also a particularly harsh attack on obscurantist language which James lifts without question. Since Sanctorius is cited, as under *cathartica* and *cutis*, this may be through Quincy's translation. Another mention, this time of his dispensatory, occurs under *cicuta*, and he is quoted again under *mel*.[168] It goes without saying that there may be any number of unacknowledged quotations from all or any of these authors.

We have now seen sufficient to understand James's methods of compilation, which are typical of eighteenth century reference works. Sources are gathered, the extracts supplied with a relevant context, changes made, albeit inconsistently, to accommodate the extracts in the new work, some attempt is made to supply acknowledgements, although these may not be distinguishable from further references to the same subject matter elsewhere, and editorial and compositorial changes are made where necessary. Little in such composite entries may have originated with the compiler.

9.11 Johnson writes for *A medicinal dictionary*

Much scholarly ink has been spilt over Johnson's actual contribution to the dictionary. *The Times Literary Supplement* published letters on the authorship of the dedication on December 20, 1928 and January 4, 1929, the first of these by the novelist G. P. R. James (1799–1860), who had controversially claimed to have the manuscript in his grandfather's hand (Hazen 1973: 73). Scholars do generally agree on stylistic grounds, however, that Johnson wrote the dedication. Martin explains the life of Boerhaave thus: Johnson was asked by Edward Cave to write a biography of Boerhaave, who had recently died. Martin comments that "Again, he simply took a Latin eulogium on the physician published in Leiden and wrote another translation and an abridgement". This was first published anonymously in 1739, then reappeared slightly changed in the *Medicinal dictionary*, and still later in the *Universal magazine* for 1743. This material also fed into some of James's later publications as well (Martin 2008: 158).

Hazen's 1936 discussion of Johnson's contributions to the medical biographies in the *Medicinal dictionary* typifies the general tone of the scholarship on this matter. He finds it tempting to regard the list of lives at the end of the preface as a list of

---

168 Many Quincy references were found manually, not by the ECCO word search; another by eliminating the swash italic Q from the search term.

Johnsonian contributions, but rejects this conclusion on the grounds that Boerhaave is not included, and that "in defending his method of dealing with the biographical part Dr James happened to mention a list of articles by Johnson" (Hazen 1936: 457–458). The fact is, however, that listing Johnsonian contributions had nothing whatever to do with this list, the purpose of which was to explain to the disgruntled subscribers why the letter A was so long. The lives of the ancients had been promised in the proposals, and so must be included. In short, the search for Johnsonian contributions has obscured the function of this section of the preface and the problems raised by the nature of this publication.

9.12 Conclusion

The most realistic assessment of James's career is not that he worked as a publisher's hack, but that he amassed a great deal of material for the dictionary, which was duly published, and then published as much as possible of what was left out of that text. It seems possible that he had a team translating and transcribing for him, including Schwanberg and Maitland, and probably others. It also seems clear that he had the money to employ such a team. James was no innovator, either in medical or lexicographical terms. The dictionary stands far to the encyclopaedic end of the spectrum, but James seems not to have grasped the essential point about systematic, principled compression in encyclopaedias. His activities were seemingly driven more by profit and reputation than principle and an almost obsessive comprehensiveness. He was certainly a medical mercenary. It might be better to see James's work not so much in the light of subsequent English medical dictionaries, but in terms of the massive *Dictionnaire des sciences médicales* published by C.L.F. Panckoucke in no less than sixty volumes (see Adelon). Panckoucke had worked with Diderot, and continued his work after the master's death.

To conclude, Robert James seems to have been caught between the Scylla of recording and preserving knowledge and the Charybdis of compressing and managing it. To take Yeo slightly out of context, he seems to have regarded his dictionary as both a place where he could store "a stable body of knowledge from major ... authors" (106), and as a file into which new knowledge could be inserted, but not as a store which had to be severely edited, pruned, and cut down to make it more compendious and accessible. The inevitable result was an overgrowth which the readers could benefit from intellectually only with difficulty or even manage physically. James insisted on keeping as much as possible, while the extremely compendious and forward-looking dictionary by Quincy continued both to sell and to be re-edited, prolonging its career for more than a century as James's own languished largely unsold for decades on the bookseller's shelves. James's dictionary may have provided discovery for the practitioner, but doing so in haste would have been all but impossible.

10 "Careful" John Barrow (fl. 1735–1773?)

John Barrow, whose life is at best shadowy, published his *Dictionarium medicum universale: or, a new medicinal dictionary* in 1749. The ODNB offers a perfunctory account of Barrow which shows that, having begun life as a mathematics teacher, he subsequently compiled many reference and historical books working as a publisher's hack. Taylor (1966: 169) suggests a last floruit date of 1774, and the will of a John Barrow, described as "Gentleman of Fleet Street", who died in 1773, lodged in the National Archives (PROB 11/991/260) may identify our author. Barrow's description of himself on the title page of his *Dictionarium medicum universale* is as a "chymist", which does not quite square with the generally accepted account of him as a mathematics teacher and expert in navigation. It seems possible that he knew Robert James, since he may be the chemist who was on the panel deputed to determine the composition of James's fever powder when the patent for it was challenged, and may have been a patient of James in 1747 (Anon: 61; James 1748: 14).

Barrow's name was associated with a number of reference works, histories, and other compendia through the middle of the century. For some he appears to have been the compiler and for others an editor. These works included the *Dictionarium polygraphicum* (1735) and *Navigatio Britannica* of 1750, and *A new and universal dictionary of arts and sciences* (1751).

[169] His background in mathematics is often mentioned, as is the care he takes over his work. The brief introduction to the *Dictionarium polygraphicum*, probably by Barrow (Yeo 2001: 64), takes up the familiar notions of the practicality of the dictionary format and the desire to obviate the need for a much larger number of books: "We have cast this work into the form of a Dictionary, because we have judged such a disposition the most methodical of any" (Preface). Barrow also appreciates that such a text must be concise and to the point: "and as we are sensible that clearness of expression is essential … we have always endeavoured to treat our subject with … perspicuity" (Preface). Thus he points out that his material has been "digested into … an easy and regular series of instructions" and that "the expence of purchasing, and the tedious fatigue of consulting a vast number of volumes on these subjects will be rendered unnecessary" (Preface).

10.1 The *Dictionarium medicum universale*

The sub-title of Barrow's medical dictionary, "a new medicinal dictionary", signals its close relation to the earlier dictionary by Robert James. The preface claims that James's dictionary is the only such work to have explained the meaning of both

---

169 Loveland takes a somewhat more skeptical and cautious view of his career; see 2007: 172.

https://doi.org/10.1515/9783110639186-010

ancient and modern medical terms, but Barrow at no point declares that his work is a compendium of James's, as indeed it is. By contrast, he makes continual mention of his reliance on the "best authors"; in fact, this means those used by James himself and those which provided the limited number of additions he makes to James's work. Barrow claims that his etymologies and derivations are from the best authors, but again they are James's. By far the most extensive change to James's dictionary is the deletions which Barrow makes. Given Barrow's work over many years as a publisher's hack and editor, this looks like an attempt to extract some market value from James's unsuccessful and probably hugely expensive dictionary. Barrow's medical dictionary had only a brief life; there was a second edition printed for T. Longman, and C. Hitch; and A. Millar, 1754, preserved in an apparently unique copy in the Philson Library of the University of Auckland in New Zealand. The second edition makes no change from the first.[170]

Detailed examination shows that Barrow's dictionary word-list is simply a cut-down version of James's, and that his entries themselves are James's by and large with all the encyclopaedic and scientific material expunged.[171] Barrow essentially retained the linguistic information and deleted the rest, making his entries characteristically very short, the longest being *generatio*, which exceptionally runs for eight and a bit pages. James's spellings are retained, with the proviso about errors explained below. We must also recall however that Barrow also used other resources, such as for *adiposa vena*, which is verbatim from John Quincy, and that in using James, he incorporated James's debts as well.

The dictionary is characterized by short, markedly lexical entries, which makes the eight-page entry for *generatio* stand out as exceptional, this alone representing no less than 1.37 percent of a 584 page work, By contrast, *animal* gets a mere nine half-column lines, *arteria* barely two pages, and *aqua* and its derivatives only nineteen lines. The entry for *nervus* (nerve) takes up nearly five pages, and *oculus* (the eye) almost four, while *hepar* occupies two full pages, and the intestines (*intestina*) not quite two and a half. His usual practice is to consolidate entries for the major organs and other parts into a single entry, usually of about this length, as in *nasus* (nose) and *lympha* (the lymph glands). The entry for *vena* with its sub-entries is also extremely long, if it is to be taken as a single entry. Barrow's presentation seems to vacillate somewhat between treating it a as a single entry, and listing all the various veins as individual head-words.

Barrow does however make changes to James, including omitting many headwords and creating new ones from James's text, particularly for botanical and anatomical entries. A botanical entry in James with a number of sub-headings or italicised binomials in the text may, for instance, provide Barrow with several new head-

---

170 I am most grateful to Stephen Innes of the Philson Library for comparing the editions.
171 For further insights into Barrow's methods, see Loveland 2007, especially 175–186.

words. It is not always easy to see either logic or consistency in what he does, but some patterns are apparent. While many obscure plant-names are deleted, others are created, particularly from entries on plants with many well-known species. Barrow seems to remove plants, minerals, fish and objects which have no obvious medical relevance, such as *aries*, a ram, or *croumata*, musical tones; there is also a tendency to remove diminutives irrespective of meaning. A curious change occurs under the massive entry in James for *anatomy* (anatome) where Barrow's dictionary has only the brief gloss "Anatomy, or the dissection of a body," but James is in fact even briefer, simply glossing it "Anatomy".

Barrow claims to have specified the use of each official plant as well as how to detect adulterated drugs. He also fulfils his promise to explain usage as we see under entries like *faba*, *lilium album*, *moschus*, and *raphanus*. He makes specific mention of including the terms used by Paracelsus and his followers, but most of this comes via James, an example being *ressella*, a Paracelsian term meaning "that which removes heat", a rather rambling entry in James which Barrow improves somewhat.

The names of people are quite consistently omitted, some examples being Boerhaave, Eristratus, Galenus, Hippocrates, Mesue, Nicolaus Myrepsis, and Paracelsus. This does not apply however to words describing particular types of people. *Sedigitus* (someone who has six fingers) has been omitted, while others such as *moneres* (a melancholic person wanting solitude), *orchotamus* (one who performs castration), and *scorpiodectos* (a person stung by a scorpion) remain. Some of the names of plants, stones, and other simples have been omitted, as have some names of medicines, possibly because they were seen as outdated, but Barrow's medical knowledge does not seem to have been great—he is in fact the only medical lexicographer since Traheron represented in this book who is not known to have had medical training. He does seem to have omitted some terms with no very obvious medical relevance, such as *æglia* (shield), *carmin* (a pigment derived from cochineal), *flagellatio* (flagellation), *intritum* (minced meat), or *schoenobata* (walking, dancing on a rope/running a race), and others. On the other hand, it is unclear why *aurea alexandrina* (an opiate or antidote), *cerusiana* (a compound medicine), *lithocolum* (making a stone pass the urinary passage) or *selinusia terra* (a medicinal earth) should have been omitted.

Barrow makes a total of 142 additions to James's word-list. An analysis of these shows that 48 were sourced from John Quincy. Of these, 26 could be described as verbatim, allowing for the odd minor omission, addition, or other change, while another 20 showed some degree of reliance on him. At least four were paraphrases. Only one, *extraneous*, had been genuinely re-edited, being both shortened and recast into a numbered entry from a text-only entry. Eighty-two were clearly not from Quincy, and a few more could not be determined one way or the other, as the entries were too laconic to be confident that Quincy had to be the source. Thus dependence on Quincy among these additions runs at about 37 percent, and there is still a considerable number to source. Two, *gastrocnemii* and *metacarpius*, were ascribed to the anatomy by Jacques-Bénigne Winslow (1733 I, III: 478), and were found to be used verbatim. It is of still more interest to note that twenty-two of these head-words are unambiguously in English form.[172] Of these, only five, *cutaneous diseases*, *digester*, *hetrogenous* [sic], *parasitical plants* and *technical* were not from Quincy. One, *odoriferous*, had only a one-word gloss, so that the possible sources are many.

Other terms which are in James are also to be found verbatim in Quincy, including *depressores labii superioris*, *generatio*, and *genio-hyoides*. The entry for *generatio* ends with an ascription to Keill, not to Quincy. James uses a great deal of what is in Quincy in this entry, although there is other material, but there is no ascription to Keill. Most of *genio-hyoides* in James is from Quincy, with some minor adjustments.

We can also learn something from the overall patterns and a macro-analysis of Barrow. His deletions from James are high in A, sometimes running at over fifty percent early in that letter, but they decline as he moves into B, and are at their lowest at about COR-. The fifty percent rate is exceeded eight times early in A, but only three times in the rest of the alphabet. The rate then varies at a relatively low level before picking up somewhat and being spread more evenly from about REM-. By contrast, the rate of additions is almost nil early in A, begins to pick up about ANC- and rises slowly to a peak at about LAB-, culminating in a very large block of additions for *lapis*. From there it declines gradually until a final increase, again about REM-. In short, it is roughly the inverse of the deletions graph for the first two-thirds of the alphabet, but tends to mirror it thereafter. This may suggest that Barrow was over-zealous in his omissions early in the task, anxious to keep the work within limits and unwilling to add, but eventually found a balance. The demands of the publishers concerning length may well also have been a factor.

---

172 These are adenography, cephalic vein, culmiformis plants, cutaneous diseases, digester, equivocal generation, essential oils, essential properties, essential salts, etherial oil, expressed oils, extraneous, gelatinous, hetrogenous [sic], intumescence, odoriferous, obstuents [sic], parasitical plants, radicle, technical, and vegitables.

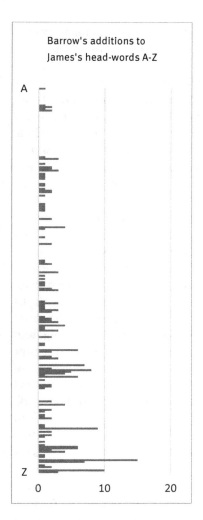
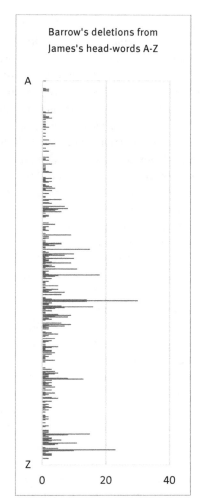

Fig. 7: The overall pattern of Barrow's deletions from and additions to James.

Recalling Barrow's claims about his care as an editor, we see that the head-words in his dictionary contain about 380 discrepancies from James, the great majority being errors of various kinds. Even allowing for some variation in endings and shifts of head-words from Latin to Greek and vice-versa, this is a considerable number. Simple typographical error accounts for some, such as *gymnastica—gymnatica* in Barrow (henceforth B); *ferrum equinum—ferru equinum* in B, and *plinthitis—plinthtis* in B; *va-nus—varus* in B. We also find *mimosa—minosa* in B, which might have been spotted by a reader with more learning, as might *fungus esculentus—fungus escunentus* in B. *Papever* (B) for *papaver* is also an obvious mistake, and a particularly egregious error is *isopipon* (B) for James's *isopyron*.

Some other obvious errors include letter doubling, such as in *trepanatio—trepannatio* in B and *grumus—grummus* in B; misreadings such as *matzatli—matzatti* in B; some of these seem quite ignorant, including *erigerum—erioerum* in B and *diglosson—diglossom* in B, where surely a reader or editor with a competent knowledge of medical terminology would have picked up the discrepancies. On some occasions, the reverse occurs, and a more familiar form is read into the original, e.g., *superligula—superlingua* in B; *gastroepiploica—gastroepiplotica* in B. Other errors include *masculinitas—masculinatus* in B again, an obvious error in Latin, as with *germinatio—germenatio* in B; *calendula palustris—galendula palustris* in B. Syllabic doublings also occur as with *gerocomice—gerocomcomice* in B. The omission or addition of 'r' seems very frequent, as in *idechtrum—idechtium* in B or *glischrocholos—glischrochrolos* in B. Other elisions also occur, such as *rododendion—rododenion* in B; *pareira brava—preira brava* in B, while one example of an omission which might have been picked up by a more expert eye is *pampiniforme corpus—pampiforme corpus* in B. Another source of error appears to be eye-skip, as with *mochlica—mochlia* in B, where the transcriber's or compositor's eye may have skipped to the previous entry (also *mochlia*). Two curious examples of repetition are that *epaphæresis* is repeated after *eperlanus* with nearly the same definition, and that *metacarpus* is entered a second time after *metatarsius*. The overall picture then is one of careless editing, compositing, and checking despite Barrow's protestations; this in a work in which the presswork is poor in any case. The publishers, Longman, Hitch and Millar, were certainly capable of better. The fact that most of these errors did not trigger a change in the alphabetical order where that would have been appropriate suggests haste and slipshod work. Loveland hints that the dictionary may not in fact be Barrow's since he does not sign it "Dr John Barrow" (207: 172), but the range of errors give us no reason to think that the compiler had to have been a physician, and Barrow's appellations vary across his works.

The question of James's definitions and the way they are used in Barrow is a large one which lies somewhat beyond the immediate scope of the present study. To cite a few instances, however, Barrow's definition of *bdellium* is: "the name of a gum of a reddish-brown colour, deeper than myrrh, and of a tougher and more tenacious consistence". This definition, which is not from Quincy, is not found until the second page of the James entry. *Acrochordon* represents only the paraphrased bare bones of James's entry. *Vena azygos* is simply the first part of James's entry verbatim, inappropriately taking over a first-person reference as well: "I have seen this vein extremely large, resembling the trunk of the inferior Cava"—a passage which James takes from Winslow's *An anatomical exposition* II, 35, a nice example of a migratory first person.

There are also entries which bear little or no relation to either Quincy or James. That for *incubus* contains only a very brief verbal echo of Quincy in the notion that something sits or rides upon the patient, the rest of the entry being unrelated to James's much longer one offering a detailed description of the symptoms, such as numbness, paleness, sweating, and a sense of suffocation. He also suggests the circumstances under which it occurs, the dangers which it poses to the patient, and its relation to epilepsy. He cites the medical observations of Jodocus Lommius, first published in 1560 in Antwerp and a work which was still frequently re-issued in the eighteenth century, as well as citing Paulus Ægineta and Cœlius Aurelianus. Another instance is that Barrow reduces his entry for *mania* to a brief derivation and the single-word gloss "madness", whereas James's entry runs for almost eighteen full columns, and includes a long section on melancholy, at which point the page-heading shifts from MAN to MEL, and then back to MAN to complete the entry. *Melancholia* has a separate entry further on which, rather than repeating what appeared under *mania*. describes a species of this complaint, erratic melancholy.[173] Barrow does associate erratic melancholy with lycanthropy as later medical lexicographers such as Parr do, but James makes the connexion clear under *lycanthropy*. In short, Barrow misses this obvious lexical connexion altogether by not attending to James's entries sufficiently, while James might have considered the rationalisation of his entries more carefully.

Barrow's dictionary had no further perceptible influence on the medical lexicon or its interpretation and dissemination. The list has a heavy bias towards plants and minerals, rather than diseases or anatomy, which to some extent reflects his reliance on James, and it almost seems that he has an agenda about preserving knowledge of Greek and Arabic terms in the medical lexicon. All in all, it seems not unfair to say that in lexicographical terms Barrow is to James as Johan Scapula's abridgment, the *Lexicon græcolatinum* of 1580, was to Estienne's massive Greek-Latin dictionary, the *Thesaurus graecæ linguæ* of 1572, with the proviso that where Scapula's dictionary became a standard and was widely used, Barrow's disappeared into obscurity fairly quickly, and probably deservedly.

---

173 There are almost verbatim extracts from this entry in Bryan Cornwell 1787: 95–96.

11 George Motherby (1731–1793)

George Motherby's medical dictionary is apparently best remembered for quite incidental matters such as being the first to list the word placebo,
[174] and for being an illustrated dictionary; circumstances which are not at all unusual in the subsequent records of such works. It has generally been neglected, but there is a much fuller and more recent account of Motherby's lexicographical work in a recent work by Elisabetta Lonati (2017). Little is known of Motherby's life, but he is usually mentioned as living in Highgate, visited Königsberg in about 1770 where he practised variolation, and his death occurred in Beverley in 1793 (Duncan 1794: 480–481).

A new medical dictionary was first printed by J. Johnson and others in 1775. A second edition of the work appeared in 1785, and a third in 1791, this time expanded by "George Wallis, M. D. S. M. S. Lecturer on the Theory and Practice of Physic, London", the work now incorporating six additional copperplate engravings. Wallis identified himself as the reviser of Motherby on the title-page of his own *The art of preventing diseases*, which appeared in 1793. A fourth edition appeared in 1795, once again corrected by Wallis. His own work, retitled as *The complete family physician* was issued in the same year, with Wallis's description appropriately updated to identify him as the editor of the "last" version of Motherby. The fifth edition of Motherby appeared in 1801.

The author's intentions are set out in the preface, which claims that this volume will end each article by citing a selection of references to "the most eminent writers on the subject" ([iii]), a means of facilitating the reader's access to information. While arguing that "systematic productions" are most illuminating in the learning process, alphabetical order is best suited to rapid reference and refreshing the practitioner's memory ([iii]). He then embarks upon a lengthy account of the virtues of both the ancient writers and the "Arabians", while acknowledging the great strides made by the moderns, including Vesalius, Harvey, and Boyle. The preface concludes with an account of the content of the entries, which stresses convenience in searching as well as concision and clarity, and rejects "wanton variety" in naming. Motherby commits himself to using "that name which is most in use" (vi), apparently irrespective of its etymology or derivation and cutting through the familiar question of whether a term was 'barbarous' or not, as well as the linguistic probity of the form used. Motherby is thus at pains to assist the busy practitioner in the pressing demands on his time rather than stressing his learning and comprehensiveness.

Motherby's dictionary seems to have established itself quite quickly and to have shared the market in the last quarter of the eighteenth century with the revamped Quincy in the form which it took with the appearance of its ninth and tenth editions.

---

174 See Shapiro./Shapiro (1997).

https://doi.org/10.1515/9783110639186-011

It was then superseded in the early nineteenth by the rapid appearance of at least three major works–the Edinburgh dictionary (Morris 1807), that by Bartholomew Parr (1809), and the Hooper revisions of Quincy, all of which lie beyond the chronology of this book.

The work appears priced at seven guineas in the catalogue of William Bent published in 1779, and again in a sale catalogue for several libraries issued by Henry Payne in 1780, "new and very neat", for £1.11.6. Motherby and his dictionary get a lengthy mention in a long footnote on pages 137–139 of the treatise on rheumatism and gout by Thomas Dawson (ca. 1725–1782), published in 1781, in which he claims to have been somewhat misinterpreted by Motherby, albeit inadvertently. The Bodleian Library announced in 1782 that it had purchased a copy for £1.10.0 (Bodleian Library 1782: 1). The 1782 treatise by Sir John Elliot, M.D. (1736–1786) contains a puff at the end for Motherby's dictionary which picks up on the familiar notion that a dictionary of this kind is a substitute for a number of individual volumes by quoting the *Critical review* assessment (see below). Thomas Prosser (fl. 1782), while pointing out an error in the dictionary, does claim that it is a work "of acknowledged merit" (2). Taking no expression of displeasure as a positive, mentions of Motherby generally seem to be approving (see Moffat 1785?: xiv). John Burrows reprints a letter he received from Motherby "the author of the Medical Dictionary", addressed from Highgate and dated August 1785, in his *New practical essay on cancers* (1785: 107–108). The letter approves Burrows' treatment of scirrhous cancers, and refers several patients to him.

The dictionary also appears regularly in sale catalogues during the 1780s, including the libraries of several physicians, such as Sir Richard Jebb (1729–1787), whose collection seems to have included a large number of dictionaries of various kinds, not just medical ones. Copies in the libraries of divines, however, are overwhelmingly the most numerous. On the other side of the Atlantic, copies had been acquired by the Library Company of Philadelphia by 1789 (Library Company of Philadelphia 1789: 261), the Pennsylvania Hospital by 1790, where it was not for lending (Pennsylvania Hospital 1790: 5, 8), and the New York Society Library by 1793 (New York Society Library 1793: 58). His work had also penetrated into the pages of less scholarly works, appearing in *The new family herbal; or, domestic physician* by the surgeon William Meyrick in 1790, and being cited at least six times.

In 1786, the second edition was now being sold by Johnson for two guineas bound, as witness the advertisement in *Elements of the branches of natural philosophy connected with medicine* by Sir John Elliot. By 1788, *The new royal cyclopædia, and encyclopædia* describes him as "the learned and judicious Dr. Motherby" (s.v. *derivative*), in discussing the word chemistry (Howard 1788), while a treatise on the effects of particular treatments on tropical diseases by John Peter Wade (d. 1802) published in 1792 incorporates a case from Motherby; s.v. *jecur*; (309–310).

The surgeon Jesse Foot, a declared and vocal enemy of John Hunter, made use of the authority ascribed to dictionaries in taking exception to Hunter's use of the word trance for the then more normal ecstasy. Foot asks

> What author has defined it ... Where, I ask his admirers, am I to look for the information which he was in possession of ... I have never read a medical case which authenticates, a Trance, and know not where to find one:—neither Motherby, nor Wallis after him, have given the word a place, even in their medical dictionaries (Foot 1794: 125–126),

thus conceding Motherby and Wallis authority in this matter, but conveniently over-looking the fact that such a term was unlikely to appear as a head-word for precisely the reason he offers. The small surgical dictionary produced by Benjamin Lara (1770–1848), which has been examined in detail in Chapter eight on surgical dictionaries, also mentions Motherby in positive terms and indicates its reliance on him (1796: 4). Meanwhile, sporadic references to Motherby continued up to the end of the century.

11.1 Reception of Motherby's dictionary

We do have the advantage of three contemporaneous reviews of Motherby's diction-ary, one written shortly after its first publication, as well as two of Wallis's revision. The review of the first edition (by Johnson [pseudonym]) is largely given over to citing the lengthy entry for asthma as an example of the best of the dictionary, but it does still offer some useful general comments. The provision of the long quote seems to assume that the reader will immediately know why it is good, since the actual reasons are not enumerated. While not all that extensive, the review alludes to the value of "a system digested in the form of a Dictionary" (327), praises the work for the fullness and accuracy of the entries, as well as for being up to date, and recommends it to "the gentlemen of the faculty" (*Critical review* 44, 1777: 333). The number of works pub-lished on the various branches of medicine makes it all but impossible to keep up with them, and the review praises Motherby, the "judicious author" (328), for his work. It also points out that he had the expert assistance of people "conversant in the different provinces of physic" (318), which the reviewer sees as essential in such an undertaking. Previous works of this kind, the reviewer asserts, had suffered from be-ing the work of a single individual, a shortcoming which Motherby has avoided. While this is not strictly true, as we have seen in the case of James, it is true that James had not sought expert medical assistance as far as we know, concentrating simply on assistance in translation and importing the expertise and repute of those already pub-lished. This is a major reason, according to the reviewer, for the superiority of Motherby's work. It is also claimed that Motherby's dictionary can also be used as a substitute for volumes which the practitioner has no opportunity to consult for him-self, another familiar virtue which harks back to the advantages of such compilations outlined by Ephraim Chambers and others.

The second, signed Robinson [pseudonym], appeared in 1785. It is again a positive review, concentrating on the material changes and additions to the dictionary and omitting the author's intentions and methods since they were originally mentioned in the first review. The review does however nicely sum up the usefulness of a dictionary of this kind as a ready reference guide when time and resources are short: "The chief use of a dictionary is, to explain, in a familiar manner, the terms of the art, and to assist the practitioner, who wants immediate assistance, and cannot turn to the more elaborate systems, or is unable from his situation to procure them" (476). The review mentions several material improvements, notably the use made of Cullen.

The third review (1791: 30–37), which reads more like a review article and is again signed Johnson [pseudonym], is longer and far more explicit about the advantages of the dictionary. It also provides such things as a historical review and assessment of medical dictionaries, something unexampled up to this period, and rare even for lexical dictionaries. It also draws some distinctions which have proved useful in the history of lexicography, including that between a lexicon and a glossary in pointing out that the earliest classical medical dictionaries such as those by Erotian and Galen are largely glossaries explaining hard words in Hippocrates. The reviewer also makes the point that medical dictionaries down into the sixteenth century remained "little more than explanations of words" (30), ascribing the addition of medical information to a dictionary to Blancard (Blanchard). As the history of medical lexicography is explicated, the reviewer posits two types of dictionary, the one consisting of "naked definitions" and the other of "minute discussions", Blancard generally representing the one, and James the other. He finds that Motherby's compilation sits somewhere in between these extremes (32).

Evidence of the positive reception of Motherby appears across the Atlantic in Samuel Stearns's *The American herbal* of 1801, where he is quoted a number of times, generally approvingly. In commenting on Motherby in his preface, however, he perhaps inadvertently identifies precisely what a medical lexicographer must do to contain the scope of his material: "Dr. *Motherby* published an excellent medical dictionary; but in treating of diseases, he breaks off, as it were in the midst of the story, and directs to the perusal of other authors" (14). Stearns's expectation of a more encyclopaedic narrative could not be met.[175]

11.2 Motherby's sources

Since Motherby's work was generally well-received, and he made obvious attempts to ensure that it was up to date, it is of interest to determine the source of his entries.

---

175 Stearns has a single reference to Robert James (s.v. *snipe*), and one to Quincy, whom he spells 'Quinsey', s.v. *sun-dew*.

Looking at the number of entries in each letter in Motherby by comparison with those in James and Barrow offers some clues.

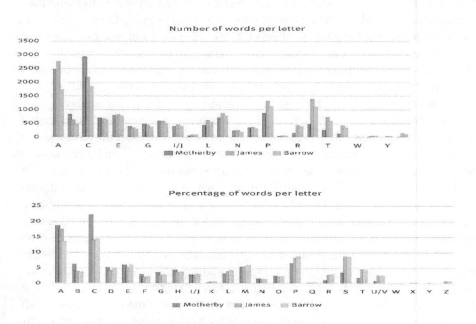

Fig. 8: Letter frequencies and percentages in Motherby, James, and Barrow

Charting these numbers shows a striking pattern. First, the similarity of the word-lists suggests a dependent relation between these dictionaries. The word-lists are largely aligned after the first three letters, the letter A being larger in James and B and C in Motherby being rather larger than James. There is a slight excess in Motherby in the letter D, but the letters move in close synchrony down to I/J, at which point Motherby begins to lag. This discrepancy becomes very noticeable from Q to the end of the alphabet and is extreme in S, where Motherby has only about 30 percent of the entries in James. It looks like a classic case of 'alphabet fatigue' (see Osselton 2007), and may simply have to do with the compiler's state of health.

The raw numbers of each are Motherby 13157, James 15651, and Barrow 12654. Expressed as percentages, the chart shows that James is reduced overall, but considerably so in A, B, C, P, R, and S, by and large the largest letters in Latin. Correspondingly, Motherby has increased somewhat, especially early in the alphabet. Motherby's decline in the latter half of the alphabet is still apparent, however.

The actual entry texts show that while Motherby is quite heavily dependent on the James/Barrow word-list (see examples in Lonati 2017: 62–63), he does exploit their entry-text rather more freely and flexibly, cutting James's text extensively, and being prepared to make his own additions, sometimes by way of bringing his entries up to date. Neither does he necessarily accept their definitions, again demonstrating that entries in medical dictionaries are not necessarily treated as a head-word/definition wholes. Motherby's methods may be illustrated by a couple of examples. James defines *abductio* as:

> A species of fracture, when a Bone near the joint is so divided transversely, that the extremities of the fractured Bone recede from each other.
> These fractures are said by Galen to be made χαυληδòν, that is, in the manner the stalk of a plant is broken.
> Abductio, in Celsius Aurelianus signifies a Strain. It is mentioned as one of the causes of Ischiadic and Psoadic pains... Morbor. Chymicorum, l. v. c. 1. Item vehemens Abductio vel raptus in Exercito factus.

This is reduced by Barrow simply to the first sentence in James, to which he adds a derivation from Latin "(of ab from, and duco, L. I draw)". Motherby, however, retains the allusion to Celsus, as well as offering a 'proper' meaning:

> a species of fracture, when a bone near the joint is so divided transversely that the extremities recede from each other. Celsius Aurelianus uses this word for a strain. Abductio properly signifies, leading from or drawing away.

Gas is a significant entry, especially since as Motherby was preparing this entry, the chemistry of gases and the terminology applied to them was undergoing a revolution which put paid to the phlogiston theory and established new terms such as hydrogen and oxygen.[176] James declares that gas:

> is a Term coin'd by Helmont, and signifies, in general, a Spirit incapable of Coagulation; such as proceeds from fermented Wine. In particular, it has various Significations; thus Gas vitale is the Spirit of our Life, the Light and the Balsam which preserves from Corruption, Complex. & Mist. N. 42. The Gas pingue Sulphureum is what is suddenly mortal, being lethiferous Exhalations, arising principally in Caves and Mines. Gas sulphuris, the Gas or Spirit of Sulphur, is made by burning Sulphur under a glass Bell, set over a Vessel of Water, till the Water is sufficiently impregnated with the sulphur. The Gas Sylvestre is that invisible and incoercible Spirit, which arises from vegetable Juices under Fermentation. See Alcohol, and Bufo. Helmont makes several other Distinctions of Gas; as the Gas Ventosum, which is mere Air; the Gas siccum, which is Sublimate, de Flatibus, N. 4. the Gas Salium, and the Gas Fructuum, which are mere elementary Water, Complex. & Mist. N. 37, 38.

By comparison, the entries in Barrow and Motherby are much shorter. Barrow writes:

> a Term coined by Helmont, and signifies a spirit incapable of coagulation, or the most volatile part of any thing

---

176 For more on phlogiston, see Woodcock 2005.

thus quoting most of James's first sentence, but making a small definitional addition. Motherby has:

> From geist, which in the German language is spirit. The word gas is an invention of Helmont's; in general it is a spirit incapable of coagulation, such as rises from fermenting liquors, &c. it is now called fixed air.[177]

Thus Motherby paraphrases part of James, but makes an important addition. Joseph Priestley's *Experiments and observations on different kinds of air*, the work Motherby mentions, appeared in 1774, although Priestley had already used the term fixed air in his *Directions for impregnating water with fixed air* published in 1772. Motherby, who also derived his etymology for gas from Priestley's *Experiments and observations on different kinds of air* (1774: 3) a work expanded upon in 1779, certainly kept his reading up to date.

In the case of *lympha*, Barrow adds a little to the definition ("properly water, but, in anatomy it signifies a fine fluid separated in the body from the mass of blood, and contained in peculiar vessels"), then deletes a quote from Keill in James, and a long paragraph on the use of lymph, but quotes the next three paragraphs verbatim, deletes the next four on the dispositions of the lymphatics, then uses the rest with at least one minor deletion as well. Motherby's approach is radically different, offering only one short paragraph, which ends with a reference to Boerhaave. This paragraph does not occur in James or Barrow or, for that matter, Quincy or Blancard.

The position seems to be that Motherby relies on the James/Barrow word-list, but weeds it out and makes some additions. Motherby also takes over some of James's etymologies, as shown by Lonati (2017: 62–63). He relies less on the James/Barrow text, however, and is happy to change it completely at times. Now and then there is some loose paraphrase, particularly of James, but this is by no means a dominant percentage of his text. More research remains to be done, a task now begun by Lonati (2017), but sampling suggests that Motherby's verbatim reliance on these dictionary sources may be no more than ten to fifteen percent. This dictionary then represents a step forward in both contemporaneous relevance and scope since it often incorporates quite recent findings and literature and is larger and more comprehensive than Quincy but not nearly so unwieldy as James.

11.3 Motherby and contemporaneous medical writing

The extent to which George Motherby kept up with recent developments is also of interest. The entry for puerperal fever shows that he was at least in this case very up-to-date. Appearing under the head-word PUERPERALIS FEBRIS, this has been chosen

---

177 See Priestley 1774: 3.

not as necessarily representative of Motherby's lexicographical practice, but as illustrating how he dealt with a relatively recent medical concept in *A new medical dictionary*. This entry is particularly, indeed, strikingly up-to-date. Whether this is typical of the rest of the dictionary must however await further research. I will refer throughout to 'puerperal fever', despite the various appellations it receives in the primary sources, including childbed fever, *sepsis puerperalis*, *febris lochialis*, and milk fever, and despite the fact that this designation has been attacked as misleading from time to time (Loudon 2000: 8–10).[178]

The name itself derives from the Latin *puerperium*, or a woman's 'lying -in', despite the fact that the disease almost always appears a few days after the delivery. The term was apparently first used by Francois Mauriceau (1637–1709) in 1668 in Latin, and is first recorded in English in a work by Edward Strother (1675–1737) in his *Criticon februm* of 1716 (Loudon 2000: 14–15). The concept of this disease and its name are however essentially phenomena of the mid-eighteenth century, despite having been sporadically mentioned before that, so that Motherby could not cite older and classical authorities, as he often did.

Hippocrates thought that the cause was the suppression of the lochia (the postpartum discharge) (Lea 1910: 1), a view which proved to be very persistent. The disease was widely recognized as a scourge by the mid to late eighteenth century, seemingly with the appearance of the lying-in hospitals (maternity hospitals) about the middle of the century.[179] While these institutions probably increased the incidence of contagion, they also provided the opportunity for observation of the nature and course of the disease by trained professionals (Loudon 2000: 16–17), although what they saw was often determined by what they expected to see.

The disease itself had a high mortality rate and inflicted terrible suffering on its victims. It began with violent shivering fits within a few days of the birth, proceeded to intense visceral pain, usually because of peritonitis, a symptom which often ended with a brief period of relief as the victim became gangrenous (Loudon 2000: 5–6). Septicaemia was frequently a cause of death. Relatives and physicians alike thought that the hapless sufferer would recover, but death was inevitable in such circumstances.

Theories about the cause other than suppression of the lochia abounded throughout the eighteenth century. These varied from the influence of putrid miasmas, Paré's notion of cold air getting into the uterine cavity, inflammation of the womb (Mercatus) (Lea 1910: 1), 'translation of the milk', a notion deriving from the observation of streptococcal pus in post-mortem examinations which conveniently but erroneously linked the complaint with milk fever, and other far-fetched notions (Loudon 2000: 18–19). Milk metastasis was first suggested by Nicolas Puzos (1686–1753; see Lea 1910:

---

178 For a near-contemporary list, see Giambattista Borsieri de Kanilfeld 1800–1803 vol. 2, 178.

179 Such as Queen Charlotte's and Chelsea Hospital, 1732, and the British Lying-in Hospital 1749.

1–2), and was widely accepted. Willis and Sydenham in the late seventeenth century continued to accept the Hippocratic view. Most agreed in the eighteenth century that it was epidemic in nature, but the discovery that it was linked with the occurrence of erysipelas had to wait until the observations of these diseases passing between patients, midwives, nurses and physicians by Alexander Gordon in 1795. Gordon had to admit that he had been responsible for some cases himself (Loudon 2000: 24). The disease was widely recognised as contagious by the 1840s, and the final connection was established by Ignaz Semmelweiss in Vienna, who adopted the practice of scrupulous disinfection, drastically reducing the rate of infection (Lea 1910: 4–5).

What then does Motherby make of this disease, recently identified in the sense that a name (or names) had been ascribed to it? His entry is copious, citing five authorities for his information. These are:

Thomas Denman (1773): *Essay on the puerperal fever*
Nathaniel Hulme (1772): *A treatise on the puerperal fevers*
John Leake (1772): *Practical observations on the child-bed fever*
Charles White (1773): *A treatise on the management of pregnant and lying-in women*
Thomas Kirkland (1774): *A treatise on child-bed fevers*

The list clearly represents most of the available and up-to-date knowledge on the subject. We should recall that Motherby's dictionary was printed in the year immediately following Kirkland's publication. There are other references to Kirkland as well, under a number of head-words and on various topics, including *calidum innatum*, *cerebrum*, *fractura*, *irritabilis*, *luxation*, and *lycoperdon vulgare*.

References to authorities are either in-text or appear at the end. Lists of authors cited at the end of a longer article, such as *arthritis*, *antithenar*, *bronchialis glandulæ*, *cardialgia*, are supplementary and frequently not those cited in the article itself. Thus under *castratio*, Sharp, Le Dran and Heister are cited at the end, but the text mentions Barnard, Gooch, and Hunter. This is only a tendency, however, there being exceptions; St Yves is mentioned both in the text of the entry for *cataracta* and at the end.

11.4 Later editions and Wallis's revisions

The second edition of Motherby makes some obvious changes. A typographical improvement is that the meanings of Latin and Greek words are now in italics, and the second edition uses italics in the texts for the head-words or its gloss where the first edition did not, although this is not consistent. Hence under *mania* "madness" is italicised in the text, as is *mania* itself.

Words for things with no apparent medical use or relevance are kept. *Bronte*, claimed by James to have no relevance to medicine has been retained. Motherby's entry *algoides*, a plant mentioned by John Ray, comments on its lack of any medical use.

Authorities have been brought up to date, and deference paid to the most significant. An obvious addition is the use of Linné as an authority. *Alkakengi, brunella, cepa, mandragora, psyllium, ptarmica, trifolium paludosum*, among many others, all make use of Linné. Another new authority is William Cullen, again frequently mentioned, as under *cachexia, comata, mania* and *ptyalismos*.

Many entries show some editing, in general adding to the text in a variety of ways; *alkakengi* adds a note on species with medical use; *allantois* adds a brief comment on William Hunter at the end; *coma* has further explanation of difference between this and apoplexy added at the end; the entry *combustio* has a variant form added; under *comedones* there is now a cross-reference. The entry for *complexus minor* now shows a considerably expanded description. *Conarium* has a small addition concerning the meaning of this term; *conceptio* adds a reference (Hamilton: *Outlines of the theory and practice of midwifery*, 1784), as Motherby was clearly very conscious of recent medical literature; *lobelia* adds further information.

There are some strikingly radical changes in the letter P. *Psoas* has been hugely increased to become a substantial entry with much surgical information on the *psoas abscess* alluding to Hunter, Pott, and Fordyce; *psoas parvus* is largely re-written and expanded; *psoriasis* is expanded, re-written and an etymology added; *psorophthalmia* expanded; and *psydracia* is now about three times the original length; how extensive these substantial re-workings are through the whole dictionary must await more detailed research than the present study permits. *Pterygion* has a gloss added, while *pterygoharyngæi* has both a new etymology and an additional gloss, and *pubis ossa* adds over a page on a surgical alternative to caesarean section ('symphysis of the pubes') and includes several new references. *Pudendagra* adds a comment on various possible definitions of this term.

Etymologies have been added to *aliformis allantoides, lochia, pterogoideus processus*, and *pudendagra* and no doubt many others. Additional head-words include *algor, comata, coma vigil, compressus, locales, lochiorrhœa, manducatores musc., mangostan, psophos, ptoses, ptosis, trichoma*, and *trigonella*. The only deletion noted thus far is *bronchos*. Motherby's second edition is thus, by comparison with reworkings of earlier medical dictionaries, thoroughgoing and responsive to current medical knowledge and trends.

The third edition, appearing in 1791, was under Wallis's editorship. As the preface to this new edition states, Motherby, now obviously ill, was no longer confident of memory and his ability to complete the work of revision. Wallis helpfully remarks that Motherby had already begun work on this edition (1791: vii), which strongly suggests that the second edition revision must also have been his work. Wallis also mentions that he and Motherby had had 'various conversations' about the revision, so that Wallis felt he could put Motherby's intentions into effect, a job to which Wallis expresses his fidelity (1791: vii).

Some changes are specified in this preface. He has omitted the lives of ancient authorities in the expectation that they are already well-known and that such 'defalcation' will be compensated by the addition of more immediately useful material (1791: 8). Additions include 'the powers and virtues of Medicines' and a more detailed account of 'medicated springs'. In general, Wallis also wishes to expunge whatever is not medically relevant (1791: vii-viii), although *algoides* and *bronte* have both survived this purge, and entries with no mention of a medical application are still everywhere to be found.

He also undertakes to rework the index. Motherby's previous 'index' had been like a glossary without page references, in which the 'gloss' was the head-word in the main dictionary. Navigation between words within the index is thus awkward. *Barrenwort* takes the reader to *epimedium*, but not vice-versa. The various synonyms are now subsumed under the relevant head words, leaving an English only index with page numbers. Wallis offers the example of *mercury*, for which he lists twelve synonyms and claims that there are even more (1791: viii-ix). Wallis also points out that an English index is more use where competence in other languages cannot be taken for granted. An exception is made for terms that are very similar in English to the other language bar the ending, which are not included.

Previous research has shown that Motherby relies on a range of acknowledged sources, both ancient and modern, the list headed by a long way by the physician and chemist William Lewis, and the botanist John Ray. These are followed by Boerhaave, Hippocrates, Galen, and Celsus, and other moderns such as the surgeons John Hunter and Lorenz Heister (see McConchie 2009). By the third edition, as we have seen, Linné and Cullen are prominent as well. To consider just one of these sources, the often-mentioned William Hunter,[180] is usually sourced merely as 'Dr. Hunter says/thinks/defines/observes/uses the term....', with no works cited. Hunter is often the first and sometimes the only authority mentioned in an entry; e.g., *antithenar*, *diarthrosis*, and *perichondrium*. There is also an instance of Hunter being cited for lexicographical comment: 'Hunter uses the term cellular as the generical name, and the terms reticular and adipose for expressing the two species'. Such mentions are not all that common, however, since most references to him are strictly medical, and anatomical in particular. Motherby mentions James now and then, as under *algema*, *allantois*, *Asclepiades*, *cachexia*, *emphysema* and *yaws*, and a singleton allusion to Quincy was found in *scrofula*.

These sources he offers not simply as references to his own content, but frequently as a range of reading suggestions for the professional to select from (Lonati 2017: 64). Looking at the allusions to modern writers, at least two trends are apparent—Motherby tended to avoid general, popularising works, and preferred moderns who were born towards the end of the seventeenth century and later, in which light

---

180 Always referred to as 'Dr. Hunter', whereas his brother is invariably 'Mr. J(ohn) Hunter'.

it interesting that no mention of Barrow was found. Motherby takes due note of a good deal of recent work, while still exploiting the authority of the classics, although he apparently makes no reference at all to Linnaeus (McConchie 2009: 128–132). More detailed analysis of some of Motherby's entries and his striking use of very recent material such as publications on puerperal fever appears in McConchie 2011a.

12 Epilogue

This book has shown, I hope, that English medical dictionaries prior to 1800 were disparate in character and even idiosyncratic. Although there was little distinction for most of the sixteenth century between them and medical glossaries, they were later distinguished from these glossaries and maintained that distinction thereafter, glossaries gradually becoming restricted and very conventional, not to say vestigial. Medical dictionaries failed to agree on a core medical lexicon to a surprising extent early on, and the fundamental medical lexicon was not gathered into comprehensive works until well into the eighteenth century. Throughout our period, they were compiled by lexicographers who felt little compunction about imposing their own agendas on their work. At the same time, they show an increasing but inconsistent concern with reflecting recent developments in medicine and with being comprehensive. All were in various ways subject to the constraints and financial aims of the publishing industry. They also remained for the most part stubbornly Latin/Greek-English lexicons despite sporadic attempts to make them more obviously monolingual. We have seen that Boorde, Culpeper, and Quincy shared the 'promotion of English' agenda for medical learning and practice, but that others silently resisted it. Latin and Greek terminology dominated, except of course in the actual text of the entries where English equivalents appeared more freely, up until the end of the eighteenth century. Indeed it is not uncommon to discover that the only use of the Latin/Greek term is a headword which never appears elsewhere in the dictionary, the English equivalent being uniformly preferred. A remnant of the Arabic terminology persisted as well.

The inclusion of ancient knowledge slowly and haltingly gives way to contemporary knowledge. Continental sources of lexicographical information are gradually replaced by English resources and a greater proportion of English authorities, but this change is glacially slow before the third quarter of the eighteenth century. Medical lexicographers begin to require assistants and the outside expert knowledge of specialist areas. None of these changes is linear or consistent, however.

Two constant and abiding notions which have kept reappearing have been the dictionary as a teaching aid and as a memory aid and a ready reference for immediate problems. A further general impression is that these works support the status quo at the lexical level rather than disseminating a new view of the medical lexicon. This need not be true of the definitions however; in fact, James, despite his conservatism, does incorporate reference to recent work, and Motherby had attempted a large if inconsistently applied introduction of new information. The medical dictionaries of this period are increasingly a way of sensing the trends of the times, especially since they tend to aim for inclusiveness in their word-lists and, in the latter part of the eighteenth century, increasingly attempt to be up-to-date where possible. Just as they were claimed to replace multi-volume collections, they perforce provide a snapshot of current medical thinking in a way that few if any other kinds of publication can match.

https://doi.org/10.1515/9783110639186-012

So many questions are raised by this area of research. One concerns the influence of continental medical dictionaries (Rivière, Blancard), and whether the English ones exerted any influence in reverse (James may have, given that he was translated into two other vernacular languages; Burnet certainly did, but in Latin). Connexions with the continent seem not to have been close—why was this so? A work like Henri-Simon-Pierre Gissey's *Dictionnaire des alimens vins et liqueurs* of 1750, despite there being nothing like it in English, was never translated. Perhaps the cultural gulf was too great, despite the work mentioning things English a number of times, and even praising English beer (s.v. *biere*). One might also wonder why there was no continental translation of Quincy. Perhaps his word-list was too obviously anglicized; after all, a medical dictionary or glossary emanating from anywhere in Europe might be expected to have an obviously Latin/Greek word-list, and to be familiar even if many items were not shared between any two of them.

The question of whether to use the vernacular in medical works was also crucial, and demands further detailed research on these dictionaries themselves as well as in relation to the medical publications of the time. Both Thomas Elyot and Robert Recorde in the first half of the sixteenth century had mounted a defence of the use of English in their medical works. Traheron's translation of Vigo, furnished with an extensive glossary, must have done much to promote the vernacular along with these explicit and spirited defences. It is nevertheless striking that as medical lexicography developed, support for this view of the vernacular remained sporadic. We have to wait until the work of Nicholas Culpeper and John Quincy to see it re-emerge. Meanwhile, medical dictionaries themselves become somewhat more bi- and trilingual, with Latin/Greek word-lists, down into the eighteenth century rather than less, the number of Latin and Greek head-words in the generality of dictionaries surveyed here in fact slightly increasing if the use made of Blancard is any guide. This clearly requires further investigation. Presumably Greek and even Latin were falling out of use in practice, so why would this happen? Is there any corresponding or countervailing increase in the number of English lemmas? The present impression is that these dictionaries are if anything becoming increasingly Latin/Greek-English, not less, which seems counter-intuitive. This may be the result of increasing anxiety about the perceived status of the medical profession and its increasingly irrelevant tripartite division into physicians, surgeons and apothecaries along with their perceived gradations in learning and status, although this is conjectural. A detailed study of the flurry of medical dictionaries appearing at the end of the eighteenth century and in the early decades of the nineteenth may reveal much on this score, but this must remain the subject of another book.

Another issue which has vexed scholarship is the inter-relations between dictionaries and the detailed changes in entries, or the lack of it, between them. To summarize briefly, these changes come into the following categories: typographical, insertion and deletion, and grammatical. The typographical changes are often minor and to do with spelling and punctuation, and may thus simply reflect a different printing house style and minor changes in the language and its orthography over time. Omissions of unnecessary words and phrases and of material no longer required or too long to incorporate also occur. Omission of material may occur for content reasons such as irrelevance and outdatedness. Insertion of new material is usually done for the reverse reasons—being up to date, personal data, (cases, observations, etc.), and insertion of new information and discoveries, whether medical or linguistic. Changes in source of information are often involved. Grammatical changes may range from revisions so minor as to be hard to distinguish from typographical changes to revisions severe enough to shift meaning. These considerations will apply to the relations between all or any of the dictionaries covered in this book. The result of such changes or the lack of them has often been seen in dictionary research in terms of plagiarism or the lack of it, but it is important to consider not just the result but the process involved, as this will produce a more insightful account of dictionary inter-relations.

Finally, adverting to the head-piece from Motherby with which this volume began, the sheer size of a medical dictionary is also significant. Quincy's was an octavo, but James and Motherby are folios and James came in three massive volumes, hardly a format to be stuffed into a physician's bag when visiting patients or the satchel of a clergyman minstering to the sick of his parish. Barrow's is also an octavo. The distinction between a vademecum and a compendium of the medical part of the circle of knowledge could be critical.

Bibliography

Notes on conventions

Very long titles have been silently shortened where appropriate. Locations of publishers and booksellers places of business have been silently deleted. Information which appears only in a colophon appears in square brackets, as do uniform titles.

Primary references

Adelon (1812–1822) = :*Dictionaire des sciences médicales, par une société de médecins et de chirurgiens*. Ed Adelon, Alard et al. 60 vols., Paris: C. L. F. Panckoucke.

Aikin, John (1780): *Biographical memoirs of medicine in Great Britain from the revival of literature to the time of Harvey. By John Aikin, Surgeon*. London: for Joseph Johnson.

Alpinus, Prosper (1601): *De praesagienda vita et morte aegrotantium libri septem*. Venice: apud hæredes Melchioris Sessæ.

Alston, Charles (1740): *Index plantarum, præcipue officinalium, quæ, in horto medico Edinburgensi, a Carolo Alston, M. & B. P. medicinæ studiosis demonstrantur*. Edinburgi: apud W. Sands, A. Brymer, A. Murray & J. Cochran.

Alston, Charles (1752): *Index medicamentorum simplicium triplex*. Edinburgi: typis W. Sands, A. Murray, & J. Cochran.

Amory, Thomas (1766): *The life of John Buncle: Esq; containing various observations and reflections, made in several parts of the world, and many extraordinary relations*. London: for J. Johnson and B. Davenport.

Anon. (1739): *The Ladies dispensatory: or Every woman her own physician. Treating of the nature, causes, and various symptoms, of all the diseases, infirmities, and disorders, natural or contracted, that most peculiarly affect the fair sex, in all their different situations of life, as maids, married women, and widows*. London: for James hodges and John James.

Anon. (1754?): *An answer to a late scurrilous pamphlet, published by one Baker and his accomplices respecting Dr. James's powder, and sold at a public-house in the liberties of the Fleet*. London: for J. Bouquet.

Anon. (1767): *The family guide to health; or, a general practice of physic: in a familiar way*. London: for J. Fletcher and B. Collins.

Bahia (Brazilian State) (1656): [The skilful physician] *Secretaria das Minas e Energia. Diretoria de Distribuição The skilful physician containing directions for the preservation of a healthful condition, and approved remedies for all diseases and infirmities (outward or inward) incident to the body of man*. London: Printed by Tho. Maxey for Nath. Ekins.

Bailey (1728) = Bailey, N.: *An universal etymological English dictionary: comprehending the derivations of the generality of words in the English tongue, either ancient or modern, from the ancient British, Saxon, Danish, Norman, and Modern French, Teutonic, Dutch, Spanish, Italian; as also from the Latin, Greek, and Hebrew languages, each in their proper characters 4th edition*. London: for J. Darby et al.

Baker, Walter (1754): *The affidavits and proceedings of Walter Baker, administrator to the late Baron Schwanberg, upon his petition presented to the King in Council, to vacate the patent obtained by Dr. Robert James for Schwanberg's powder*. London: printed, and there published for Physicians, Surgeons, and Apothecaries, and all others whom it may concern.

https://doi.org/10.1515/9783110639186-013

[Banckes's herbal] [1525]: *Here begynnyth a newe mater, the whiche sheweth and treateth of ye ver-tues [and] proprytes of herbes, the whiche is called an herball.* [London]: Imprynted by me Ry-charde Banckes.

Banester, John (1589): *An antidotarie chyrurgicall, containing great varietie and choice of all sorts of medicines that commonly fal into the chyrurgions vse.* Imprinted at London: By Thomas Orwin for Thomas Man.

Baret (1574) = Baret, John: *An aluearie or triple dictionarie, in Englishe, Latin, and French.* [London: Henry Denham].

Barnes, (satirist) (1541?): *The treatyse answerynge the boke of berdes. Compyled by Collyn Clowte, dedycatyd to Barnarde barber dwellynge in Banbery.* [London: R. W[yer].

Barrough, Philip (1583): *The methode of phisicke conteyning the cavses, signes, and cvres of invvard diseases in mans body from the head to the foote.* Imprinted at London: By Thomas Vau-troullier.

Barrow (1735) = Barrow, John: *Dictionarium polygraphicum: or, the whole body of arts regularly di-gested* vol. 1, London: for C. Hitch, C. Davis, and S. Austen.

Barrow (1749) = Barrow, John: *Dictionarium medicum universale: or, a new medicinal dictionary. Containing an explanation of all the terms used in physic ... botany, &c. ... The whole collected from the original authors, by J. Barrow, chymist.* London: for T. Longman, and C. Hitch; and A. Millar.

Barrow, John (1750): *Navigatio Britannica: or a complete system of navigation in all its branches, both with regard to theory and practice. ... To which is added, the method of surveying and drawing maps or charts ... By J. Barrow.* London: for W. and J. Mount and T. Page.

Barrow (1751) = Barrow, John: *A new and universal dictionary of arts and sciences ... With an intro-ductory preface ... And illustrated with a great number of copper-plates, engraven by the best hands.* London: for the proprietors.

Barrow (1754) = Barrow, John: *Dictionarium medicum universale: or, a new medicinal dictionary. Containing an explanation of all the terms used in physic ... botany, &c. ... The whole collected from the original authors, by J. Barrow.* 2nd edition, London: for T. Longman, and C. Hitch; and A. Millar.

Behr, Georg Heinrich (1738): *Lexicon physico-chymico-medicum reale.* Argentorati: sumptibus Jo-hannis Beckii.

Bell, Benjamin (1783–1788): *A system of surgery.* 6 vols., Edinburgh: Charles Elliot/London: G. Rob-inson.

Bent, William (1779): *A general catalogue of books in all languages, arts, and sciences, that have been printed in Great Britain, and published in London, since the year M.DCC. to the present time. The whole alphabetically and classically disposed under the several branches of litera-ture, with their sizes and prices.* London: [s.n.].

Bielfeld, Jacob Friedrich, Freiherr von (1771): *The elements of universal erudition, containing an ana-lytical abridgment of the sciences, polite arts, and belles lettres. Translated from the last edi-tion printed at Berlin by W. Hooper, M.D.* 3 vols., London: for G. Scott et al.

Blancard (1679) = Blancard, Steven: *Lexicon Medicum, Græco-Latinum.* Amsterdam: Ex Officina Jo-hannis ten Hoorn; Typis Viduae Petri Boeteman.

Blancard (1684) = Blancard, Steven: *A physical dictionary; in which, all the terms relating either to anatomy, chirurgery, pharmacy, or chymistry, are very accurately explain'd.* London: Printed by J.D.

Blancard (1690) = Blancard, Steven (1690): *Steph. Blancardi lexicon novum medicum, Græco-Lati-num, cæteris editionibus longè perfectissimum.* Lugduni Batavorum: Cornelium Boutesteyn [et] Jordaanum Luchtmans.

Blancard (1693) = Blancard, Steven (1693): *The physical dictionary. Wherein the terms of anatomy, the names and causes of diseases, chyrurgical instruments and their use; are accurately describ'd*. London: Printed for S. Crouch.

Blancard (1697) = Blancard, Steven (1697): *The physical dictionary. Wherein the terms of anatomy, the names and causes of diseases, chyrurgical instruments and their use, are accurately described*. London: Printed for S. Crouch.

Blancard (1708) = Blancard, Steven (1708): *The physical dictionary. Wherein the terms of anatomy, the names and causes of diseases, chyrurgical instruments, and their use, are accurately described*. 5th edition, London: For Samuel Crouch and John Sprint.

Blancard (1726) = Blancard, Steven (1726): *The physical dictionary. Wherein the terms of anatomy, the names and causes of diseases, chirurgical instruments, and their use, are accurately described*. 7th edition, London: For John and Benjamin Sprint and Edward Symon.

Blount (1656) = Blount, Thomas: *Glossographia: or a dictionary, interpreting all such hard words whether Hebrew, Greek, Latin, Italian, Spanish, French, Teutonick, Belgick, British or Saxon; as are now used in our English tongue*. London: Tho. Newcomb.

Bodleian Library (1782*): A catalogue of books purchased for the Bodleian Library in 1782; with an account of monies collected for that purpose*. [Oxford, s.n.].

Boerhaave, Herman (1741*): A new method of chemistry; including the history, theory, and practice of the art: translated from the original Latin of Dr. Boerhaave's Elementa chemiæ, as published by himself. By Peter Shaw, M.D.* London: for T. Longman.

Bonet Théophile (1684): *A guide to the practical physician:shewing, from the most approved authors, both ancient and modern, the truest and safest way of curing all diseases, internal and external, whether by medicine, surgery, or diet*. London: for Thomas Flesher.

Boorde, Andrew (1542): *Hereafter foloweth a compendyous regyment or a dyetary of helth, made in Mouñtpyllier, compyled by Andrew Boorde of physycke doctour*. [London]: Imprynted by me Robert Wyer.

Boorde, Andrew (1545): *A pronostycacyon or an almanacke for the yere of our lorde, M. CCCCC. xlv. made by Andrewe Boorde of physycke doctor an Englyshe man of the vniversitie of Oxforde*. (London]: s.n.

Boorde (1547) = Boorde, Andrew: *The breuiary of helthe, for all maner of syckenesses and diseases the whiche may be in man, or woman doth folowe. Expressynge the obscure termes of Greke, Araby, Latyn, and Barbary in to Englysh concerning phisicke and chierurgye / compyled by Andrewe Boord of phisicke doctour an Englysh man*. [Imprynted at London by Wylllyam Myddelton].

Boorde, Andrew (1547?): *The pryncyples of astronamye the whiche diligently perscrutyd is in maner a pronosticacyon to the worldes end complyd by Andrew Boorde of phisick doctor*. [Enprynted at London: by Robert Coplande].

Boorde, Andrew (1550): *The boke for to lerne a man to be wyse in buyldyng of his howse for the helth of body & to holde quyetnes for the helth of his soule, and body*. [London: Imprynted by me Robert Wyer].

Boorde, Andrew [1555?]: *The fyrst boke of the introduction of knowledge. The whych dothe teache a man to speake parte of all maner of languages, and to know the vsage and fashion of al maner of countreys ... Made by Andrew Borde, of physycke doctor*. [Imprinted at London by me William Copland].

[Boorde, Andrew] (1626): *The first and best part of Scoggins iests: full of witty mirth and pleasant shifts, done by him in France, and other places: being a preseruatiue against melancholy. Gathered by Andrew Boord, Doctor of Physicke*. London: Printed [by Miles Flesher] for Francis Williams.

Borsieri de Kanilfeld, Giambattista (1800–1803): *The institutions of the practice of medicine; delivered in a course of lectures.* Trans. William Cullen Brown. 5 vols. Edinburgh: for Thomas Cox.

Buchan, William (1769): *Domestic medicine; or the family physician.* Edinburgh: Balfour, Auld and Smellie.

Buchan, William (1788): *Domestic medicine: or, a treatise on the prevention and cure of diseases by regimen and simple medicines.* Tenth ed., London/Edinburgh: Strahan, A. Cadell. T., Balfour, J. et al.

Buchan, William (1795): *Domestic medicine: or, a treatise on the prevention and cure of diseases by regimen and simple medicines.* Philadelphia: Thomas Dobson.

Buffon, Georges Louis Leclerc, comte de (1780–1785): *Natural history: general and particular, by the Count de Buffon, translated into English.* [pt.4] Edinburgh: for William Creech.

Bullein, William (1562): *Bulleins bulwarke of defe[n]ce againste all sicknes, sornes, and woundes, that dooe daily assaulte mankinde, whiche bulwarke is kepte with Hillarius the gardiner, Health the phisician, with their chyrurgian, to helpe the wounded soldiors.* Imprinted at London: By Ihon Kyngston.

Bullokar, John (1616): *An English expositor teaching the interpretation of the hardest words vsed in our language.* London: Printed by Iohn Legatt.

Bulstrode, Richard, Sir (1715): *Miscellaneous essays: Viz. I. Of company and conversation. ... XIII. Of old age. ... By Sir Richard Bulstrode, ... Publish'd, with a preface, by his son Whitlocke Bulstrode, Esq.* London: for Jonas Browne.

Burnet, Thomas (1681): *Telluris theoria sacra: orbis nostri originem & mutationes generales, quas aut jam subiit, aut olim subiturus est, complectens : libri duo priores de diluvio & paradiso.* Londini : Typis R.N. impensis Gualt. Kettilby.

Burnet, Thomas (1659a): *Currus iatrikus triumphalis. In quo conclusæ iacent ter trinæ principes difficultates medicæ, ad Apollinarem lauream consequendam seorsim singulari certamine, non sine gloria deuictae & prostratae: in totius orbis celeberrimo Monspeliensium Medicorum campo martio medico.* Monspelii: apvd Danielem Pech.

Burnet, Thomas (1659b): *Qvæstiones qvatuor cardinales pro svprema Apollinari daphne conseqvend. Thomas Burnet, Sir M.D.* Monspelii: apud Danielem Pech.

Burnet (1673) = Burnet, Thomas: *Thesaurus medicinæ practicæ, ex præstantissimorum tum veterum tum recentiorum medicorum observationibus, consultationibus, consiliis & epistolis, summa diligentia collectus ordineq[ue] alphabetico dispositus. Studio & opera Thomæ Burnet Scoto-Britanni, M. D. & medici regis ordinarii.* Londini: excudebat G. R[awlins] pro Roberto Boulter.

Burnet (1678) = Burnet, Thomas: *Thesavrvs medicinæ practicæ. Ex præstantissimorum medicorum observationibus, consultationibus, consiliis, & epistolis, summa diligentia collectus ordineq[ue] alphabetico dispositus.* Genevae: Joh. Herm. Widerhold.

Burnet, Thomas (1685): *Hippocrates contractus in quo magni Hippocratis ... opera omnia, in brevem epitomen, summa diligentia redacta habentur. Studio & opera Thomæ Burnet.* Edinburgi: excudebat J. Reid.

Burnet (1687) = Burnet, Thomas: *Thesavrvs medicinæ practicæ ex præstantissimorum medicorum observationibus, consultationibus, consilijs & epistolis summa diligentia collectus ordineque alphabetico dispositus et à Daniele Pverario ... avctus observationibus selectissimis.* Venetiis: typis Gasparis Storti.

Burnet (1691) = Burnet, Thomas: *Le trésor de la pratique de medecine, ou le dictionaire medical: contenant l'histoire de toutes les maladies; et leurs remedes choisis dans les observations, consultes, conseils & ordonnances des plus habiles medecins: le tout recueilli par Mr. Thomas Burnet. Enrichi des remarques de Mr. Dan. Puerarivs. Traduit de latin en françois par Mr N.P.D.M.* A Lyon: chez Hilaire Baritel.

Burnet (1694) = Burnet, Thomas: *Thesavrus medicinæ practicæ. Ex præstantissimorum medicorvm observationibus, consultationibus, consilijs, & epistolis, summa diligentia collectus, ordineque alphabetico dispositus: et à Daniele Pverario... auctus observationibus selectissimis.* Venetiis: Typis Gasparis Storti.

Burnet (1698) = Burnet, Thomas: *Thesaurus medicinæ practicæ ex præstantissimorum medicorum observationibus, consultationibus, consilijs, & epistolis, summa diligentia collectus, ordine alphabetico dispositus ... Editio novissima.* Genevæ: Sumptibus J. Ant. Chouët & Davidis Ritteri.

Burnet (1703) = Burnet, Thomas: *Thesaurus medicinæ practicæ thesauri, medicinæ practicæ, breviarium; cum indice remediorum, qua inibi continentur: authore Thoma Burneto.* Edinburgi: typis Georgii Mosman Bibliopolae.

Burnet (1733) = Burnet, Thomas: *Thesaurus medicinae practicae. Ex praestantissimorum medicorum observationibus, consultationibus, consiliis, & epistolis, summa diligentia collectus, ordine alphabetico dispositus, & in octodecim libros divisus. Editio novissima, pluribus ipsius auctoris additamentis, aliis omnibus hactenus vulgatis, longe auctior.* Venedig: Hieronymus Savioni.

Burrows, John (1785): *A new practical essay on cancers ... With a dissertation on the disorders occasioned by the milk ... To which are annexed accounts of cures.* 4th edition. London: for the author.

Butler, Samuel (1770): *Hudibras: in three parts. Written in the time of the late wars. With large annotations by Zachary Grey, LL.D.* 3 vols. Edinburgh: S. Crowder, C. Ware and T. Payne.

Caius, John (1576): *Of Englishe dogges, the diuersities, the names, the natures, and the properties. A short treatise written in Latine by Iohannes Caius of late memorie, Doctor of Phisicke in the Vniuersitie of Cambridge; and newly drawne into Englishe by Abraham Fleming student.* London: Richard Jones.

Calepinus, Ambrosius (1502): *Dictionarium latinum.* Reggio Emilia: Dionysius Berthoch.

Castelli (1598) = Castelli, Bartolomeo: *Lexicon medicvm Graecolatinum Bartolomæi Castelli Messanensis stvdio, ex Hippocrate, et Galeno desvmptvm.* Messanæ: Typis Petri Breæ.

Castle, George (1667): *The Chymical Galenist: a treatise, wherein the practise of the ancients is reconcil'd to the new discoveries in the theory of physick.* London: by Sarah Griffin for Henry Twyford and Timothy Twyford.

Cawdrey (1604) = Cawdrey, Robert: *A table alphabeticall, conteyning and teaching the true writing, and vnderstanding of hard vsuall English wordes, borrowed from the Hebrew, Greeke, Latine, or French, &c. With the interpretation thereof by plaine English words, gathered for the benefit & helpe of ladies, gentlewomen, or any other vnskilfull persons.* At London: Printed by I. R[oberts] for Edmund Weauer.

Chambers (1728) = Chambers, Ephraim: *Cyclopædia: or, an universal dictionary of arts and sciences; containing the definitions of the terms, and accounts of the things signify'd thereby, in the several arts, both liberal and mechanical, and the several sciences, human and divine ... Compiled from the best authors, dictionaries, journals, memoirs, transactions, ephemerides, &c. in several languages.* 2 vols., London: James and John Knapton et al.

Chambers (1738) = Chambers, Ephraim (1738): *Cyclopædia: or, an universal dictionary of arts and sciences; containing the definitions of the terms, and an account of the things signified thereby, in the several arts, both liberal and mechanical, and the several sciences, human and divine ... Extracted from the best authors, dictionaries, journals, memoirs, transactions, ephemerides, &c. in several languages.* 2 vols., London: D. Midwinter et al.

Chambers (1778–1788) = Chambers, Ephraim (1778–1788): *Cyclopædia: or, an universal dictionary of arts and sciences ... By E. Chambers, F.R.S. With the supplement, and modern improvements, incorporated in one alphabet..* Abraham Rees (ed.) 4 vols., London: for Strahan et al.

Cheyne, George (1735): *The English malady: or, a treatise of nervous diseases of all kinds; as spleen, vapours, lowness of spirits, hypochondriacal, and hysterical distempers, &c.* 6th edition, London: for G. Strahan and J. Leake.

Child, Samuel (1798): *Every man his own brewer. A practical treatise, explaining the art and mystery of brewing porter, ale, twopenny, and table-beer.* London: for J. Ridgway.

Chomel (1725) = Chomel, N.: *Dictionaire Oeconomique: or, the Family Dictionary ... done into English from the second edition, lately printed at Paris.* London: for D. Midwinter.

Cocker (1715) = Cocker, Edward: *Cocker's English dictionary, containing, an explanation of the most refined and difficult words and terms in divinity, philosophy, law, physick, mathematicks, navigation, husbandry, military discipline, with other arts and sciences.* 2nd edition, John Hawkins (ed.) London: for T. Norris, C. Brown and A. Bettesworth.

Cornwell, Bryan (1787): *The domestic physician or guardian of health.* London: for the author.

Cruso (1701) = Cruso, John: *Medicamentorum Ευπορiστον thesaurus.* Londini: Impensis Sam. Smith & Benj. Walford.

Cruso (1771) = Cruso, John: *A treasure of easy medicines, briefly comprehending approved and specific remedies for almost all disorders of the human body.* London: W. Faden et al.

Culpeper, Nicholas (1649): see Royal College of Physicians of London.

Culpeper, Nicholas (1651): *A directory for midwives: or, a guide for women, in their conception, bearing, and suckling their children.* London: Peter Cole.

Culpeper, Nicholas (1652): *The English physician or an astrologo-physical discourse of the vulgar herbs of this nation.* London: William Bentley.

Culpeper, Nicholas (1654): *A new method of physick: or, A short view of Paracelsus and Galen's practice ... Written in Latin by Simeon Partlicius, phylosopher, and physitian in Germany. Translated into English by Nicholas Culpeper.* London: Peter Cole.

Culpeper, Nicholas/Cole, Abdiah (1668): *Bartholinus anatomy; made from the precepts of his father, and from the observations of all modern anatomists, together with his own ... published by Nich. Culpeper and Abdiah Cole.* London: Printed by John Streater.

Dancer, Daniel (1797): *Biographical curiosities; or, various pictures of human nature. Containing original and authentick memoirs of Daniel Dancer, Esq. An Extraordinary Miser. &c. &c.* London: for James Ridgway.

Dawson, Thomas (1781): *Cases in the acute rheumatism and the gout; with cursory remarks, and the method of treatment.* London: for J. Johnson; and P. Elmsly.

de Volder, Burchard (1698): *Oratio de rationis viribus, et usu in scientiis: dicta publice cum Rectoris Academiae Lugd. Bat. munere abiret.* Leiden: apud Fredericum Haaringium.

Dorneus (1584) = Dorneus, Gerardus: *Dictionarium Theophrasti Paracelsi.* Francoforti: s.n.

Douglas, James. (1724): *Index materiæ medicæ: or, A catalogue of simple medicines that are sit to be used in the practice of physick and surgery. Containing I. The officinal name of each in Latin, with the accent and genitive case. II. A short botanical description fo the species that is commonly used. III. The name in Greek and English. IV. The part that is most in use. V. The names of the dispensatory, or shop preparations and compositions. To which are added two tables, in the first the simple medicines are reduced under general heads. And, in the second, they are classed according to theri principal vertues.* London: for George Strahan.

Duncan, Andrew (1794): *Medical Commentaries ... collected and published by Andrew Duncan.* London: printed for Charles Dilly.

Duddell (1729) = [Duddell, Benedict?]: *Prosodia chirurgica: being a lexicon calculated for the use of young students in surgery. Wherein all the terms of art are accounted for, their most received sense given; An exact definition of them from the best Greek authors: their pronunciation, as to quantity, determined by proper marks over each syllable.* London: for T. Corbett.

Duddell (1732) = [Duddell, Benedict?]: *Prosodia chirurgica: or, a memoria technica, calculated for the use of old practitioners, as well as young students in surgery. Being a lexicon; wherein all the terms of art are accounted for.* 2nd edition, London: for Charles Corbett, and Richard Chandler.

Dyche/Pardon (1735) = Dyche, Thomas/Pardon, William (1735): *New General English Dictionary.* London: for Richard Ware.

Elliot, Sir John (1782): *Elements of the branches of natural philosophy connected with medicine. Viz. chemistry, optics, sound, hydrostatics, electricity and physiology.* London: for J. Johnson.

Elliot, Sir John (1786): *Elements of the branches of natural philosophy connected with medicine. Viz. chemistry, optics, acoustics, hydrostatics, electricity, and physiology ... The second edition, corrected, with additions.* London: for J. Johnson.

Elyot (1538) = Elyot, Sir Thomas: *The dictionary of syr Thomas Eliot knyght.* Londini: In ædibus Thomæ Bertheleti typis impress.

Elyot, Sir Thomas (1534, i.e., 1539?): *The castel of helth, gathered and made by Syr Thomas Elyot knyghte, out of the chiefe authors of physyke, wherby euerye manne maye knowe the state of his owne body, the preseruation of helth, and how to instructe welle his physytion in skynes that he be not deceyued.* [Londini: in ædibus Thomæ Bertheleti].

Estienne (1564) = Estienne, Henri: *Dictionarivm medicum, vel, expositiones vocum medicinaliū, ad verbum excerptæ ex Hippocrate, Aretaeo, Galeno, Oribasio, Rvfo Ephesio, Aetio, Alex. Tralliano, Pavlo Aegineta, Actvario, Corn. Celso. Cum latina interpretatione. Lexica duo in Hippocratem huic dictionario praefixa sunt, vnum, Erotiani, nunquā antea editū: alterū, Galeni.* S.l.: Excudebat Henricus Stephanus, illustris viri Huldrici Fuggeri typographus.

Estienne (1572) = Estienne, Henri: *Thesaurus graecae linguae.* [Lutetiæ Parisiorum]: Henricus Stephanus.

Eutropius (1564): *A briefe chronicle, where in are described shortlye the originall, and the successiue estate of the Romaine weale publique, the alteratyon and chaunge of sondrye offices in the same ... Englished by Nicolas Havvard.* London: Thomas Marsh.

Fielding, Henry (1742): *The history of the adventures of Joseph Andrews, and his friend Mr. Abraham Adams.* 2nd edition, 2 vols., London: for A. Millar.

Florio (1598) = Florio, John: *A worlde of wordes, or most copious and exact dictionarie in Italian and English.* London: Arnold Hatfield for Edw. Blount.

Florio (1611) = Florio, John: *Queen Anna's nevv vvorld of words, or dictionarie of the Italian and English tongues,] [c]ollected, and newly muc[h augmented by] Iohn Florio, reader of the Italian vnto the Soueraigne Maiestie of Anna, crowned Queene of England, Scotland, France and Ireland, &c. And one of the gentlemen of hir Royall Priuie Chamber. Whereunto are added certaine necessarie rules and short obseruations for the Italian tongue.* London: Melch. Bradwood [and William Stansby], for Edw. Blount and William Barret.

Foesius, Anutius (1561): *Pharmacopœia medicamentorum omnium.* Basel: apud Thomam Guerinum.

Foot, Jesse (1794): *The life of John Hunter.* London: for T. Becket.

Fothergill, John (1783): *The works of John Fothergill, M. D. Member of the Royal College of Physicians, and Fellow of the Royal Society, of London; and of the Royal College of Physicians in Edinburgh; and corresponding Member of the Royal Medical Society of Paris 3 vols.*, ed. John Coakley Lettsom. London: for Charles Dilly.

Freind, John (1719): *A letter to the learned Dr. Woodward. By Dr. Byfielde.* London: for James Bettenham.

Freind, John (1725–1726): *The history of physick; from the time of Galen, to the beginning of the sixteenth century. Chiefly with regard to practice. In a discourse written to Doctor Mead.* 2 vols., London: for J. Walthoe.

Fuchs, Leonhard (1539) *De medendis singvlarvm hvmani corporis partivm. A summo capite ad imos usque pedes passionibus ac febris libri quatuor, nunquam antea in lucem editi.* Basileæ: s.n.

Gerard, John (1597): *The herball or generall historie of plantes. Gathered by Iohn Gerarde of London Master in Chirurgerie.* Imprinted at London: by [Edm. Bollifant for Bonham Norton and] Iohn Norton.

Gerard, John (1633): *The herball or generall historie of plantes. Gathered by John Gerarde of London master in chirvrgerie; Very much enlarged and amended by Thomas Johnson citizen and apothecarye of London.* London: Adam Islip, Joyce Norton and Richard Whitakers.

Gesner, Konrad (1576): *The newe iewell of health, wherein is contayned the most excellent secretes of phisicke and philosophie ... Gathered out of the best and most approued authors, by that excellent doctor Gesnerus ... Faithfully corrected and published in Englishe, by George Baker, chirurgian.* London: Henry Denham.

Gissey (1750) = Gissey, Henri-Simon-Pierre: *Dictionnaire des alimens vins et liqueurs, leurs qualités, leurs effets, relativement aux différens âges, & aux différens tempéramens.* Paris: Chez Gissey, Bordelet.

Glasse, Hannah (1747): *The art of cookery, made plain and easy; which far exceeds any thing of the kind ever yet published.* London: for the author.

Good, John Mason (1796*): The history of medicine, so far as it relates to the profession of the apothecary, from the earliest accounts to the present period: the evils to which the profession and the public have been of late years equally exposed; and the means which have been devised to remedy them. Published at the request of the Committee of the General Pharmceutic Association of Great Britain.* 2nd edition, London: for C. Dilly.

Gorraeus (1564) = Gorraeus, Joannes: *Definitionum Medicarum Libri XXIIII literis græcis distincti.* Lutetiae Parisiorum: apvd Andream Wechelvm.

Gorton (1826–1828) = Gorton, John: *A general biographical dictionary: containing a summary account of the lives of eminent persons of all nations.* 2 vols., London: Hunt & Clarke.

Grey, Zachary (1754): *Critical, historical, and explanatory notes on Shakespeare, with emendations of the text and metre.* 2 vols., London: for the author.

Guillemeau, Jacques [1587]: *A worthy treatise of the eyes; contayning the knowledge and cure of one hundreth and thirtene diseases, incident vnto them: first gathered & written in French, by Iacques Guillemeau, chyrurgion to the French King, and now translated into English.* London: R Waldegrave for T. Mann and W. Brome.

Hale, Rich./Tyson, Edward (1700): The humane allantois fully discovered and the reasons assigned why it has not hitherto been Found out, even by those who believed its existence. *Phil. Trans.* 22, 260–276 835–850.

Halle, John, see Lanfranc of Milan.

Haller, Albrecht von (1776–1788): *Bibliotheca medicinæ practicæ qua scripta ad partem medicinæ practicam facientia a rerum initiis ad a. MDCCLXXV recensentur.* 4 vols., Bernæ: E. Haller.

[Harris, John] [1702]: *Lexicon technicum magnum; or, an universal English dictionary of arts and sciences: explaining not only the terms of art, but the arts themselves.* London: for D. Brown, T. Goodwin, J. Walthoe, etc.

Harris (1704) = Harris, John: *Lexicon technicum: or, an universal English dictionary of arts and sciences: explaining not only the terms of art, but the arts themselves.* London: for D. Brown et al.

Haward, Nicholas (1564): *A briefe chronicle, where in are described shortlye the originall, and the successiue estate of the Romaine weale publique, the alteratyon and chaunge of sondrye offices in the same.* London: Thomas Marshe.

Hoffmann, F. (1705): *Dissertatio inauguralis medica de morbis certis regionibus & populis propriis.* Halæ Magdeburgicæ: Chr. Henckel.

Holme, Randle (1688): *The academy of armory, or, a storehouse of armory and blazon. Containing the several variety of created beings, and how born in coats of arms, both foreign and domestick: with the instruments used in all trades and sciences, together with their terms of art. Also the etymologies, definitions, and historical observations on the same, explicated and explained according to our modern language.* Chester: Printed for the author.

Hooper (1817) = Hooper, Robert; *A new medical dictionary, containing an explanation of the terms in anatomy, chymistry, physiology, pharmacy, practice of physic, surgery, materia medica, midwifery, and the various branches of natural philosophy connected with medicine.* Philadelphia: M. Carey & son, Benjamin Walker, and Edward Parker.

Howard, George Selby (1788): *The new royal cyclopædia, and encyclopædia; or, complete, modern and universal dictionary of arts and sciences.* London: for Alex. Hoggs.

Hutchinson, Benjamin (1799): *Biographia medica; or, historical and critical memoirs of the lives and writings of the most eminent medical characters that have existed from the earliest account of time to the present period.* 2 vols., London: for J. Johnson.

Ingram, Dale (1751): *Practical cases and observations in surgery.* London: for J. Clarke.

Ivimey, Joseph (1811–1830): *A History of the English Baptists.* 3 vols., London: Printed for the author.

James, Robert (1741a*): A new method of preventing and curing the madness caused by the bite of a mad dog. Laid before the Royal Society, in February last, 1741.* London: the Society of booksellers for promoting of learning.

James, R[obert] (1741b): *Proposals for printing a medicinal dictionary designed as a body of physic and surgery both with regard to theory and practice. Compiled from the best writers ancient and modern: with useful observations.* [London: the society of booksellers for promoting learning].

James (1742–1745) = James, R[obert*]: A medicinal dictionary; including physic, surgery, anatomy, chymistry, and botany, in all their branches relative to medicine. Together with a history of drugs.* 3 vols., London: for T. Osborne.

James, Robert (1746a*): A dissertation on endemial diseases; or, those disorders which arise from particular climates, situations, and methods of living; together with a treatise on the diseases of tradesmen … The first by the celebrated Frederick Hoffman, Professor of Physick at Hall in Saxony, and Physician to the late and present King of Prussia. The second by Bern. Ramazini, Professor of Physick at Padua: newly translated with a preface and an appendix by Dr. James.* London: Thomas Osborne and J. Hildyard.

James, Robert (1746b): *Health's improvement: or, rules comprizing and discovering the nature, method and manner of preparing all sorts of foods used in this nation. Written by that ever famous Thomas Moffet, Doctor in Physick … To which is now prefix'd … an introduction, by R. James, M.D.* London: T. Osborne.

James, Robert (1746c): *The modern practice of physic; as improv'd by the celebrated professors, H. Boerhaave, and F. Hoffman, physician to the late and present King of Prussia: being a translation of the aphorisms of the former, with the Commentaries of Dr. Van Swieten.* 2 vols. London: for J. Hodges.

James, R. (1746d): *The presages of life and death in diseases. By Prosper Alpinus, Professor of Medicine and Philosophy in the University of Padua. Translated from the last Leyden edition, revised and published by Gaubius, at the request of Dr. Boerhaave.* 2 vols., London: for G. Strahan et al.

James, R[Robert] (1746e): *A treatise on tobacco, tea, coffee, and chocolate: written originally by Simon Pauli ; and now translated by Dr. James.* London: for T. Osborne, J. Hildyard, M. Bryson et al.

James (1746–1748) = James, Robert: *Dictionnaire universel de medecine, de chirurgie, de chymie, de botanique, d'anatomie, de pharmacie, d'histoire naturelle, &c. traduit de l'Anglois de M. James par Mrs Diderot, Eidous & Toussaint*. 6 vols., Paris: Briasson, David l'aîné, Durand.

James, R[obert] (1747): *Pharmacopoeia universalis: or, a new universal English dispensatory … With a copious index to the whole*. London: for J. Hodges and J. Wood.

James, R[obert] (1748): *A dissertation on fevers and inflammatory distempers. Wherein a method is proposed of curing, or at least of removing the danger usually attending, those fatal disorders*. London: for J. Newbery.

James, Robert (1752): *Discorso istorico del sig. dottor James sopra la medicina. Tradotto dalla lingua inglese*. In Venezia: presso Giambattista Pasquali.

James (1753) = James, R[obert]: *Dizionario universale di medicina di chirurgia, di notomia, di chimica, di farmacia, di botanica, d'istoria naturale &c. del Signor James … tradotto dall' originale inglese dai signori Diderot, Eidous e Toussaint*. 11 vols., Venezia: Giambatista Pasquali.

John XXI, Pope (1550?): *The treasurie of healthe conteynyng many profitable medycines, gathered out of Hypocrates, Galen and Auycen, by one Petrus Hyspanus & translated into Englysh by Humfre Lloyde*. [Imprynted at London by Wyllyam Coplande].

Johnson [pseudonym] (1777): Review of A New Medical Dictionary; or, General Repository of Physic. By G. Motherby, M. D. Folio. 1l. 11s. 6d. in boards. *The Critical Review; or, Annals of Literature* 44, 327–333.

Johnson [pseudonym] (1791): Review of Wallis's edition of A New Medical Dictionary. *The Critical Review; or Annals of Literature*: ser. 2,3, 30–37.

Johnson, Robert (1684): *Enchiridion medicum: or a manual of physick. Being a compendium of the whole art*. London: J. Heptinstall for Brabazon Aylmer.

Johnson, Samuel (1745): [Bibliotheca Harleiana] *This day is published, price five shillings, the fifth and last volume of Bibliotheca Harleiana: or, A catalogue of the remaining part of the library of the late Earl of Oxford*. London: T. Osborne.

Johnson (1755) = Johnson, Samuel: *A dictionary of the English language in which the words are deduced from their originals, and illustrated in their different significations by examples from the best writers*. 2 vols., London: for J. and P. Knapton et al.

Johnson, Thomas (1634): *The workes of that famous chirurgion Ambrose Parey translated out of Latine and compared with the French. by Th: Johnson*. London: Th. Cotes and R. Young.

Johnson (1652) = Johnson, William: *Lexicon chymicum. Cum obscuriorum verborum, et rerum hermeticarum, tum phrasium Paracelsicarum in scriptis ejus. Et aliorum chymicorum, passim occurrentium, planam explicationem continens*. Londini: excudebat G. D. Impensis Gulielmi Nealand.

Keill, James (1703): *The anatomy of the humane body abridg'd: or, a short and full view of all the parts of the body*. 2nd, revised ed., London: for Ralph Smith and William Davis.

Keill, James (1708): *An account of animal secretion, the quantity of blood in the humane body, and muscular motion*. London: for George Strahan.

Keill, James (1718): *Tentamina medico-physica, ad quasdam quæstiones, quæ oeconomiam animalem spectant, accommodata. Quibus accessit medicina statica Britannica*. Londini: Geo. Strahan and W., and J. Innys.

Keir (1771) = [Keir, James]: *A dictionary of chemistry. Containing the theory and practice of that science; its application to natural philosophy, natural history, medicine, and animal economy… Translated from the French. With, notes, and addition, by the translator*. London: for S. Bladon.

Keir (1789) = Keir, James: *The first part of a dictionary of chemistry, &c. By J. K., F. R. S. and S. A. Sc.* Birmingham: by Pearson and Rollason. For Elliot and Kay and Charles Elliot.

Kelly, John (1741): *The Levee. A farce. As it was offer'd to, and accepted for representation by the master of the Old-House in Drury-Lane, but by the Inspector of Farces denied a licence.* London: for the Society of Booksellers for promoting Learning.

Kettilby, Mary (1724): *A collection of above three hundred receipts in cookery, physick and surgery; for the use of all good wives, tender mothers, and careful nurses.* 3rd ed., London: for Mary Kettilby.

Knight, Thomas (1731): *A vindication of a late Essay on the transmutation of blood, Containing The true Manner of Digestion of our Aliments, and the Aetiology: or, An Account of the Immediate Cause of Putrid Fevers or Agues.* London: for the author.

Knox, Vicesimus (1789): *Liberal education: or, a practical treatise on the methods of acquiring useful and polite learning.* 2 vols., London: for Charles Dilley.

Lanfranc, of Milan (1565): *A most excellent and learned vvoorke of chirurgerie, called Chirurgia parua Lanfranci Lanfranke of Mylayne his briefe: reduced from dyuers translations to our vulgar or vsuall frase, and now first published in the Englyshe prynte by Iohn Halle chirurgien. Who hath thervnto necessarily annexed. A table, as wel of the names of diseases and simples with their vertues, as also of all other termes of the arte opened.* London: Thomas Marshe.

Lara, Benjamin (1791): *An essay on the injurious custom of mothers not suckling their own children; with some directions for chusing a nurse, and weaning of children, &c. &c.* London: for William Moore.

Lara (1796) = Lara, Benjamin: *A dictionary of surgery; or, the young surgeon's pocket assistant.* London: for James Ridgway.

Library Company of Philadelphia (1789): *A catalogue of the books, belonging to the Library Company of Philadelphia.* Philadelphia: by Zachariah Poulson, Junior.

Linné, Carl von (1783; 1782–1785): *A system of vegetables, according to their classes genera orders species with their characters and differences* 2 vols., By a botanical society, at Lichfield. London: for Leigh and Sotheby.

Linné, Carl von/Elmgren, Johannes (1762): *Termini Botanici, Quos Concensu Experient, Fac. Medicæ in Reg. Acad. Upsaliensi, præside ... D:no. doct. Carolo Linnæo ... examinandos sistit Johannes Elmgren Smolandus.* Upsaliæ: Evalt Ziervogel?

Littleton (1677) = Littleton, Adam: *Dictionarium Latino-barbarum. Cui præmittitur præfatiuncula, docens quo pacto barbaries in Latinitatem irrepserit.* London: Typis J.C. Impensis Johannis Wright, & Richardi Chiswel.

Littleton (1703) = Littleton, Adam: *Linguæ latinæ liber dictionarius quadripartitus. Dr. Adam Littleton's Latine dictionary, in four parts: I. An English-Latine. II. A Latine-Classical. III. A Latine-proper. IV. A Latine-barbarous. Representing I. The English words and phrases before the Latin ... II. The Latin-classic before the English; ... III. The Latin-proper names of those persons, people or countries that frequently occur ... IV. 1. The Latin-barbarous ... 2. The law-Latin.* 4th edition, London: for W. Rawlins et al.

Llwyd, Humphrey (1573): *The breuiary of Britayne. As this most noble and renowmed iland, was of auncient time deuided into three kingdomes, England, Scotland and Wales ... Writen in Latin by Humfrey Lhuyd of Denbigh, a Cambre Britayne, and lately Englished by Thomas Twyne, Gentleman.* [Imprinted at London: by Richard Iohnes].

Lommius, Jodocus (1560): *Medicinalium observationum libri tres.* Antverpiae : Ex Off. Christophori Plantini.

Luisini, Luigi (1736): *Aphrodisiacus. Containing a summary of the ancient writers on the venereal disease ... With a large preface, by Daniel Turner, of the College of Physicians in London.* London: John Clarke.

Macer, Floridus (1543?): *A newe herball of Macer, translated out of Laten in to Englysshe.* [London: Imprynted by me Robert Wyer].

Marescot, Michel (1599): *A trve discovrse, vpon the matter of Martha Brossier of Romorantin, pretended to be possessed by a deuill. Translated out of French into English, by Abraham Hartvvel.* London: John Wolfe.

Markham, Gervase (1614): *Cheape and good husbandry for the vvell-ordering of all beasts, and fowles, and for the generall cure of their diseases.* London: Printed by T[homas] S[nodham] for Roger Iackson.

Marten, Benjamin (1720): *A new theory of consumptions: more especially of a phthisis, or consumption of the lungs.* London: for R. Knaplock et al.

Martin (1749) = Martin, Benjamin: *Lingua Britannica reformata or, a new English dictionary.* London: J. Hodges et al.

Martin, Benjamin (1755): *The general magazine of arts and sciences, philosophical, philological, mathematical, and mechanical.* Vol. 5, London: W. Owen.

Martyn, Thomas (1793): *The language of botany: being a dictionary of the terms made use of in that science, principally by Linneus.* London: B. and J. White.

Maubray, John (1724): *The female physician, containing all the diseases incident to that sex, in virgins, wives, and widows.* London: for James Holland.

Mead, Richard (1719a): *The life and adventures of Don Bilioso de L'Estomac. Translated from the original Spanish into French; done from the French into English. With a letter to the College of Physicians.* London: J Bettenham for T. Bickerton.

[Mead, Richard] (1719b): *A serious conference between Scaramouch and Harlequin, concerning three and one. With a dedication to two eminent meetings within the bills of mortality. By Momophilus Carthusiensis.* London: for J. Roberts.

Medical register for the year 1780, the (1780): London: for Fielding and Walker.

Mesue [Yuhanna ibn Masawaih] (1549): *Mesve et omnia qvae cvm eo imprimi consueverunt.* Venetis: apud Iuntas.

Meyrick, William (1790): *The new family herbal; or, domestic physician: enumerating, with accurate descriptions, all the known vegetables which are any way remarkable for medical efficacy; with an account of their virtues in the several diseases incident to the human frame.* Birmingham: Thomas Pearson.

Miller, Joseph (1722): *Botanicum officinale; or a compendious herbal: giving an account of all such plants as are now used in the practice of physick. With their descriptions and virtues.* London: for E. Bell et al.

Miller (1724) = Miller, Philip: *The gardeners and florists dictionary, or a complete system of horticulture ... To which is added, a catalogue of curious trees, plants and fruits.* 2 vols., London: by H. P. for Charles Rivington.

Miller (1731) = Miller, Philip: *The gardeners dictionary: containing the methods of cultivating and improving the kitchen, fruit and flower garden. As also, the physick garden, wilderness, conservatory, and vineyard.* London: for the author; and sold by C. Rivington.

Milman, Francis, Sir (1786): *Dr. Milman's animadversions on the nature and on the cure of the dropsy, translated from the Latin into English, By F. Swediaur, M. D.* London: at the Logographic Press for W. Richardson.

Moffat, John (1785?): *Aretæus, consisting of eight books, on the causes, symptoms and cure of acute and chronic diseases; translated from the original Greek.* London: at the Logographic Press, by J. Walter for W. Richardson.

Moffat, Thomas, see James, Robert (1746b).

Molini, Peter (1765): *A catalogue of Latin, French and Italian books, (among which are several new physical ones) to be sold cheap.* [London]: s.n.

Morris/Kendrick (1807) = Morris, Robert/Kendrick, James et al. (eds.): *The Edinburgh medical and physical dictionary: containing an explanation of the terms of art in anatomy, physiology, pathology, therapeutics, surgery, midwifery, pharmacy, materia medica, botany, chemistry, natural history, &c. ... to which is added, a copious glossary of obsolete terms.* Edinburgh: Bell & Bradfute; and Mundell, Doig, & Stevenson.

Motherby (1775) = Motherby, G[eorge]: *A new medical dictionary; or, general repository of physic. Containing an explanation of the terms, and a description of the various particulars relating to anatomy, physiology, physic, surgery, materia medica, pharmacy, &c. &c. &c. Each article, according to its importance, being considered in every relation to which its usefulness extends in the healing art.* London: for J. Johnson.

Motherby (1785) = Motherby, G[eorge]: *A new medical dictionary; or, general repository of physic. Containing an explanation of the terms, and a description of the various particulars relating to anatomy, physiology, physic, surgery, materia medica, chemistry, &c. &c. &c. Each article, according to its importance, being considered in every relation to which its usefulness extends in the healing art.* 2nd edition, London: for J. Johnson; G. G. J., and J. Robinson et al.

Motherby (1791) = Motherby, G[eorge]: *A new medical dictionary; or, general repository of physic. Containing an explanation of the terms, and a description of the various particulars relating to anatomy, physiology, physic, surgery, materia medica, chemistry, &c. &c. &c. Each article, according to its importance, being considered in every relation to which its usefulness extends in the healing art.* 3rd edition [edited] by George Wallis, M. D. S. M. S., London: for J. Johnson; G. G. J. and J. Robinson et al.

Motherby (1795) = Motherby, G[eorge]: *A medical dictionary; or, general repository of physic. Containing an explanation of the terms, and a description of the various particulars, relating to anatomy, physiology, physic, surgery, materia medica, chemistry, &c. &c. &c. Each article, according to its importance, being considered in every relation to which its usefulness extends in the healing art.* 4th edition, London: Printed for J. Johnson, G. G., and J. Robinson; T. N. Longman et al.

Motherby (1801) = Motherby, G[eorge]: *A medical dictionary; or, general repository of physic. Containing an explanation of the terms, and a description of the various particulars, relating to anatomy, physiology, physic, surgery, materia medica, chemistry, &c. &c. &c. Each article, according to its importance, being considered in every relation to which its usefulness extends in the healing art.* 5th edition, London: Printed for J. Johnson et al.

[Mylner of Abyngton] (1532–1534): *Here is a mery iest of the mylner of Abyngton with his wyfe and his doughter, and two poore scholers of Cambridge.* [London: W. de Worde].

[N., N.] (1719): *An account of Dr. Quincy's examination of Dr. Woodward's state of physick and diseases. In a letter to the Free-Thinker.* London: J. Roberts ... and A. Dodd.

Nedham, Marchamont (1665): *Medela medicinæ. A plea for the free profession and a renovation of the art of physick, out of the noblest and most authentick writers ... tending to the rescue of mankind from the tyranny of diseases, and of physicians themselves, from the pedantism of old authors and present dictators.* London: for Richard Lownds.

New York Society Library (1793): *The charter, bye-laws, and names of the members of the New-York Society Library: with a catalogue of the books belonging to the said library.* New-York: T. & J. Swords.

Nott (1723) = Nott, John: *The cook's and confectioner's dictionary: or, the accomplish'd housewife's companion ... With an explanation of the terms us'd in carving. Revised and recommended by John Nott, Cook to his Grace the Duke of Bolton.* London: C. Rivington.

Parr (1809) = Parr, Bartholomew: *The London Medical Dictionary; including under distinct heads every branch of medicine.* 3 vols., London: for J. Johnson et al.

Payne, Henry (1780): *A catalogue of several valuable collections of books, comprehending a variety of articles ... including, among other purchases, the library of the Rev. Emanuel Langford, deceased ... now selling by Henry Payne.* [London: for Henry Payne].

Pennsylvania Hospital (Philadelphia, Pa.) (1790): *A catalogue of the books belonging to the medical library in the Pennsylvania Hospital.* Philadelphia: Zachariah Poulson, Junior.

Phillips (1658) = Phillips, Edward: *The new world of English words.* London: E. Tyler for Nath. Brooke.

Pierce, Robert (1697): *Bath memoirs: or, observations in three and forty years practice, at the Bath, what cures have been there wrought.* Bristol: for H. Hammond.

Pitcairn, Archibald (1715): *The works of Dr. Archibald Pitcairn; wherein are discovered the true foundation and principles of the art of physic.* London: for E. Curll, J. Pemberton, and W. Taylor.

Pitcairn, Archibald (1718*): The philosophical and mathematical elements of physick ... Translated from the correctest impression of the Latin, and compared with the best manuscripts; some of which were transcribed from the original, under the doctor's direction and approbation.* London: for Andrew Bell and John Osborn.

Pitcairn, Archibald (1745): *The philosophical and mathematical elements of physick ... Translated from the correctest impression of the Latin, and compared with the best manuscripts; some of which were transcribed from the original, under the doctor's direction and approbation. By John Quincy, M.D.* 2nd edition, London: for W. Innys et al.

Postlethwayt, Malachy (1749): *A dissertation on the plan, use, and importance of the Universal Dictionary of Trade and Commerce.* London: for John and Paul Knapton.

Prevost, Jean (1656): *Medicaments for the poor; or, physick for the common people containing, excellent remedies for most common diseases, incident to mans body ... Translated into English, and something added, by Nich. Culpeper, student in physick, and astrology.* London: Peter Cole.

Priestley, Joseph (1772): *Directions for impregnating water with fixed air; in order to communicate to it the peculiar spirit and virtues of Pyrmont water, and other mineral waters of a similar nature.* London: for J. Johnson.

Priestley, Joseph (1774): *Experiments and observations on different kinds of air.* London: for J. Johnson.

Priestley, Joseph (1779): *Experiments and observations relating to various branches of natural philosophy; with a continuation of the observations on air.* London: for J. Johnson.

Prosser, Thomas (1782): *An account and method of cure of the bronchocele, or, derby-neck.* 3rd edition, London: for J. Kerby.

Pulteney, Richard (1781): *A general view of the writings of Linnæus.* London: for T. Payne and B. White.

Pulteney, Richard (1790): *Historical and biographical sketches of the progress of botany in England, from its origin to the introduction of the Linnæan system.* 2 vols., London: for T. Cadell.

Quincy, John (1712, 1720), see Santorio, Santorio.

Quincy, John (1713): *A poem to the memory of the Reverend Mr. Joseph Stennett.* London: A. Baldwin, J. Noon, and T. Harrison.

Quincy, John (1718): *Pharmacopœia officinalis & extemporanea: or, a compleat English dispensatory, in four parts.* London: for A. Bell, T. Varnam, J. Osborn and W. Taylor.

Quincy, John (1719a): *An examination of Dr Woodward's State of physick and diseases.* London, for Andrew Bell et al.

Quincy (1719b) = Quincy, John: *Lexicon physico-medicum; or, a new physical dictionary, explaining the difficult terms used in the several branches of the profession, and in such parts of philosophy as are introductory thereunto. To which is added, some account of the things signified by such terms: collected from the most eminent authors; and particularly those who have wrote upon mechanical principles.* 2nd ed., London: for Andrew Bell, William Taylor and John Osborn.

Quincy, John (1720): *Pharmacopœia officinalis & extemporanea: or, a compleat English dispensatory, in four parts.* London: for E. Bell, W.Taylor, and J. Osborn.

Quincy (1722a) = Quincy, John: *Lexicon physico-medicum; or, a new physical dictionary; explaining the difficult terms used in the several branches of the profession, and in such parts of philosophy as are introductory thereunto. To which is added, some account of the things signified by such terms: collected from the most eminent authors; and particularly those who have wrote upon mechanical principles.* 2nd ed., London: for E. Bell, W. Taylor and J. Osborn.

Quincy, John (1723): *Prælectiones pharmaceuticæ: or a course of lectures in pharmacy, chymical and Galenical.* London: for E. Bell, J. Senex, and W Taylor.

Quincy (1775) = Quincy, John: *Lexicon physico-medicum: or, a new medicinal dictionary; explaining the difficult terms used in the several branches of the profession, and in such parts of natural philosophy as are introductory thereto: with an account of the things signified by such terms. Collected from the most eminent authors.* 9th edition, London: for T. Longman.

Quincy (1787) = Quincy, John: *Lexicon physico-medicum; or, a new medicinal dictionary. Explaining the difficult terms used in the several branches of the profession, and in such parts of natural philosophy, as are introductory thereto. With an account of the things signified by such terms. Collected from the most eminent authors. The tenth edition, with new improvements from the latest authors.* London: for T. Longman.

Ramazzini, Bernard (1705): *A treatise on the diseases of tradesmen.* London: for Andrew Bell et al.

Ramazzini, Bernard (1750): *Health preserved, in two treatises. I. On the diseases of artificers, which by their particular callings they are most liable to. With the method of avoiding them, and their cure. By Bern. Ramazini ... II. On those distempers, which arise from particular climates, situations and methods of life. With directions for the choice of a healthy air, soil and water. By Frederick Hoffman, M. D ... Translated and enlarged, with an appendix, by R. James, M. D. Author of the Medicinal Dictionary.* London: for John Whiston and John Woodyer.

Recorde, Robert (1547): *The urinal of physick.* London: Reynolde Wolfe.

Renou, Jean de (1657): *A medicinal dispensatory, containing the vvhole body of physick discovering the natures, properties, and vertues of vegetables, minerals, & animals: the manner of compounding medicaments, and the way to administer them. ... now Englished and revised, by Richard Tomlinson of London, apothecary.* London: Jo: Streater and Ja: Cottrel.

Renou (1657) = *A physical dictionary, or, an interpretation of such crabbed words and terms of art, as are derived from the Greek or Latin, and used in physick, anatomy, chirurgery, and chymistry. Published for the more perfect understanding of Mr. Tomlinson's translation of Rænodæus dispensatory and whatever other books of physick and surgery are extant in the English tongue.* London: G. Dawson.

Reuss, Jeremias David (1791–1804): *Das gelehrte England oder Lexikon der jeztlebenden Schriftsteller in Grosbritannien, Irland und Nord-Amerika nebst einem Verzeichnis ihrer Schriften. Vom Jahr 1770 bis 1790.* 2 vols., Berlin und Stettin: bey Fried. Nicolai.

Rider (1589) = Rider, John: *Bibliotheca scholastica. A dovble dictionarie, penned for all those that would haue within short space the vse of the Latin tongue, either to speake, or write.* [Oxford]: Ioseph Barnes.

Ridgway, James [1800]: *James Ridgway respectfully acquaints the public, that he continues to supply the London newspapers ... The following new publications ... are now ready to be delivered.* [London: James Ridgway].

Rivers, David (1798): *Literary memoirs of living authors of Great Britain.* 2 vols., London: for R. Faulder.

Rivière, Lazare (1646): *Lazari Riverii consiliarii, et medici regii atqve in Monspeliensi universitate medicinæ professoris, observationes medicæ & curationes insignes. Quibus accesserunt, observationes ab aliis communicatæ.* Londini: typis Milonis Flesher.

Rivière, Lazare (1655): *The practice of physick in seventeen several books wherein is plainly set forth the nature, cause, differences, and several sorts of signs together with the cure of all diseases in the body of man / by Nicholas Culpeper ... Abdiah Cole ... and William Rowland ... being chiefly a translation of the works of that learned and renowned doctor, Lazarus Riverius.* London: Printed by Peter Cole.

Rivière, Lazare (1657): *The universal body of physick in five books; comprehending the several treatises of nature, of diseases and their causes, of symptomes, of the preservation of health, and of cures.* London: for Philip Briggs.

Rivière, Lazare (1661): *The practice of physick, wherein is plainly set forth, the nature, cause, differences, and several sorts of signs: together with the cure of all diseases in the body of man. With ... A physical dictionary.* London: Peter Cole and Edward Cole.

Rivière, Lazare (1668): *The practice of physick in seventeen several books wherein is plainly set forth the nature, cause, differences, and several sorts of signs : together with the cure of all diseases in the body of man by Nicholas Culpeper ... Abdiah Cole ... and William Rowland ... with a physical dictionary, explaining the hard words used in these books.* London: J. Streator.

Robertson, Robert (1777): *A physical journal kept on board His Majesty's ship Rainbow, during three voyages to the coast of Africa, and West Indies, in the years 1772, 1773, and 1774.* London: for E. and C. Dilly et al.

Robinson [pseudonym] (1785): Review of A New Medical Dictionary; or, General Repository of Physic and Surgery. By G. Motherby, M. D. Folio. The Second Edition. 2l. 2s. *The Critical Review; or, Annals of Literature* 59, 476–477.

Royal College of Physicians of London (1632): *Pharmacopœia Londinensis, in qva medicamenta antiqva et nova vsitatissima, sedulò collecta, accuratissime examinata, quotidianâ experientia confirmata describuntur.* London: for Iohn Marriott.

[Royal College of Physicians of London] (1649): *A physicall directory, or, a translation of the London dispensatory made by the Colledge of Physicians in London ... By Nich. Culpeper Gent.* London: for Peter Cole.

Royal College of Physicians of London. (1721): *The dispensatory of the Royal College of physicians in London. With some notes ... by John Quincy. M.D.* London : Printed by W. Bowyer, for R. Knaplock, B. Took, D. Midwinter et al.

Sadler, John (1657): *Enchiridion medicum: an enchiridion of the art of physick. Methodically prescribing remedies in such an order, that it may be accounted to the sick-man a sanctuary, and to the studious a library ... translated, revised, corrected and augmented by R.T.* London: by J.C. for R. Moone.

Salmon (16–?) = Salmon, William: *The family-dictionary; or, houshold companion: wherein are alphabetically laid down exact rules and choice physical receipts for the preservation of health, prevention of sickness, and curing the several diseases, distempers, and grievances, incident to men, women, and children ... By J.H.* [s.l., s.n.].

Salmon, William (1694): *Pharmacopœia Bateana: or, Bate's dispensatory. Translated from the second edition of the Latin copy, published by Mr. James Shipton.* London: for S. Smith and B. Walford.

Salmon, William (1705): *The family-Dictionary: or, houshold companion ... The third edition, enlarged, with several hundreds of excellent receipts.* London: H. Rhodes.

Salmon (1710) = Salmon, William: *The family dictionary: or, houshold companion ... with above eleven hundred additions, intersperst through the whole work.* 4th. ed., London: H. Rhodes.

Santorio, Santorio (1614): *De statica medicina: aphorismorvm sectionibus septem comprehensa.* Venetiis: Apud Nicolaum Polium.

Santorio, Santorio (1676): *Medicina statica: or, rules of health, in eight sections of aphorisms. Originally written by Sanctorius chief professor of physick at Padua English'd by J. D.* London: for John Starkey.

Santorio, Santorio (1712): *Medicina statica: Being the aphorisms of Sanctorius, translated into English with large explanations. Wherein is given a mechanical account of the animal oeconomy, and of the efficacy of the non-naturals, either in bringing about or removing its disorders: also with an introduction concerning mechanical knowledge, and the grounds of certainty in physick. By John Quincy*. London: for William Newton.

Santorio, Santorio (1720): *Medicina statica: being the aphorisms of Sanctorius, translated into English with large explanations. The second edition. To which is added Dr. Keil's Medicina statica britannica, with comparative remarks, and explanations ... By John Quincy, M.D.* London: for W. and J. Newton et al.

Scapula (1580) = Scapula, Joannis: *Lexicon Graecolatinum novvm in qvo ex primitivorvm & simplicivm fontibus derivata atque composita*. Basileæ: ex officina Herguagiana, per Evsebivm Episcopivm.

Scogan, John (1613): *Scoggins iestes. Wherein is declared his pleasant pastimes in France, and of his meriments among the fryers: full of delight and honest mirth*. London: Raph Blower.

Scultetus, Johannes (1674): *The chyrurgeons store-house furnished with forty-three tables cut in brass, in which are all sorts of instruments ... useful to the performance of all manual operations ... English'd by E. B.* London: for John Starker.

Securis, John (1566): *A detection and querimonie of the daily enormities and abuses cōmitted in physick, concernyng the thre parts therof: that is, the physitions part, the part of the surgeons, and the arte of poticaries*. [Londini: In aedibus Thomae Marshi].

Simon Genuensis (1473): *Synonyma medicinae seu clavis sanationis* Milan: Antonius Zarotus.

Smith, John (1656): *A compleat practice of physick. Wherein is plainly described, the nature, causes, differences, and signs, of all diseases in the body of man. VVith the choicest cures for the same*. London: Printed by J. Streater, for Simon Miller.

Smollett, Tobias (1771): *The expedition of Humphry Clinker*. 3 vols., London: W. Johnson and B. Collins

Society for the Relief of Widows and Orphans of Medical Men (London, England) (1788?): *Laws of the Society for the Relief of Widows and Orphans of Medical Men, in London, and its vicinity*. [London]: s.n.

Society of Apothecaries, London [1737]: *A catalogue of the several members of the Society of Apothecaries, London, this present first of September, 1737*. [London]: s.n.

Society of Apothecaries, London [1738]: *A catalogue of the several members of the Society of Apothecaries, London, this present fifth of September, 1738*. [London]: s.n.

Society of Apothecaries, London [1742]: *A catalogue of the several members of the Society of Apothecaries, London, this present seventh of September, 1742*. [London]: s.n.

Society of Apothecaries, London [1746]: *A catalogue of the several members of the Society of Apothecaries, London, this present second of September, 1746*. [London]: s.n.

Society of gentlemen (1754): *A new and complete dictionary of arts and sciences; comprehending all the branches of useful knowledge, with accurate descriptions as well of the various machines, instruments, tools, figures, and schemes necessary for illustrating them*. 3 vols., London: for W. Owen.

Southcomb, Lewis (1750): *Peace of mind and health of body united: or, a discourse, shewing the distinction between a wounded conscience, convicted by a sense of sin, and a wounded spirit, proceeding from a disordered body*. London: for M. Cooper.

Sparrow, John (1731): *The mechanical dissertation upon the lues venerea. Proving not only the Possibility, but Certainty of Curing that Disease, without the hazard of Salivation*. London: for Richard King.

S[parrow], J. (1739): *Observations in Surgery: containing one hundred and fifteen different cases with particular remarks on each, for the improvement of young students. Written originally in*

French, by Henry-Francis Le Dran, of the academy of arts, sworn surgeon at Paris ... Translated by J. S. Surgeon ... To which is added, a new chirurgical dictionary ... explaining the terms of art contained in the body of the book, and likewise all such as properly belong to physick and surgery. London: for J. Hodges.

Spooner, Thomas, of Lemon Street (1721): *A compendious treatise of the diseases of the skin, from the slightest itching humour in particular parts only, to the most inveterate itch, stubborn scabbiness, and confirmed leprosy.* 4th edition, London: T. Child et al.

Stearns, Samuel (1801): *The American herbal, or, Materia medica : wherein the virtues of the mineral, vegetable, and animal productions of North and South America are laid open, so far as they are known : and their uses in the practice of physic and surgery exhibited : comprehending an account of a large number of new medical discoveries and improvements, which are compiled from the best authorities with much care and attention, and promulgated for the purpose of spreading medical light and information in America.* Walpole [N.H.]: for Thomas & Thomas, and the author.

Sterne, Laurence (1766): *The life and opinions of Tristram Shandy, gentleman.* Vol. 9. 2nd edition, London: for T. Durham.

Strother, Edward (1716): *Criticon febrium: or, a critical essay on fevers; with the diagnosticks and methods of cure, in all the different species of them.* London: for Charles Rivington.

Strother, Edward (1729): *Practical observations on the epidemical fever, which hath reign'd so violently for these two years past.* London: C. Rivington.

Sydenham, Thomas (1676): *Observationes medicae circa morborum acutorum historiam et curationem.* Londini: typis A[ndrew] C[larke], impensis Gualteri Kettilby.

T., A. (1607): *Rich storehouse, or, treasurie for the diseased.* London: Ralph Blower.

Tabernæmontanus, Jacobus Theodorus (1590): *Eicones Plantarvm seu Stirpivm, Arborvm Nempe, Frvcticvm, Herbarvm, Fructvvm ... Quæ Partim Germania Sponte Producit.* Frankfurt: Nicolao Bassaeo.

Tanner, John (1659): *The hidden treasures of the art of physick; fully discovered.* London: for George Sawbridge.

Tomlinson, Richard (1657): *A medicinal dispensatory, containing the whole body of physick: discovering the natures, properties, and vertues of vegetables, minerals, & animals, the manner of compounding medicaments, and the way to administer them ... and now Englished and revised, by Richard Tomlinson of London, apothecary.* London: by Jo. Streater and Ja. Cottrell.

Traheron, Bartholomew (1543): *The most excellent workes of chirurgerye, made and set forth by maister John Vigon, heed chirurgië of our tyme in Italie, translated into English. Whereunto is added an exposition of straunge termes and vnknowen symples, belongyng to the arte.* [London]: Edward Whitchurch.

Turner, Daniel (1722): *The art of surgery: in which is laid down such a general idea of the same, as is founded upon reason, confirm'd by practice, and farther illustrated with many singular and rare cases medico-chirurgical.* 2 vols., London: for C. Rivington.

Turner, William (1538): *Libellus de re herbaria novvs, in quo herbarum aliquot nomina Greca, Latina, & Anglica habes, vna cum nominibus officinarum, in gratiam studios[qu]e iuuentutis nunc primum in lucem æditus.* Londini: Apvd Ioannem Byddellum.

Turner, William (1551): *A new herball, wherin are conteyned the names of herbes in Greke, Latin, Englysh, Duch Frenche, and in the potecaries and herbaries Latin, with the properties degrees and naturall places of the same.* Imprinted at London: by Steven Mierdman.

Turner, William (1562): *The seconde part of Vuilliam Turners herball wherein are conteyned the names of herbes in Greke, Latin, Duche, Frenche, and in the apothecaries Latin, and somtyme in Italiane, wyth the vertues of the same herbes.* Imprinted at Collen: by Arnold Birckman.

Turton (1797) = Turton, William: *A medical glossary: in which the words in the various branches of medicine are deduced from their original languages. Properly accented, and explained.* London: Printed for J. Johnson.

Wade, John Peter (1792): *Nature and effects of emetics, purgatives, mercurials, and low diet, in disorders of Bengal and similar latitudes.* London: for J. Murray.

Wallis, George (1793): *The art of preventing diseases, and restoring health, founded on rational principles, and adapted to persons of every capacity.* London: for G. G. J. and J. Robinson.

Wallis, George (1795?): *The complete family physician, or the art of preventing diseases, and restoring health, founded on rational principles, and adapted to persons of every capacity.* 2nd edition, London: by G. Sidney.

Wallis (1759) = Wallis, Thomas: *The farrier's and horseman's complete dictionary.* London: for W. Owen and E. Baker.

Warton, Thomas (1774): *The history of English poetry, from the close of the eleventh to the commencement of the eighteenth century.* 4 vols., London: J. Dodsley et al.

Webster, Noah (1807): *A letter to Dr. David Ramsay, of Charleston, (S.C.) Respecting the Errors in Johnson's Dictionary, and Other Lexicons.* New Haven: Oliver Steele.

Wilkes, John = EL (1810–1829) = *Encyclopædia Londinensis; or, Universal Dictionary of Arts, Sciences, and Literature.* London: for the proprietors by J. Adlard.

Wilkins John (1648): *Mathematicall magick.* London: by M. F[lesher] for Sa. Gellibrand.

Wilkins, John (1668): *An essay towards a real character, and a philosophical language.* London: for Sa. Gellibrand, and for John Martyn.

Winslow, Jacques-Bénigne (1743): *An anatomical exposition of the structure of the human body. Translated from the French original, by G. Douglas, M.D.* 2 vols., 2nd edition, London: R. Ware et al.

Wirsung, Christof (1598): *Praxis medicinae vniuersalis; or a generall practise of physicke … translated … by Iacob Mosan Germane, Doctor in the same facultie.* Imprinted at London: By Edmund Bollifant.

Woodall, John (1617): *The svrgions mate, or a treatise discouering faithfully and plainely the due contents of the svrgions chest … with certaine characters, and tearmes of arte.* London: Edward Griffin for Laurence Lisle.

Woodward, John (1718): *The state of physic: and of diseases.* London: for T. Horne

Würtz, Felix (1656): *An experimental treatise of surgerie in four parts … faithfully the second time translated into Neather Dutch, out of the twenty eighth copy printed in the German tongue, and now also Englished and much corrected, by Abraham Lenertzon Fox.* London: Printed by Gartrude Dawson.

Secondary references

Adams, J. N. (1995): *Pelagonius and Latin veterinary terminology in the Roman empire.* Leiden: Brill.

Adamska-Salaciak, Arleta (2016): Explaining meaning in bilingual dictionaries. In: Durkin, Philip *The Oxford handbook of lexicography* Oxford: Oxford University Press, 144–160.

Alcock, N. W./Cox, Nancy (2000): *Living and working in seventeenth-century England: An encyclopedia of drawings and descriptions from Randle Holme's original manuscripts for The academy of armory (1688).* The British Library. CD-ROM.

Allsopp, C. B. (1957): Physical methods in medical diagnosis: An evening discourse delivered during the Bristol conference. In: *British journal of applied physics* 8, supplement 6, S40–S47.

Andrews, Jonathan (1990): A respectable mad-doctor? Dr Richard Hale, F. R. S. (1670–1728) In: *Notes and records of the Royal Society of London* 44.2, 169–204.

Andrews, Jonathan (2008): Hale, Richard (1670–1728). In: *Oxford dictionary of national biography*, online edn., Oxford University Press [<http://www.oxforddnb.com/view/article/11906>; last access: September 23, 2013].

Anon.(1837) Cyclopædiæ and dictionaries of medicine and surgery. *Medico-chirurgical Review* 53, July 1, 129-143.

Baigent, Elizabeth (2004): Barrow, John (fl. 1735–1774). In: *Oxford dictionary of national biography*, Oxford University Press [<http://www.oxforddnb.com/view/article/1543>; last access: October 18, 2013].

Baigent, Elizabeth (2004): Motherby, George (bap. 1731, d. 1793). In: *Oxford dictionary of national biography*, Oxford University Press [<http://www.oxforddnb.com/view/article/19418>; last access: May 6, 2008].

Baines, Edward Jun. (1835): *History of the cotton manufacture in Great Britain*. London: Fisher, H., Fisher, R., and Jackson, P.

Barry, J. (1987): Publicity and the public good: presenting medicine in eighteenth-century Bristol. In: Bynum/Porter, 29–39.

Bazerman, Charles (2011): Church, state, university and the printing press: Conditions for the emergence and maintenance of autonomy of scientific publication in Europe. In: *Languages of science in the eighteenth century*. Gunnarsson, Britt-Louise (ed.) Berlin/Boston: De Gruyter Mouton, 25–44.

Beattie, Lester M. (1935): *John Arbuthnot: Mathematician and satirist*. Cambridge, Mass: Harvard University Press.

Bisaccia, C. et al. (2011): Nephrology in A medicinal dictionary of Robert James (1703–1776). In: *Journal of nephrology* 24 May-June; suppl. 17: S37–S50. doi: 10.5301/JN.2011.6466.

Bocast, Alexander K (2016): *Definition in Chambers's* Cyclopaedia: *Chambers on Definition*. McLean, VA: Berkeley Bridge Press

Boswell, James (1791/1953): *Boswell's Life of Johnson*. Geoffrey Cumberlege (ed.) new ed., Oxford standard authors, London: Oxford University Press.

Brack, O. M. (2008): Osborne, Thomas (bap. 1704?, d. 1767). In: *Oxford dictionary of national biography*, online edn., Oxford University Press [<http://www.oxforddnb.com/view/article/20885>; last access: October 26, 2013].

Brack, O. M., Jr. (2009): The Works of Samuel Johnson and the canon. In: Clingham/Smallwood, 246–261.

Brock, Helen (2004) Douglas, James (*bap. 1675, d. 1742*). In: *Oxford dictionary of national biography*, online edn., Oxford University Press [<https://doi-org.libproxy.helsinki.fi/10.1093/ref:odnb/7899>; last access: December 12, 2018].

Brown, P. S. (1987): Social context and medical theory in the demarcation of nineteenth-century boundaries. In: Bynum/Porter, 216–233.

Brown, Theodore M. (1987): Medicine in the shadow of the *Principia*. In: *Journal of the history of ideas* 48.4, 629–648.

Burnby, Juanita G. L. (1983): A study of the English apothecary from 1660 to 1760. In: *Medical history* supplement no. 3, London: Wellcome Institute for the History of Medicine.

Burnett, Charles (1988): Scientific speculations. In: *A history of twelfth-century Western philosophy*. Dronke, Peter (ed.), Cambridge: Cambridge University Press.

Burr, Charles W. (1929): Dr. James and his medical dictionary. In: *Annals of medical history*. NS 1, 180–190.

Bynum, W. F. (1980): Health, disease and medical care. In: Rousseau/Porter (eds.) Cambridge: Cambridge University Press, 211–253.

Bynum, W. F./Porter, Roy (eds.) (1987): *Medical fringe & medical orthodoxy 1750–1850*. London: Croom Helm.

Cain Christopher M./ Russom, Geoffrey (2007): *Studies in the history of the English language III: Managing chaos : strategies for identifying change in English*. Berlin/New York : Mouton de Gruyter.

Carruthers, Mary J. (1990): *The book of memory: A study of memory in medieval culture*. Cambridge: Cambridge University Press.

Charpy, Jean-Pierre (2011): Les premiers dictionnaires médicaux en langue anglaise: glissements diachroniques du spécialisé au non spécialisé. In: *ASp - La revue du GERAS*, 59, 25–42.

Clark, Sir George (1964–1972): *A history of the Royal College of Physicians of London*. 3 vols., Oxford: Clarendon Press for the Royal College of Physicians.

Clingham, Greg/Smallwood, Philip (2009): *Johnson after 300 years*. Cambridge: Cambridge University Press.

Colman, Andrew M. (2009): *A dictionary of psychology*. 3rd edition. Oxford: Oxford University Press.

Considine, John/Iamartino, Giovanni (eds.) (2007): *Words and dictionaries from the British Isles in historical perspective*. Newcastle: Cambridge Scholars Publishing.

Considine, John (2008): *Dictionaries in early modern Europe: Lexicography and the making of heritage*. Cambridge: Cambridge University Press.

Considine, John (2014): English dictionaries as sources for work in English historical linguistics: An overview. In: *Studia linguistica Universitatis Iagellonicae Cracoviensis* 131, 27–41.

Cook, Harold J. (1986): *The decline of the old medical regime in Stuart London*. Ithaca/London: Cornell University Press.

Corley, T. A. B. (2004): James, Robert (bap. 1703, d. 1776) In: *Oxford dictionary of national biography*, Oxford University Press [<http://www.oxforddnb.com/view/article/14618>; last access: August 25, 2013].

Craig, W. S. (1976): *History of the Royal College of Physicians of Edinburgh*. Oxford: Blackwell Scientific Publications.

Debus, Allen G. (2001): *Chemistry and medical debate: Van Helmont to Boerhaave*. Canton, MA: Science history Publications.

Demaitre, Luke (2013): *Medieval medicine: The art of healing, from head to toe*. Santa Barbara: Praeger.

Diderot, Denis (s.a.): *The Encyclopedia of Diderot & D'Alambert*. S.l.: Michigan Publishing [<http://quod.lib.umich.edu/d/did/index.html>; last access: January 19, 20+19].

Doig, Kathleen Hardesty/Medlin, Dorothy (eds.) (2007): *British-French exchanges in the eighteenth century*. Newcastle: Cambridge Scholars Press.

Donato, Maria Pia/Mazzei, Valentina (2014): *Sudden death: Medicine and religion in eighteenth-century Rome* Burlington: Ashgate.

Drake, Miriam A. (ed.) (2003): *Encyclopedia of library and information science*. 2nd ed., New York: Marcel Dekker.

Dyer, Peter (2007): Randle Holme and 17th century brewing, malting and coopering terminology. In: *Journal of the brewery history society* 126, 62–73.

Emmerson, Joan Stuart (1965): *Translations of medical classics: A list*. Newcastle upon Tyne: University Library.

Erasmus, Desiderius of Rotterdam (2005): *On copia of Words and ideas (De utraque verborum ac rerum copia)*. King, Donald B./Rix, H. David (ed.) Milwaukee: Marquette University Press.

Erler, Mary C. (2008): Copland, Robert (fl. 1505–1547). In: *Oxford dictionary of national biography*, online edn., Oxford University Press [<http://www.oxforddnb.com/view/article/6265>; last access: April 23, 2014].

Eyles, V. A. (1965): John Woodward, F.R.S. (1665–1728): Physician and geologist. In: *Nature* 206.4987, 868–870.

Fay, Isla (2015): *Health and the city: Disease, environment and government in Norwich, 1200–1575.* Woodbridge: York Medieval Press.

Feingold, Mordechai (2004): *The Newtonian moment: Isaac Newton and the making of modern culture.* New York/Oxford: New York Public Library/Oxford University Press.

Fichtner, Gerhard (2009): *Wissenschaftshistorische Bibliographie 1975–2009 (mit ausgewählten Rezensionen).* Tübingen: Institut für Ethik und Geschichte der Medizin [<http://www.iegm.uni-tuebingen.de/Hirschmueller/MWHB/mwhb.pdf>; last access: January 26, 2019].

Fissell, Mary E. (2007): The marketplace of print. In: Jenner/Wallis, 108–132.

Fletcher P. E. (2002): The life of Andrew Boorde, c1490–1549.In: *Adverse drug reactions and toxicological reviews* 21.4, 243–252.

Foster, Brett (2008): "The goodliest place in this World": Early Tudor reactions to papal Rome. In: Papazian 2008, 27–56.

French, Roger/Wear, Andrew (eds.) (1989): *The medical revolution of the seventeenth century.* Cambridge: Cambridge University Press.

Furdell, Elizabeth Lane (2001): *The royal doctors, 1485–1714: Medical personnel at the Tudor and Stuart courts.* Rochester, NY: University of Rochester Press.

Furdell, Elizabeth Lane (2002): *Publishing and medicine in early modern England.* Rochester NY: University of Rochester Press.

Furdell, Elizabeth Lane (2004): Boorde, Andrew (c.1490–1549). In: *Oxford dictionary of national biography*, online edn., Oxford University Press [<http://www.oxforddnb.com/view/article/2870>; last access: March 9, 2014].

Furnivall, F. J. (ed.) (1870): *The fyrst boke of the introduction of knowledge made by Andrew Borde, of physycke doctor. A compendyous regyment; or, a dyetary of helth made in Mountpyllier ... Barnes in defence of the berde.* London: Trübner, for the EETS.

Griffiths, Jeremy/Pearsall, Derek (eds.) (1989): *Book production and publishing in Britain 1375–1475.* Cambridge: Cambridge University Press.

Guerra, F. (1962*): American medical bibliography 1639–1783: A chronological catalogue, and critical and bibliographical study of books, pamphlets, broadsides, and articles in periodical publications relating to the medical sciences.* New York: L. C. Harper.

Guerrini, A. (1985): James Keill, George Cheyne, and Newtonian physiology, 1690–1740. In: *Journal of the history of biology* 18.2, 247–266.

Guerrini, A. (1987): Archibald Pitcairne and Newtonian medicine. In: *Medical history* 31.1, 70–83.

Guerrini, A. (1989): Isaac Newton, George Cheyne and the Principia medicinae. In: French/Wear 1989, 222–245.

Guerrini, Anita (2008): Mead, Richard (1673–1754). In: *Oxford dictionary of national biography*, Oxford University Press [<http://www.oxforddnb.com/view/article/18467>; last access: September 9, 2013].

Gunnarsson, Britt-Louise (ed.) (2011): *Languages of science in the eighteenth century.* Berlin/Boston: De Gruyter Mouton.

Guthrie, Douglas (1943): The "Breviary" and "Dyetary" of Andrew Boorde (1490–1549), physician, priest and traveller. In: *Journal of the Royal Society of Medicine* 37.9, 507–509.

Hadju, Steven I. (2005): Entries on laboratory medicine in the first illustrated medical dictionary. In: *Annals of clinical & laboratory science* 35.4, 465–468. [<http://www.annclinlabsci.org/content/35/4/465.full>; last access: January 26, 2019].

Hanson, Craig Ashley (2009): *The English virtuoso: Art, medicine, and antiquarianism in the age of empiricism.* Chicago/London: University of Chicago Press.

Harrison, J. F. C. (1987): Early Victorian radicals and the medical fringe. In: Bynum/Porter 1987, 198–215.

Hazen, Allen T. (1936): Samuel Johnson and Dr. Robert James. In: *Bulletin of the institute of the history of medicine* 4.6, 455–465.

Hazen, Allen T. (1973): *Samuel Johnson's prefaces and dedications*. Port Washington: Kennikat Press.

Helmstaedter, G. (2005): The impact of Thomas Linacre on German medicine and the role of pharmacists: Linacre, medicine and Michael Barth's works (1530–1560). In: *Pharmacy in history* (Lond.) 35.3, 47–49.

Holme, Randle (1905): *The academy of armory, or a storehouse of armory and blazon: Printed from Harleian MSS. 1920–2180 in the British Museum.* Jeayes, I. H. (ed.) London: for the Roxburghe Club.

Howard-Jones, N. (1951): John Quincy, M.D. [d.1722], apothecary and iatrophysical Writer. In: *Journal of the history of medicine and allied sciences* 6 spring, 149–175.

Hueget-Termes, Teresa (2008): Islamic pharmacy and pharmacology in the Latin west: An approach to early pharmacopoeias. In: *European review* 16.2, 229–239.

Jacyna, L. S. (1983): Images of John Hunter in the nineteenth century. In: *History of science* 21.51, 85–108.

Jarcho, Saul (1982): Blankaart's dictionary: An index to 17th century medicine. In: *Bulletin of the New York Academy of medicine* 58, 568–577.

Jenner, Mark S. R./Wallis, Patrick (2007): *Medicine and the market in England and its colonies c. 1450–c.1850.* Houndmills, Basingstoke: Palgrave Macmillan.

Johnson, Samuel (2006): *The lives of the most eminent poets: With critical observations on their works.* Lonsdale, Roger (ed.), 4 vols., Oxford: Clarendon Press.

Jones, Peter Murray (2011): Medical literacies and medical culture. In Taavitsainen/Pahta 2011, 30–43.

Kaminski, Thomas (1987): *The early career of Samuel Johnson.* New York: Oxford University Press.

Kassell, Lauren (2013): Forman, Simon (1552–1611). In: *Oxford dictionary of national* biography, online edn., Oxford University Press [<http://www.oxforddnb.com/view/article/9884>; last access: January 15, 2014].

Kennedy, Krista (2016): *Textual curation: Authorship, agency, and technology in* Wikipedia *and* Chambers's Cyclopædia. Columbia, S.C.: University of South Carolina Press.

King-Hele, Desmond (ed.) (1981): *The letters of Erasmus Darwin.* Cambridge: Cambridge University Press.

Kopperman, Paul E. (ed.) (2012): *Theory and practice in eighteenth century British medicine: "Regimental practice" by John Buchanan, M. D. An eighteenth-century medical diary and manual.* Farnham: Ashgate.

Lancashire, Ian (2002): 'Dumb significants' and early modern English definition. In: Jens Brockmeier/Min Wang/David R. Olson, eds. Literacy, narrative and culture London/New York: Routledge, 131–154.

Lancashire, Ian (2004): Lexicography in the early modern period: The manuscript record. In: *Historical dictionaries and historical dictionary research: papers from the International Conference on historical lexicography and lexicology at the University of Leicester, 2002.* Coleman/McDermott, (eds.) Tübingen: Max Niemayer, 19–28.

Lancashire, Ian (2007): The two tongues of early modern English. In: *Managing chaos: Strategies for identifying change in English studies in the history of the English language III*: Cain/Russom, (eds.) Berlin: Mouton de Gruyter, 105–142.

Langdon-Brown, Sir Walter (1946): Some chapters in Cambridge medical history. *Medical history* Cambridge: Cambridge University Press.

Lea, Arnold W. W. (1910): *Puerperal infection* London: Oxford University Press.

Leong, Elaine/Pennell, Sara (2007): Recipe collections and the currency of medical knowledge in the early modern 'medical marketplace'. In: Jenner/Wallis 2007, 133–152.

Levine, J. M. (2004): Woodward, John (1665/1668–1728). In: *Oxford dictionary of national biography*, Oxford University Press [<http://www.oxforddnb.com/view/article/29946>; last access: September 14, 2013].

Lonati, E. (2007): Blancardus' *Lexicon medicum* in Harris's Lexicon technicum: A lexicographic and lexicological study. In: Considine/Iamartino 2007, 91–108.

Lonati, Elisabetta (2017): *Communicating medicine: British medical discourse in eighteenth-century reference works*. Milan: di/segni.

Loudon, Irvine (1986): *Medical Care and the General Practitioner, 1750–1850*. Oxford: Clarendon Press.

Loudon, Irvine (1987): "The vile race of quacks with which this country is infested". In: Bynum/Porter 1987, 106–128.

Loudon, Irvine (2000): *The tragedy of childbed fever*. Oxford: Oxford University Press.

Loveland, Jeff (2007): Two partial English-language translations of the *Encyclopédie*: The encyclopedias of John Barrow and Temple Henry Croker. In: Doig/Medlin 2007, 168–187.

Lynch, Beth (2008): Darby, John (d. 1704) In: *Oxford dictionary of national biography*, Oxford University Press, online edn. [<http://www.oxforddnb.com/view/article/67087>; last access: December 9, 2013].

Martin, Peter (2008): *Samuel Johnson: A biography*. London: Weidenfeld and Nicholson.

Martin, R. J. J. (1988): Explaining John Freind's *History of physick*. In: *Studies in history and philosophy of science* 19, 399–418.

Maxted, Ian (2008): Newbery, John (bap. 1713, d. 1767). In: *Oxford dictionary of national Biography*, online edn., Oxford University Press [<http://www.oxforddnb.com/view/article/19978>; last access: August 25, 2013].

McArthur, Tom (1998): *Living words: Language, lexicography and the knowledge revolution*. Exeter: University of Exeter Press.

McConchie, R. W. (1997): *Lexicography and physicke: The record of sixteenth-century English medical terminology*. Oxford: Clarendon Press.

McConchie, R. W. (2009):Propagating what the ancients taught and the moderns improved': The sources of George Motherby's A new medical dictionary; or, a general repository of physic, 1775. In: *Selected proceedings of the 2008 Symposium on new approaches in historical English lexis (HEL-LEX 2)*. Somerville, MA: Cascadilla Press, 124–133.

McConchie, R. W. (2011a): Converting 'this uncertain science into an art': Innovation and tradition in George Motherby's A new medical dictionary; or, general repository of physic, 1775. In: *Adventuring in dictionaries: New studies in the history of lexicography*. Considine, John (ed.) Newcastle: Cambridge Scholars Publishing, 126–148.

McConchie, R. W. (2011b): Compounds and code-switching: Compositorial practice in William Turner's Libellus de re herbaria novvs, 1538. In: *Scribes, printers, and the accidentals of their texts* Thaisen/Rutkowska, (eds.) Frankfurt am Main: Peter Lang, 177–190.

McConchie, Rod/Curzan, Anne (2011): Defining in early modern English medical texts. In: *Medical writing in early modern English*, Taavitsainen/Pahta (eds.) Cambridge: Cambridge University Press, 74–92.

McConchie, Roderick (2012): Sixteenth-century English books and authors in the National Library of Russia, St Petersburg: A preliminary survey. In: *Western European manuscripts and early printed books in Russia: Delving into the collections of the libraries of St Petersburg studies in variation, contacts and change in English*. Vol. 9, Kahlas-Tarkka/Kilpiö, eds. Research Unit for Variation, Contacts and Change in English (VARIENG), Helsinki: University of Helsinki.

McConchie, R. W. (2013): "The most discriminating plagiarist": The unkindest cut (and paste) of all. In: *Selected proceedings of the 2012 Symposium on new approaches in English historical lexis (HEL-LEX 3)* edited by McConchie/Juvonen/Kaunisto/Nevala/Tyrkkö Somerville, MA: Cascadilla Press, 107–119.

McConchie, Roderick/Tyrkkö, Jukka (2018): *Historical dictionaries in their paratextual context*. Berlin: De Gruyter.

McDermott, Anne (2005): Johnson's definitions of technical terms and the absence of illustrations. In: *International journal of lexicography*, 18.2, 173–187.

McKerrow, R. B./Ferguson, F. S. (1932): *Title-page borders used in England & Scotland 1485–1640*. London: Oxford University Press for the Bibliographical Society.

McKitterick, David (1992): Thomas Osborne, Samuel Johnson and the learned of foreign nations: A forgotten catalogue. In: *The book collector* 41, 55–68.

Moore, Norman (2010): Quincy, John (d. 1722). Rev. Michael Bevan. In: *Oxford dictionary of national biography*, online edn., Oxford University Press [<http://www.oxforddnb.com/view/article/22965>; last access: September 14, 2013].

Morris, G. C. R. (2008): Molins, William (1617–1691 In: *Oxford dictionary of national biography*, online edn., Oxford University Press [<http://www.oxforddnb.com/view/article/18910>; last access: December 6, 2013].

Mortimer, Ian (2007): The rural medical marketplace in southern England c. 1570–1720. In: Jenner/Wallis 2007, 69–87.

Muldrew, Craig (2011): *Food, energy and the creation of industriousness: Work and material culture in agrarian England, 1550–1700*. Cambridge: Cambridge University Press.

Munk, William (1878): *The roll of the Royal College of Physicians of London: Comprising biographical sketches of all the eminent physicians whose names are recorded in the annals*. 2nd edition, London: for the College, Harrison.

Nokes, David (2009): *Samuel Johnson: A life*. London: Faber and Faber.

Norri (2016) = Norri, Juhani: *Dictionary of medical vocabulary in English, 1375–1550: Body parts, sicknesses, instruments, and medicinal preparations*. London: Routlege.

Osselton, N. E. (2007): Alphabet fatigue and compiling consistency in early English dictionaries. In: Considine/Iamartino 2007, 81–90.

ODNB = *Oxford dictionary of national biography* (2017): Oxford: Oxford University Press [<http://www.oxforddnb.com>; last access: December 12, 2017].

OED = *Oxford English dictionary* (2017): Oxford: Oxford University Press [<http://www.oed.com>; last access: December 1, 2017].

Papazian, Mary A. (ed.) (2008): *The sacred and profane in English renaissance literature*. Newark: University of Delaware Press.

Payne, J. F. (2004): Burnet, Sir Thomas (1638–1704). Rev. Michael Bevan. In: *Oxford dictionary of national biography*, Oxford University Press [<http://www.oxforddnb.com/view/article/4066>; last access: February 15, 2014].

Plomer, Henry R. (1922): *Dictionary of the printers and booksellers who were at work in England, Scotland and Ireland from 1668 to 1725*. London: The Bibliographical Society.

Plomer, H. R. et al. (1968): *Dictionary of the printers and booksellers who were at work in England, Scotland and Ireland from 1726 to 1775*. Oxford: for the Bibliographical Society.

Porter, Roy (1979): John Woodward: "A droll sort of philosopher" In: *Geological magazine* 116.5, 335–344.

Porter, Roy (1987): "I think ye both quacks": The controversy between Dr Theodor Myersbach and Dr John Coakley Lettsom. In: Bynum/Porter 1987, 56–78.

Poukens, Johan/Provoost, Nele (2011): Respectability, middle-class material culture, and economic crisis: The case of Lier in Brabant, 1690–1770. In: *Journal of interdisciplinary history* 42.2, 159–184.

Power, D'A. (2004): Shipton, John (1680–1748). Revised by Michael Bevan. In: *Oxford dictionary of national biography*, Oxford University Press [<http://www.oxforddnb.com/view/article/25421>; last access: February 11, 2015].

Pranghofer, Sebastian (2009): "It could be seen more clearly in unreasonable animals than in humans": The representation of the rete mirabile in early modern anatomy. In: *Medical history* 53.4, 561–586.

Reid, George William (1880): Thomas Osborne, the bookseller. In: *Notes and queries* S6-II, 48, 424–425.

Roger, Jacques (1980): The living world. In: Rousseau, G. S./Porter, Roy, 255–283.

Rousseau, G. S./Porter, Roy (1980): *The ferment of knowledge: Studies in the historiography of eighteenth-century science*. Cambridge: Cambridge University Press.

Rowlinson, J. S. (2007): John Freind: Physician, chemist, Jacobite, and friend of Voltaire's. *Notes and records of the Royal Society of London* 61.2, 109–127 , [<http://rsnr.royalsocietypublishing.org/content/61/2/109.full#sec-2>; last access: January 26, 2019].

Rydén, Mats/Helander, Hans/Olsson, Kerstin (eds.) (1999): *William Turner Libellus de re herbaria novus 1538: Edited with a translation into English*. Uppsala: Swedish Science Press.

Schäfer, Jürgen (1989): *Early modern English lexicography*. 2 vols., Oxford: Clarendon Press.

Schofield, Robert E. (1963): *The Lunar Society of Birmingham: A social history of provincial science and industry in eighteenth-century England*. Oxford: Clarendon Press.

NSSL = Sedgwick, Leonard W./Power, Henry (1879–1892): *Lexicon of medicine and the allied sciences*. 5 vols., London: New Sydenham Society.

Shapiro, Arthur K./Shapiro, Elaine (1997): *The powerful placebo: From ancient priest to modern physician*. Baltimore/London: Johns Hopkins University Press.

Shapiro, Rebecca (2018) The wants of women: Lexicography and pedagogy in seventeenth-and eighteenth-century dictionaries. In McConchie/Tyrkkö (eds.), 188–209.

Slack, Paul (1979): Mirrors of health and treasures of poor men: The uses of the vernacular medical literature of Tudor England. In: Webster (ed.) 1979, 237–274.

Smith, Barbara M. D. (2013): Keir, James (1735–1820). In: *Oxford dictionary of national biography*, online edn., Oxford University Press [<http://www.oxforddnb.com/view/article/15259>; last access: February 18, 2015].

Spedding, Patrick (2009): *Patrick Spedding; research notes: Informal writing centre for the book, Monash University*. [<http://patrickspedding.blogspot.co.uk/2009/09/society-of-booksellers-1741.html>; last access: 20 November, 2017].

Stein, David M./Laakso, William (1988): Bulimia: A historical perspective. In: *International journal of eating disorders* 7.2, 201–210.

Stein, G. (1989): The emerging role of English in the dictionaries of renaissance Europe. In: *Folia linguistica historica* 22, IX.1, 29–138.

Stein, Gabriele (2014): *Sir Thomas Elyot as lexicographer*. Oxford: Oxford University Press.

Steinke, Hubert (2005): Irritating experiments: Haller's concept and the European controversy on irritability and sensibility, 1750–1790. In: *Clio medica: The Wellcome series in the history of medicine*, 76.1, 7–16.

Stolberg, Michael (s.a.): Das »Medicinal Dictionary« des Robert James' nd. Die "Definitionum medicarum libri XXIII" In: *Archiv der europäischen Lexikographie: Fach-Enzyklopädien Geschichte der Medizin* 3/1 Harald Fischer Verlag [<http://www.haraldfischerverlag.de/hfv/AEL/ael_3-1_einleitung.php>; last access: February 8, 2015].

Suarez, Michael F./Turner, Michael L. (eds.) (2009): *The Cambridge history of the book in Britain. Volume V. 1695–1830*. Cambridge: Cambridge University Press.

Taavitsainen, Irma et al. (2011): Medical texts in 1500–1700 and the corpus of early modern English medical texts. In: Taavitsainen/Pahta (eds.) 9–29.

Taavitsainen, Irma,/Pahta, Päivi (eds.) (2011): *Medical writing in early modern English*. Cambridge: Cambridge University Press.

Tarp, Sven (2013): Old wisdom: The highly relevant lexicographical knowledge obtainable from a specialized dictionary from 1774. In: *Lexikos* 23, 394–413.

Tarp, Sven (2014): The concept of "dictionaries of things" viewed through the prism of Malachy Postlethwayt's Universal dictionary of trade and commerce: unpublished conference paper 7 ICHLL Las Palmas July 9–11 2014. See abstracts on https://sites.google.com/site/ichll2014/

Tarp, Sven/Bothma, Theo (2013): An alternative approach to enlightenment age lexicography: The Universal dictionary of trade and commerce. In: *Lexicographica: international annual for lexicography* 29, 222–284.

Taylor, E. G. R. (1966): *The mathematical practitioners of Hanoverian England, 1714–1840*. Cambridge: Cambridge University Press for The Institute of Navigation.

Tedder, H. R. (2004): Copland, William (d. 1569). Rev. Mary C. Erler. In: *Oxford dictionary of national biography*, Oxford University Press [<http://www.oxforddnb.com/view/article/6266>; last access: April 23, 2014].

Thomson, St. Clair, Sir (1929): The strenuous life of a physician in the 18th century. In: *Annals of medical history* NS 1, 1–14.

Thorton, John L. (1947): Andrew Boorde's *Dyetary of helth* and its attribution to Thomas Linacre. In: *The library* s5-II.2–3: 172–173 doi:10.1093/library/s5-II.2–3, 172.

Thornton, J. L. (1948): Andrew Boorde, Thomas Linacre and the "Dyetary of helth". In: *Bulletin of the medical library association* July 36.3, 204–209.

Timbs, John (1876): *Doctors and patients; or, anecdotes of the medical world and curiosities of medicine*. London: Richard Bentley.

Tittler, Robert/Thackray, Anne (2008): Print collecting in provincial England prior to 1650: The Randle Holme album. In: *British art journal* 9.2, 3–10 [<http://www.thefreelibrary.com/Print+collecting+in+provincial+England+prior+to+1650%3a+the+Randle...-a0220059002>; last access: November 11, 2017].

Trueman, Carl R. (2004): Traheron, Bartholomew (c.1510–1558?). In: *Oxford dictionary of national biography*, Oxford University Press [<http://www.oxforddnb.com/view/article/27658>; last access: May 6, 2014].

Turberville, A. S. (ed.) (1933): *Johnson's England: An account of the life & manners of his age*. 2 vols., Oxford: Clarendon Press.

Twain, Mark (1890): "A majestic literary fossil". In: *Harper's magazine* 80.477, February, 439–445.

Tyrkkö, Jukka (2009): A physical dictionary 1657: The first English medical dictionary. In: *Selected proceedings of the 2008 Symposium on new approaches in English historical lexis (HEL-LEX 2)* edited by McConchie/Honkapohja/Tyrkkö (eds.) Somerville, MA: Cascadilla Press, 172–187.

Tyrkkö, Jukka (2018): "Weak shrube or underwood": The unlikely medical glossator John Woodall and his glossary. In: *Historical dictionaries in their paratextual context*. McConchie/Tyrkkö (eds.), 261–283.

University of Edinburgh (1846): *Nomina eorum, qui gradum medicinæ doctoris in academia Jacobi Sexti Scotorum rregis, quæ Edinburgi est, adepti sunt: ab anno MDCCV. ad annum MDCCCXLV.* Edinburgi: excudebant Neill et socii.

Voigts, Linda Ehrsam (1989): Scientific and medical books. In: Griffiths/Pearsall 1989, 345–402.

Waingrow, Marshall (ed.) (1969): The correspondence and other papers of James Boswell relating to the making of the life of Johnson. London: Heinemann.

Waingrow, Marshall (ed.) (1994–2012): *James Boswell's Life of Johnson: An edition of the original manuscript in four volumes*. New Haven/London: Edinburgh and Yale University Press.

Warbasse, James P. (1907): Doctors of Samuel Johnson and his court. In: *Medical library and historical journal* 5.3, 260–272.

Ward, John (1839) *Diary of the Rev. John Ward, A. M. Vicar of Stratford-upon-Avon, extending from 1648 to 1679*. Severn, Charles (ed.) London: Henry Colburn.

Wear, Andrew (1998) *Health and healing in early modern England: Studies in social and intellectual history*. Aldershot: Ashgate.

Webster, Charles (ed.) (1979): *Health, medicine and mortality in the sixteenth century*. Cambridge: Cambridge University Press.

Welsh, Charles (1885*): A bookseller of the last century: Being some account of the life of John Newbery, and of the books he published, with a notice of the later Newberys*. London: for Griffith, Farran, Okeden et al.

Williams, Franklin B. (1962): *Index of dedications and commendatory verses in English books before 1641*. London: The Bibliographical Society.

Williams, Jack (2011): *Robert Recorde: Tudor polymath, expositor and practitioner of computation*. London: Springer.

Wiltshire, John (1991): *Samuel Johnson in the medical world: The doctor and the patient*. Cambridge: Cambridge University Press.

Wimsatt, W. K. (1948): *Philosophic words: A study of style and meaning in the Rambler and dictionary of Samuel Johnson*. New Haven: Yale University Press.

Woodcock, Leslie V. (2005). Phlogiston theory and chemical revolutions. In: *Bulletin for the history of chemistry* 30.2, 63–69.

Wyman, A. L. (1992): Benedict Duddell: Pioneer oculist of the 18th century. In: *Journal of the Royal Society of Medicine* 85.7, 412–415.

Wyman, A. L. (2004): Duddell, Benedict (c.1695–1759x67) In: *Oxford dictionary of national biography*, Oxford University Press [<http://www.oxforddnb.com/view/article/57676>; last access: September 16, 2014].

Yeo, Richard (2001): *Encyclopaedic visions: Scientific dictionaries and Enlightenment culture*. Cambridge: Cambridge University Press.

Index

https://doi.org/10.1515/9783110639186-014

Middleton, William 29, 31
Miller, Joseph
– *Botanicum officinale* 161
Miller, Philip 161
– *Gardener's dictionary* 125, 168
Moffett, Thomas 143
Molins, William 85
Monardes, Nicholas 168
Montagu, John, Duke of 100
Motherby, George 2f., 13ff., 17, 133, 134–37
– dictionary, use of James 182–84
– mentions of Blancard 91
– *New medical dictionary*, editions 178
– *New medical dictionary*, James, use of 184
– *New medical dictionary*, reception 180f.

N. N. (pseudonym) 95
names
– confusion of 13
New Sydenham Society *Lexicon* 146
Newbery, John 141, 164
Newtonian entries
– in Blancard and Quincy 117, 116–18
Newtonian medicine 95, 102, 119
Newtonian principles 98, 103
Newtonian words 116–18
nominal forms
– in medical lexicon 70
Nott, John
– *The cook's and confectioner's dictionary* 26

OED 44, 57, 104
Osborne, Thomas 101, 146, 164

Panckoucke, Charles-Joseph 170
Paracelsus 111
Parr, Bartholomew 165
Paul, Lewis 147
Paulli, Simon 168
Paulus Ægineta 177
Philosophical transactions of the Royal Society 6
physical
– meaning of 104–5
Physical dictionary
– reissues 71–72
physical, meaning of 17–18
Pitcairn, Archibald 97, 98–99
plagiarism 167

plants
– medicinal qualities 57
polysemy
– in Quincy 107
Postlethwayt, Malachy 1
Priestley, Joseph 184
Prosodia chirurgica
– authorship 129
– structural principles 127f.
publishers
– influence of 2
puerperal fever 184–86

Quincy, John 2, 7, 19, 25, 89, 131, 140, 144, 155, 174
– authorities mentioned 105
– criticism of earlier dictionaries 103
– denunciation of alchemy 121
– dispensatory 168
– hyperbole, dislike of 116
– *Lexicon physico-medicum* 17
– *Lexicon*, innovation 103
– *Lexicon*, ninth and tenth editons 178
– *Lexicon*, notice of 95–96
– life 95–96
– medical folklore 142
– *Pharmacopœia* 111, 119
– translation of Santorio 167

Ramazzini, Bernardo 145
Ray, John 168
readers, unlearned 69
Recorde, Robert 50, 52f., 191
regional usage 24
remedies, collections of 27
Rider, John
– *Bibliotheca scholastica* 145
Ridgway, James 132f.
Rieger, Johan 159
Rivière, Lazare 60, 68
Robertson, Robert 89
Rowland, William 21, 68
Royal College of Physicians 98
Royal College of Physicians of Edinburgh 78

Salmon, William 88, 98, 140
– dispensatory 168
Santorio, Santorio 122
– *Medicina statica* 97

CPSIA information can be obtained
at www.ICGtesting.com
Printed in the USA
BVHW062321300120
570891BV00014B/7